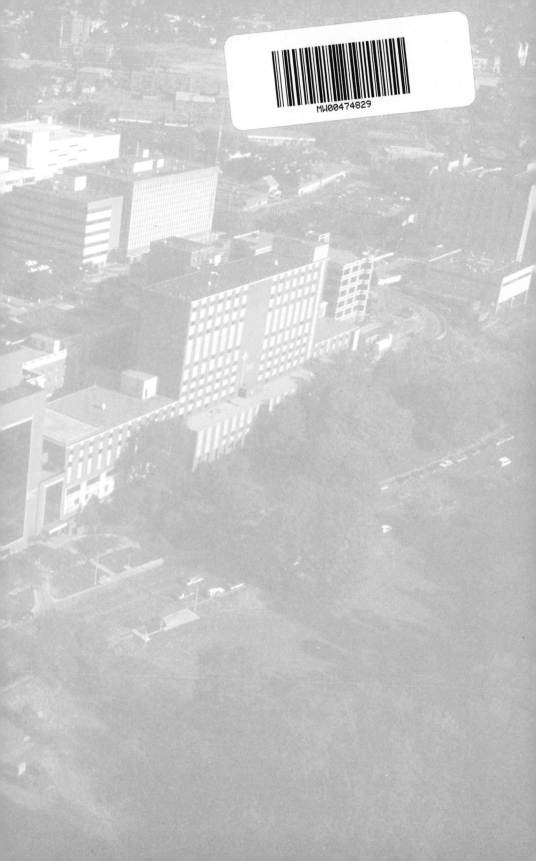

THE
PRESENCE
OF CARE

ॐ

The History of
Saint Luke's Hospital of Kansas City

ॐ

EDWARD T. MATHENY JR.

THE PRESENCE OF CARE

The History of
Saint Luke's Hospital of Kansas City

by Edward T. Matheny Jr.

SAINT LUKE'S HOSPITAL PRESS
KANSAS CITY, MISSOURI

THE PRESENCE OF CARE
The History of Saint Luke's Hospital of Kansas City

© 1997, Edward T. Matheny Jr.

ISBN: 0-9657425-0-4

Cover jacket and book design by Prime Media, Inc.

Printed in the United States of America by Walsworth Publishing Company

Saint Luke's Hospital Press
Kansas City, Missouri

To Ann, and to our family.

TABLE OF CONTENTS

"We at Saint Luke's want to disassociate ourselves from the factory concept of medicine."

– The Right Reverend Arthur A. Vogel, retired Bishop of West Missouri and former Chairman of the Board, Saint Luke's Hospital of Kansas City, who in March, 1976, suggested "The Presence of Care" as the hospital's motto.

"Do not neglect to show hospitality to strangers, for by doing so some have entertained angels without knowing it."

– Hebrews 13:2

"Take care of him and I will repay thee."

– From the parable of the Good Samaritan, as reproduced on the seal of Pennsylvania Hospital

"When did we see thee a stranger and welcome thee ... and when did we see thee sick ... and visit thee? ... 'Truly, I say to you, as you did it to one of the least of these my brethren, you did it to me.' "

– Matthew 25:38-40

PROLOGUE

S aint Luke's Hospital began as All Saints Church, an institution founded by the Church Charity Association in 1882 to meet a need in early Kansas City. A decision in a will contest formally established the linkage between All Saints, which closed its doors in 1893, and Saint Luke's, founded by the same Association nine years later.

A common thread running through the history of the hospital has been the Episcopal Church. The organizational meeting that resulted in the Church Charity Association and its hospital, All Saints, was convened by an Episcopal priest in his parish church, St. Mary's. The cornerstone for All Saints was laid by an Episcopal bishop, and the same bishop formally dedicated and opened the hospital building upon its completion. When the Church Charity Association rose again from the ashes of All Saints Hospital, the rector of Saint Paul's Episcopal Church was one of the three incorporators of the association's new hospital, Saint Luke's. And almost at once, the first bishop of the new Diocese of West Missouri assumed sponsorship of Saint Luke's.

At all times since, Saint Luke's Hospital has been affiliated with the Diocese of West Missouri. Diocesan bishops served as the hospital's president and later as its board chairman. The hospital has been the subject of reports to the annual Diocesan Convention since 1904.

Episcopal church services and Episcopal chaplains have been part of the fabric of Saint Luke's Hospital, where the church has added an extra dimension to "the presence of care."

ONE

founding father

The Reverend Henry David Jardine was a maverick Episcopal priest in cowtown Kansas City. Faced with defrocking, the rector of St. Mary's Episcopal Church died a mysterious death. But if Saint Luke's Hospital had a founding father, it was Father Jardine.

St. Mary's was organized in 1857. It today ministers to a small but devoted mission congregation of the Episcopal Diocese of West Missouri and, some believe, the restless apparition of Father Jardine. But Jardine's place in the history of Saint Luke's Hospital is real enough.

It was Father Jardine who convened a meeting of prominent Kansas City businessmen in his small, wooden church building at Eighth and Walnut streets on July 7, 1882, to discuss the need for more and better hospital accommodations in Kansas City. At the time, only tax-supported City Hospital and Sisters' Hospital, a Roman Catholic institution established by the Sisters of St. Joseph of Carondelet, served the teeming city of 56,000. Jardine's meeting led in due course to Saint Luke's Hospital, where "the presence of care" is to be found today.

Father Jardine was a paradox. His ecclesiastical appearance—notably his elaborate vestments—was a curiosity in the rough frontier community that was Kansas City in the latter part of the 19th century. But his contrasting conduct was characteristic of the time and the town.

One episode is illustrative. A drunken communicant disrupted a religious service when Jardine refused him communion. In the face of threatened retaliation, the priest proceeded with his celebration of the Mass ... fortified by a pair of six-shooters laid upon the altar.

Jardine's employment of "catholic" ritual (including incense and confession) alienated another parishioner, this time with more serious consequences. The offended communicant was the editor of a fledgling local newspaper—*The Kansas City Times*—whose subsequent investigation of Jardine uncovered a prior criminal record and two-year prison term. There were also more current allegations of child molestation, seduction, misuse of church funds, and drug abuse. The newspaper published unsavory stories about Father Jardine, and in 1885 he filed suit for libel. *The Times* defended its articles as factual, and Father Jardine lost his case.

The Episcopal bishop of Missouri, Charles Franklin Robertson, convened a nationally publicized ecclesiastical trial of charges against Jardine. The proceeding was held in St. Louis, the bishop's See city. The verdict, returned October 7, 1885, found Father Jardine guilty on three counts, two of them involving women and one the use of chloroform, a drug which Jardine had used for years to alleviate insomnia. He maintained his innocence in newspaper interviews despite the verdict and sought a new trial. But on January 10, 1886, before there could be any decision by the bishop on that issue, Jardine died.

The beleaguered priest's body was found in the sacristy of Trinity Church in St. Louis, a handkerchief wet with chloroform over his face. Most people believed he had taken his own life, although some maintained that he had been murdered and the chloroform used to disguise the crime.

Father Jardine's remains were returned to Kansas City for interment. While Jardine's body lay in state in St. Mary's Church, more than 3,000 curious Kansas Citians came to view it. Admission tickets were required for the burial service as a means of crowd control.

Because of the prevailing belief that his death was a suicide, Jardine's remains were interred in an unconsecrated plot in Union Cemetery. Thirty-five years later, church officials concluded that Father Jardine's death was not a suicide, and the body was reburied in consecrated ground in Forest Hills Cemetery.

During the century since the death of Father Jardine, there have been rumors that his spirit occasionally visits St. Mary's, now at 1307 Holmes, in a "new" building dating back to 1888 and listed on the National Register of Historic Places. These phenomena are attributed to Father Jardine's desire for rehabilitation. The priest's ghost is innocuous, however, creating noises and shadowy appearances but doing no harm.

Meanwhile, the hospital Father Jardine helped found has demonstrated, like the priest, the ability to survive its own demise.

Saint Luke's early history is an account of considerable resilience during often turbulent times. Throughout, the hospital has steadfastly clung to its fundamental mission of quality care for all patients, including many who are unable to pay.

TWO
1830-1882

early Kansas City ... its physicians, hospitals and history

S aint Luke's story is a part of the history of Kansas City in general and of its medical community in particular. This history predates Saint Luke's and, indeed, predates the city.

A plaque on the Saint Luke's campus now marks the location of the home of the Reverend Isaac McCoy, a Baptist missionary to the Shawnee Indians. The site, known as "Locust Hill," overlooked a small valley to the east drained by Mill Creek.

In 1833, Isaac McCoy's son, John Calvin McCoy, built a general store not far from the present location of Saint Luke's and filed a plat mapping out the town of "West Port"—soon to become known as "Westport." Riverboat passengers disembarked at neighboring Independence, some 14 miles to the east; their first day's travel by oxen team brought them to Westport.

In 1834, John McCoy and others purchased land near the junction of the Missouri and Kansas Rivers and founded Westport Landing. When passengers discovered that they could disembark at this more westerly point, the struggling landing began to grow. Incorporated as the Town of Kansas, it ultimately became Kansas City, engulfing Westport and dwarfing Independence in the process. When John McCoy died, he joined other Kansas City founders in Union Cemetery.

• • • • •

During Kansas City's formative years, the citizenry of Jackson County believed more in self-help than in consulting a physician. Typical was a treatise for the layman written by Dr. John A. Gunn, bulging with "do-it-yourself" remedies. According to Gunn's *Domestic Medicine or Poor Man's Friend,* should an amputation become appropriate, the operation required "nothing but firmness and common dexterity for any man to perform it well." The dilettante surgeon would need a large carving knife, pen-knife, strip of leather or linen, twelve ligatures made of waxed thread, curved awl, pincers, adhesive plasters, bandages, and sponge. Equipped with those items and Gunn's instructions " … any man, unless he be an idiot or an absolute fool," could perform the operation.

Missouri native Mark Twain was skeptical of such publications, cautioning the citizenry of that era: "Be careful when you use a 'doctor book.' You might die of a misprint."

Physicians were prominent in the early development of Kansas City. The first medical doctor to settle in the community was Dr. Benoist Troost, a former steward in Napoleon's army who arrived in 1847. Dr. Isaac Ridge, the first American medical school graduate to open a practice in Kansas City, established an office in 1849 where Main Street ended at the Missouri River levee. Ridge had great influence over neighboring Wyandotte Indians, who made him a member of their tribe and named him "Little Thunder" in recognition of his short stature and stentorian voice.

Dr. Johnston Lykins, also destined to occupy space in Union Cemetery, was Kansas City's first capitalist and served as the town's mayor in 1854. During the Civil War, Mrs. Lykins refused to take a required oath of Union allegiance and was banished to neighboring Clay County, across the Missouri River. It is said that as her boat left the landing, she called to the doctor and reminded him where his underwear was to be found, warning him against putting it on if it was damp.

· · · · ·

The Civil War created a shortage of physicians in Jackson County, as most doctors heeded a call to arms on one side or the other. Those who remained in private practice at home found their services badly needed during the Battle of Westport. Fought in October, 1864, that engagement was the largest land battle west of the Mississippi, with 29,000 men participating. Each side set up a hospital in the Harris House in Westport, which also served as the headquarters of the Kansas Militia's commander, General Curtis. A second medical facility was housed a few miles south at the 500-acre farm of John Wornall, purchased by John's father, Richard Wornall, from John Calvin McCoy in 1833.

Saint Luke's Hospital's main entrance is located on the road that, just a few blocks away, leads past the old Wornall home. Originally called "Wornall's Lane," it is now the thoroughfare Wornall Road.

Approximately 75 percent of Missouri's inhabitants were of Southern ancestry, and many of the state's traditions and sympathies lay with the South. The Confederate battle flag featured thirteen stars, representing the eleven states of the Confederacy plus two more—Missouri and Kentucky—which the Confederacy hoped would join it in secession from the Union.

The Missouri slave population was small in comparison to that of other slaveholding states. A two-block-square group of homes just to the west of Saint Luke's present location was set aside as slave quarters prior to the Civil War. The site of Penn School, built in 1868 as the first school west of the Mississippi River "for the express purpose of educating black children," lies just to the north of the hospital. Dwindling remnants of this community remain today, some of them having found work at Saint Luke's Hospital over the years. Lois Cooper, a Saint Luke's RN, remembered it as "a high-caliber black community; the blacks had been there for a long time."

The Civil War propelled medicine into modern times and in the process altered the perception and quality of hospitals. Hospitals before the Civil War were dreadful places, inhabited primarily by the destitute, who, like the poor souls consigned to Dante's *Inferno,* abandoned all hope upon entry. Hospitals were usually sponsored by religious organizations. The sick were cared for but seldom restored to health. Confinement in a hospital ward diminished a patient's survival prospects, and post-surgery death rates were higher in hospitals than at home. Florence Nightingale cautioned: "No patient should be kept in the hospital one day longer than his condition warrants." Prior to the Civil War, a physician might never have set foot in a hospital during his entire medical career.

The Civil War enhanced the reputation of hospitals, particularly the Union hospitals, whose patients were treated with considerable success. Once hospitals gained credibility, it became apparent that post-war

Jackson County was seriously deficient in its facilities. Doctors who had previously attended all of their patients at home and performed operations on kitchen tables now wanted access to hospitals.

• • • • •

The first hospital within the city limits was City Hospital, opened for the indigent in 1870. It was a time of progress on several fronts. *The Kansas City Times* began publication that same year. A new mule-powered streetcar system connected Kansas City and Westport. And the Kansas City Medical College had just been founded. A proprietary institution, it suffered from low admission standards and poor facilities. There was also a shortage of legally procured clinical material ... cadavers often were obtained by midnight forays to the public burying ground. In 1905, the college would be absorbed by the University of Kansas School of Medicine.

Although hospitals were scarce in post-war Jackson County, medical practitioners were plentiful. If anything, the county was oversupplied with men calling themselves doctors. These "doctors" were not always reputable—their numbers included unlicensed adventurers who saw opportunity in the west. Nearly 5,000 people practiced medicine in Missouri in the year 1882, but only about half were graduates of legitimate medical schools.

Legislation adopted in 1874 required a doctor to have a degree from a legally chartered medical school and register it with a county clerk, but it was so easy to establish a medical school in Missouri that the state had a plethora of such "colleges," and possession of a degree was virtually meaningless. An anatomy act was also passed in 1874, allowing medical students the use of unclaimed or donated cadavers for dissection; raids on cemeteries declined.

The Missouri State Board of Health, established in 1883, was responsible for the licensing of medical schools and introduced an admissions requirement of at least a high school degree "or equivalent." But good old American ingenuity found a way around this: there arose a brisk business in the manufacture of ambiguous "equivalent certificates." When the Board of Health countered with a compulsory examination, the Missouri Supreme Court ruled that the Board had exceeded its authority.

Finally, a Medical Practice Act was proposed, establishing a Board of

Medical Examiners. This solution had impressive support, not only in the medical community but also in the Presbyterian and Methodist churches … the latter motivated less by concern over the quality of medical care than by the growing popularity of Christian Science. The act was adopted, despite the opposition of physicians with a financial stake in the success of medical schools.

One consequence of the remedial Medical Practice Act in Missouri was an exodus of many of the state's quacks across the border to neighboring Kansas. Some Missourians claimed that this migration of medical ne'er-do-wells actually improved things on both sides of the state line. But there soon followed pressure for reform legislation in Kansas similar to that adopted in Missouri. Kansas established a state board of health and gained some measure of control over the practice of medicine there.

Post–Civil War Kansas City was a wide-open town, its gambling emporiums a lure for some of the West's most colorful characters, including Wyatt Earp, Wild Bill Hickok, and Bat Masterson. In 1881, gambling was outlawed, leading a riverboat gambler named Bob Potee to don his high silk hat, pick up his gold-tipped cane, and commit suicide by sauntering into the rushing waters of the Missouri River.

Jesse James, a frequent Kansas City visitor, was shot and killed in nearby St. Joseph, Missouri, on April 3, 1882. Three months later, on July 7, 1882, occurred the meeting hosted by Father Jardine at St. Mary's Episcopal Church.

THREE
1882-1883

All Saints Hospital ... Sisters of the Holy Cross ...
Dr. Flavel Tiffany ... osteopathy ... bankruptcy

*T*he St. Mary's gathering, although encouraged by the Episcopal Church, actually led to an independent, nonsectarian hospital whose board was composed of distinguished citizens, including the then-mayor of Kansas City, John W. Moore. The founding parent organization, formed to own and operate the hospital, was named "The Church Charity Association of Kansas City," and the Articles of Agreement of the Association were dated October 3, 1882. The Association's original charter made it clear that charity care was to be integral to its hospital, and revenue from paying patients was to be spent in support of "free wards," whose occupants would not be charged for their hospital stay or treatment.

A lot was purchased at 1005 Campbell, and in an elaborate religious ceremony, Bishop Robertson laid the cornerstone for All Saints Hospital on May 6, 1883. The fifty-bed hospital was opened on May 10, 1885, after three years of planning and fund raising. The formal dedication and opening, over which Bishop Robertson presided, predated Father Jardine's fall from grace by only a few months.

The All Saints Hospital building was a three-story structure of red brick, heated by steam and boasting a newfangled elevator. It was designed by local architect Vantyle W. Coddington, with an interior plan "drawn with full consideration for the latest knowledge of sanitary laws." George Halley, M.D., in a *Kansas City Medical Index* advertisement, promised that his surgery patients would be admitted to the new hospital … the city's most modern facility at the time.

During Father Jardine's tenure at St. Mary's, he organized a parochial sisterhood of Episcopal nuns, "The Sisters of the Holy Cross," and enlisted a Miss Brock and a Miss Ferero as novices. Miss Brock became Sister Mary Frances. Miss Ferero, who adopted the name "Sister Isabel," became the Mother Superior. When All Saints Hospital opened, the two sisters, garbed in traditional habits, took charge of nursing services aided by Father Jardine. (Thomas B. Bullene, a former mayor and founder of what became the prosperous Emery, Bird, Thayer & Company department store, assisted financially.) Sister Mary Frances died soon after the order's inception, but Sister Isabel—who demonstrated a considerable aptitude for fund raising—became the superintendent of All Saints.

The new hospital was a teaching institution, offering instruction in clinical medicine. Cases were assigned to advanced students, who were required to examine their patients and then present a diagnosis, prognosis and recommendation for treatment. Instruction was supplied by faculty from the city's medical schools, who also served as members of the hospital staff.

The All Saints admission book listed mule skinners, wheelwrights, cowboys and lamplighters as patients. Among the first patients were: a meatcutter who breathed ammonia leaked from the primitive refrigeration system of a meatpacking plant; a 17-year-old mother of three with childbed fever; and a child with tetanus from a rusty nail.

• • • • •

The hospital's physicians included an "oculist and aurist" with a florid name: Flavel Tiffany. Dr. Tiffany was also a professor of diseases of the mind and the nervous system at the University Medical College. In an 1885 advertisement in the *Kansas City Medical Index,* Dr. Tiffany offered a twelve-week course in medicine for $25. According to the *Index,* the course would pay special attention to the use of certain equipment described in the ad, and in addition a portion of the course time would be devoted to practical study of the ear and the eye. There also would be an opportunity to perform minor operations on a living "subject"—clinical experience that was and continues to be an essential element of the medical-education process. At the conclusion of the course, participants received a certificate—presumably suitable for framing and mounting on the office wall.

Later *Index* ads by Tiffany added a paragraph offering continuing medical education to practicing physicians. He advised that his post-graduate courses were designed to benefit the general practitioner who wanted to rest from the routine work of a laborious practice and also to enhance or refresh his knowledge of those special subjects that for want of time and opportunity might have been neglected during his college days.

Anesthesia was a developing art, and an article in the *Medical Record* in January, 1886, by Dr. Tiffany shared with his colleagues an unsatisfactory experience in the use of cocaine as an anesthetic during a cataract operation performed at All Saints Hospital; the popular anesthetic was not without risk and was to be used with great care.

That year, several members of the All Saints medical staff attended a meeting of the Missouri State Medical Association in St. Louis. There the Women's Christian Temperance Union proposed an educational program to acquaint school children with the evil effects of demon rum. However the supporting resolution was tabled … some of the doctors believed alcohol to be medically beneficial.

The new era brought a growing understanding of the importance of public hygiene, and 19th-century medical science led the fight for greater sanitation. It was discovered that polluted drinking water caused cholera, which occasioned many deaths in Kansas City. In a plea for cleaner streets, Dr. Herman B. Pearse, then editor of the *Kansas City Medical Index,* complained that at the intersection of East Fifteenth Street and Southwest Boulevard "the mud has been from two to six inches deep, of the consistency of gravy, filthy beyond expression from the offal cast into it and the droppings of animals that pass over it."

In addition to championing public hygiene, Dr. Pearse in 1891 presented a paper to the Jackson County Medical Society entitled "Meddlesome Midwifery," in which he maintained that for women in childbirth, any labor lasting longer than three-and-a-half hours was "unnatural." He advocated the use of forceps in such cases, to relieve the mother of further pain. Many of his colleagues vehemently disagreed with his compassionate recommendation.

One of those most influential in establishing All Saints Hospital was Dr. John Fee, who as City Physician had a substantial impact on the public health of the day. His surname notwithstanding, Fee did not show undue interest in compensation for his work … indeed he served the city for $2,200 per year, a modest sum even by the standards of that era. An article in the *Medical Index* decried the inadequacy of Dr. Fee's salary. The work of City Physician was described as onerous, and the article observed that if the occupant of the office were to do justice to the job and to himself, the position should command compensation of $3,000 per year.

The 19th century produced medical practitioners of considerable variety. Osteopathy was founded in that era by a rural Missouri doctor, Andrew Still. Dr. Still believed that diseases were due chiefly to loss of skeletal integrity, which could be restored by manipulation of the body's parts, supplemented by therapeutic measures such as the use of medicine or surgery. In 1891, Dr. Still began teaching osteopathy in Kirksville, and the next year he obtained a charter and established a school. Osteopathy, the only philosophy of health care native to the United States, won legal recognition from the state legislature in 1897 and has remained a significant force in Missouri medicine.

There were other medical sects as well: hydropaths and magnetic healers, to name two. Relief for the sick also was offered by patent-medicine manufacturers. Lydia Pinkham's Vegetable Compound, heavily laced with alcohol, was an example of the elixirs available for purchase in Missouri and elsewhere. And for decades Dr. John Sappington of Saline County, Missouri, manufactured and sold quinine pills for the relief of those suffering from malaria … the scourge of the frontier.

As the 19th century drew to a close, the advent of antiseptic surgery further reduced hospital mortality. Advances were made in immunology, with vaccines against typhoid and tetanus becoming available. There were also new diagnostic techniques and technologies. The latter included microscopic and X ray tests and electrocardiograms.

• • • • •

Meanwhile, the supporters of the new All Saints Hospital sought ways to sustain their institution financially. A benefit bazaar in 1885 produced gratifying results. The bazaar featured a popularity contest in which patrons cast ballots for their favorite clergyman, with a bookcase and some books to be awarded the winner. A Jewish rabbi garnered a number of votes. Another finalist was Father Jardine; apparently the stories in circulation about St. Mary's priest did not greatly damage his popularity. However, after careful tabulation of the votes, one R. Talbot was proclaimed the winner.

In 1893, disaster struck. A hospital board member who also acted as hospital manager authorized the expenditure of $15,000 for improvements to All Saints, intending to personally advance the funds needed to defray that expense as a gift. The improvements were effected, but the director was forced to declare bankruptcy before he was able to transfer the money. Resources were no longer available to pay for the improvements, and the hospital was compelled to close its doors at the 10th and Campbell location.

Neighboring University Medical College acquired the hospital building, renaming it University Hospital. The facility was used by the elite surgeons of Kansas City, who taught clinical techniques to the medical students there.

FOUR
1902-1903

resurrection ... Dr. Herman Pearse ...
River Market ... Sponable will

*D*r. d'Estang Dickerson, friend of Dr. Herman Pearse, was one of the more reputable physicians to make his way west after the Civil War. He was the prison physician for New York's Sing Sing Penitentiary and thereafter served as a Union Army surgeon, before establishing a medical practice in Kansas City in 1865. He preceded Dr. Fee as Kansas City's first City Physician. Dr. Dickerson died of pneumonia in 1902, bequeathing his medical equipment to his friend, Dr. Pearse—enough instruments to equip two floors of a hospital.

A member of St. Paul's Episcopal Church in Westport, Dr. Pearse consulted his pastor, the Reverend Percy Eversden, about the use to be made of the Dickerson windfall. The two men decided to open a hospital in a brick building with a slate roof at the northeast corner of Fifth and Delaware streets, a structure that had formerly housed Dr. Dickerson's Western Surgical Institute and that stood until recently in Kansas City's River Market area (then the city's tenement district). Percy Eversden declared that the location was fortuitous—social-settlement work and hospital care could now go hand-in-hand, and a free dispensary and hospital in that district would do much to relieve the overburdened and crowded City Hospital. It was his conviction that this new "free" institution could be maintained permanently.

William Rockhill Nelson published his first edition of *The Kansas City Evening Star* in 1880. By 1902 his newspaper was *The Kansas City Star,* and an article published October 2 of that year applauded the new enterprise:

> "The hospital will be dependent upon subscriptions for support. The task of raising the money for this purpose will not be confined to any denomination in the city, but an effort will be made to interest businessmen and members of all churches in the undertaking. The plan is entirely a new one in Kansas City. There are a number of private hospitals and sanitariums here, but people in poor circumstances have no place to go because of the overcrowded condition of the city hospital."

The hospital, opened October 4, 1902, contained twelve beds and was located on the second and third floors of the building. It had a kitchen, laboratory, surgery, and nurses' quarters.

The Church Charity Association was resurrected to own and operate the new institution ... named Saint Luke's Hospital. This is a popular name for church-sponsored hospitals—St. Luke, the "beloved physician" and companion of St. Paul, in whose gospel is found the parable of the Good Samaritan. A report of the first few months' operation, printed in the *Journal of the Diocese of West Missouri,* proclaimed that "to visit the sick is a divine commandment."

The first board of directors of the revived Church Charity Association consisted of the Reverend Percy Eversden, Dr. Pearse, and Mr. William A. Rule. Mr. Rule, cashier of the National Bank of Commerce and treasurer of the Church Charity Association, was a prominent member of the Kansas City community. His home, "Oaklawn," included elaborate stables for show horses.

Like All Saints Hospital, Saint Luke's accepted paying patients, and the initial financial statement of Saint Luke's Hospital reflected three months' income of $885.89. However, the revenue from paying patients was spent in support of the free beds, and expenses for the same period amounted to $886.89. The $1 deficit was covered by the Board of Directors.

A subsequent report for the seven months from October, 1902, to April, 1903, listed 588 patients treated in the free clinic, ninety-seven hospital inpatients, one death, and twenty-two referrals to other hospitals. Notably, all of the latter were patients willing and able to pay for hospital care but whom Saint Luke's could not accommodate without displacing charity cases. There were enough paying patients to generate revenues of $757.19. Cash contributions brought in another $502.10. There were also donations of clothing, linens, sewing, and other items from more than forty individuals and guilds.

• • • • •

Saint Luke's was firmly established as the successor to All Saints in a battle over a $5,000 bequest from one Sanford G. Sponable. Payment had been delayed because of a will contest. Sponable actually had bequeathed his money for the benefit of the defunct All Saints Hospital. University Hospital, having acquired All Saints' real property, claimed to be All Saints' successor with respect to this bequest. The Church Charity Association then entered the fray, bringing a lawsuit contending that in fact Saint Luke's, not University Hospital, was All Saints' true successor. In a legal brief filed in the case, the Association's attorney expressed regret that the administrator's doubts as to the proper distributee had generated an unseemly "scramble" for the funds, but that inasmuch as University Hospital had laid claim to the bequest, it became the Association's duty to contest the matter.

Saint Luke's case rested primarily on the fact that University Hospital was not the charity hospital that All Saints had been, whereas Saint Luke's clearly was. Persuaded by this argument, the court determined that Saint Luke's was indeed the reincarnation of All Saints and entitled to benefit from the Sponable bequest. Thus by judicial decree in a will contest, the All Saints Hospital of Father Jardine and his colleagues gained a new life as Saint Luke's Hospital.

The *Medical Index-Lancet* (formerly the *Kansas City Medical Index*) for July, 1903, carried an advertisement for Saint Luke's Hospital, identifying it as a general and surgical hospital for the care of the sick and stating that it received both charity and paying patients. There were two "free beds," one in the men's ward and one in the women's ward. Other indigent patients, when they could be taken, were given cots in the halls or ward or placed in pay beds.

Holidays were observed in the hospital. At Thanksgiving time in 1903, Dr. Pearse gave a live turkey, oysters, cranberries, sugar, and pears to the hospital's patients. And for Christmas that year, Mrs. Pearse contributed other foodstuffs, including mincemeat and candy, while the good doctor donated a basket of holly.

The hospital's annual report for 1903 pleaded:

> "Keep the hospital in mind. It is small now, but it is orderly, efficient, and its service first-class. Its location is ideal. We need our friends' good words and good offices to assist in filling our pay beds."

FIVE
1904-1906

the Hunter House ... Board of Directors ...
Edward Robert Atwill ... donations ... free beds

*I*n 1904, the hospital moved to a larger building known as "the Hunter House," located in a better neighborhood at 40th and Baltimore streets (4207 Central). The new site was conveniently near St. Paul's, the church of Percy Eversden and Dr. Pearse.

The Diocese of Missouri had been divided in two in 1890. The first bishop of the new Diocese of West Missouri was the Right Reverend Edward Robert Atwill, Dr. Pearse's future father-in-law, described by a contemporary as a "big, pompous sort of man." Bishop Atwill assumed sponsorship of the hospital and was largely responsible for making it a diocesan institution.

A report in an early *Journal of the Diocese of West Missouri,* covering the period May 1, 1903, to May 1, 1904, detailed the financial aspects of the hospital's activities during that early period in its existence. Donations were received in those months amounting to $171.02; charity care valued at $1,105.25 was contributed; and operating revenues were generated by patients' board, by the sale of medicines and dressings, and by the operating room.

The report listed highly diversified donations in kind, including paint, operating gowns and caps, pillowcases and sheets, screens, gasoline stoves, cots, and free delivery service. Spoons were donated by the wife of Dr. Pearse. Also contributed were magazines (copies of *Collier's Weekly*), rags, underdrawers, gifts of tea, jam and bedclothes by "St. George's girls," and medicinal spirits—two quarts of rum and two quarts of wine from a liquor dealer. To meet "constant needs," the hospital solicited fruits and vegetables and other foodstuffs, soap, flowers, and various kinds of night-wear. Also needed were surgeons' gowns and caps—the hospital's superintendent offered to furnish patterns for these items upon request.

For sanitary reasons, beards were losing favor with Saint Luke's medical personnel. German physicians denounced facial hair as a fertile source of infection during surgery, and the German emperor decreed that those who practiced medicine or surgery should cut off their whiskers. To avoid contamination of the milk supply, the New York milk commission ordered that only smooth-faced men should be employed for milking cows and delivering milk in the state.

Fund raising was incessant. A building fund was accumulating, in the hope that the Church Charity Association might some day own rather than lease its hospital premises. Meanwhile M.G. Harmon, the secretary of the Association and later the hospital's lay head, referred to the constant financial struggle as akin to the biblical "making brick without straw."

There were various endowment opportunities, ranging from a $300 donation entitling the donor to nominate a patient for free treatment in a ward for a year to a $20,000 charge for endowing a free room in per-petuity with the accompanying privileges of naming the room and nom-inating its occupants (privileges would extend to the donor's successor). Plans also were underway to endow a free bed, to be known as the "Bishop Atwill cot" … prospective donors were assured that Atwill endowment funds would be "faithfully applied and recorded."

Dr. Pearse continued his largess with donations of medical supplies. He contributed syringes, thermometers, gutta-percha tissue, gauze, absorbent cotton, chloroform, ether, needles, and plaster.

• • • • •

Membership on the Saint Luke's board was prestigious. At the turn of the century, hospital directors usually controlled access to free beds. To obtain entry, patients generally petitioned a director or the contributors who had endowed the beds. Hospital philanthropy enabled wealthy con-tributors to gain status and influence. Board memberships became important indicia of social position. Benefits enjoyed by sponsors not only helped satisfy a sense of "noblesse oblige" but also conferred power—through final decision-making authority—in the management of hospital funds, awarding of contracts, patronage in staff appointments, and admission of patients.

Despite the foregoing emoluments, the Saint Luke's board did not lose sight of its charitable mission; the people of the diocese were urged to keep Saint Luke's Hospital in mind when death threatened a "deserving poor person" in their neighborhood. They were asked to call the hospital in such cases and were assured that help would be given if at all possible. The hospital sent a free ambulance to transport patients and furnished free bed and medicine when the cause was deemed to be "just" and the hospital's means permitted.

The hospital was then paying rent of $60 per month for its Hunter House premises. The daily cost per patient of maintaining the hospital was $2.25. To help defray this expense, various charges were imposed upon paying patients for use of its facilities. The operating room cost $5 for a major operation and $3 for minor surgery. The charge for a private room was $15-20 per week and $7-10 per week for a ward bed. Private-duty nurses were available to the well-to-do at $10-15 per week. Medicines and dressings were furnished at cost.

The hospital promulgated stringent rules to be observed by its patients: prohibitions against profanity or vulgarity, loud talking, and any unnecessary disturbance or noise in the hospital or about its grounds. And it became an early smoke-free institution when it banned the use of tobacco in its wards or building.

• • • • •

In 1905, the Church Charity Association amended its articles of incorporation and bylaws. The revised articles stated that the purpose of the Association was to conduct both a charity and a pay hospital as well as other charities and to furnish gratuitous medical and surgical aid to such poor, sick, indigent, and distressed persons as might become patients of the hospital.

The Association's bylaws contained a general reservation of discretionary powers in the board of directors "to insure that nothing shall detract from the efficiency and high character of the hospital." Also, anyone contributing $5 per year became a member of the Association; a contribution of $100 entitled the donor to life membership. The hospital president, as provided in both the bylaws and the articles, was the bishop of the Episcopal diocese.

An enlarged board of directors in 1905 included a parish priest, the Reverend Theodore B. Foster, as well as Bishop Atwill. Among others listed were John Harding, a prominent attorney who the following year would become the lay head of the hospital, and B.C. Christopher, a successful businessman. Dr. Pearse also continued to serve as a director. Christopher resigned in 1905, noting that he had served on the board fourteen years (spanning the years when the hospital was inoperative). The secretary also tendered his resignation because of the clerical burdens of the office, but his objections to continued service were overcome when Mr. Rule furnished him with a typewriter.

Board committees included a "visiting committee," whose membership of two directors rotated monthly among board members in alphabetical order. It was the committee's duty to visit and inspect the hospital as often as its members thought proper.

The hospital employed a superintendent and a house physician. A superintendent of nurses doubled as principal of the nurses' training school. In addition to these executives, there were several subordinate employees.

Kansas City was home to two professional medical associations at that time—the Kansas City Academy of Medicine and the Jackson County Medical Society. Neither organization conducted dinner meetings, but after their business was concluded, members stopped at one of Kansas City's 500 saloons, paying five cents for a glass of beer and the excellent free lunch.

Medical ethics and professional image were of great concern to physicians, and there was an obsession with avoiding publicity. In 1906, Dr. Tiffany was charged by the Jackson County Medical Society with an ethical violation when he talked to a *Kansas City Star* reporter about a trip abroad and paid the reporter to mention that he left competent assistants in charge of his practice during his absence. Later, ads for abortions concerned physicians greatly. In his 1912 inaugural address, the then-president of the Jackson County Medical Society condemned "the ruthless performance of abortions in our private hospitals."

SIX
1906-1913

*the Samuel Scott House ... Auxiliary ... Nurse Keely
and the School of Nursing ... whites only ... Sidney C.
Partridge ... Hospital rules and charges ... Ursulla Burr*

*I*n 1906, the hospital moved again, to new quarters at 11th and
Euclid in a remodeled dwelling formerly owned by one Samuel
Scott. The house was purchased by Dr. Pearse for $15,000. He raised the
funds by mortgaging his home at 4515 Wornall Road, near Saint Luke's
present site. After acquiring the title to the 11th and Euclid property, Dr.
Pearse sold it to Saint Luke's for $1—a magnificent gift. It would house
Saint Luke's for the next seventeen years.

The Scott house had four upstairs rooms, with furnishings (including
crystal lights) supplied by the A.W. Peet Company. Room 19 on the front
of the house was the largest of the four. It had a beautiful Oriental rug on
the floor and was reserved for wealthy patients and their private-duty
nurses. The latter slept in the room, on a cot that fitted under the bed
when not in use.

Supplies were stored in the attic—liquid green soap, cotton, gauze,
and pads. There were not many medicines but plenty of aspirin,
whiskey, and wine.

The Saint Luke's Hospital Club, an organization of young women,
sponsored a charity ball at the New Casino, a large hall at 1023 Broadway.
Two hundred couples attended. The ball's proceeds went to maintain four
beds in the children's ward at the hospital. Also tickets were sold at $1 each

for performances of *Chimes of Norway*, an opera; profits went for hospital furnishings and maintenance.

The concerns of Saint Luke's physicians with their profession were not parochial. Dr. Jabez Jackson of the medical staff journeyed to Chickasha in the Indian Territory to participate in a meeting of the Central Oklahoma Medical Association. His broad interest in medical organizations would continue throughout his life; in 1927, he would serve as president of the American Medical Association.

Members of the hospital's medical staff attended the 1907 meeting of the American Medical Association in Atlantic City. They traveled by special train ... starting from Kansas City on the Missouri Pacific Railway to St. Louis, where they transferred to the Big Four and C&O railways. There were stops in Hot Springs and White Sulfur Springs, Virginia, and a visit to the Jamestown exposition.

Saint Luke's physicians were generous with their services. *The Diocesan Journal* for 1907 reported that all free patients accepted by the hospital received medical and surgical treatment from the doctors without charge, care representing the medical staff's contribution to the hospital's work in relief of the sick and suffering.

The treatment prescribed would be regarded as eccentric today. An article in a popular medical journal of the time advised doctors to administer a tonic of strychnine arsenate to patients suffering from chronic arthritis or rheumatism. Purging with laxatives also was believed to be beneficial; and some patients found relief in using tight rubber bands above affected joints. A panacea for consumption, constipation, gastritis, eczema, and nerve disorders was olive oil.

• • • • •

Patients undergoing such treatment were in need of tender, loving care, and Bishop Atwill appealed to the ladies of the community to form a hospital auxiliary "to visit and cheer the sick, to encourage the nurses, and to bring flowers and delicacies." The ladies responded enthusiastically, and Kansas City's first hospital auxiliary held its initial meeting in May, 1908, when seven women representing seven Episcopal parishes gathered in the parish house of downtown Grace Church for a planning session. Mrs. Andrew S. Buchanan was elected president.

From its inception, the auxiliary brought comfort and hope to Saint

Luke's patients. But it also made fund raising a central concern. The initial effort, an "author's reading" presented in a member's home, produced the sum of $35.75. Less than two years later, another $363.12 was generated through dues, musicals and rummage sales. With these funds in hand, the auxiliary assumed certain responsibilities at Saint Luke's, including care of the hospital grounds and walks. Later, using $900 generated by a county fair at the New Casino, the auxiliary was able to help maintain the hospital chapel and to purchase life memberships in the Church Charity Association for Bishop and Mrs. Atwill.

For the next decade or so, the auxiliary raised several thousand dollars through plays, dances, concerts, and bridge teas. Later, their fund-raising efforts expanded to include lectures, card parties, and "vanishing luncheons." The organization was particularly interested in children's care—a concern that endures today—and also supported a circulating library. The connection with the church was quite evident during those years. A history of the auxiliary commented that the lives of its members had been enriched by their association with the hospital.

• • • • •

Care offered by dedicated nurses was a characteristic of the new Saint Luke's Hospital. Among the first women in history to adopt nursing as a permanent vocation were the Canonesses of St. Augustine, Roman Catholic nuns who operated leper colonies in the Philippines and India. Later, handmaidens in the court of King Henry VIII of England wore velvet and brocade as they cared for the sick and wounded. There were nurses at the Battle of Bunker Hill and the Battle of Gettysburg. Civil War nurses included men, the poet Walt Whitman among them.

Nursing became more professional after the Civil War; three training schools were established in 1873. The profession received further impetus when women of refinement initiated reformation of nursing as an occupation. Doctors came to appreciate the improved care and to rely heavily upon trained nurses. By 1900, there were 432 training schools in existence in the United States.

All Saints Hospital organized a training school for nurses in 1887, but financial difficulties necessitated the school's closure two years later. In 1905, Saint Luke's Hospital established a diploma school of nursing, offering a three-year course of study with tuition rebates "for extra duty and good work." The nursing school has continued in unbroken service, providing nurses for the hospital and the community during the ensuing ninety-one years. There has been a constant need; often the demand has exceeded the supply.

When the hospital relocated in the Scott house in 1906, the superintendent of nurses was Miss Lou Eleanor Keely ... a tall, large-boned woman who was responsible for the nursing school and who commanded the respect of nurses and physicians alike.

Student nurses lived in two houses adjacent to the hospital. They were single women who tended to be between 20 and 30 years of age. They wore long-sleeved, long-skirted, high-necked blue dresses with detachable, starched, white "Betsy Ross" collars and cuffs, and a starched, long, bibbed apron. Completing the uniform were small organdy caps, black high-topped shoes and black cotton stockings.

Miss Keely conducted daily inspection, noting minutiae such as missing buttons. Perfection was required—"Miss Keely saw everything" was the comment of one graduate. Keely, "with the manner of a strict disciplinarian," insisted that nurses stand at attention when in the presence of doctors.

The training school for nurses graduated its first nurse in 1908 ... Miss Virginia Pate.

On October 12, 1908, Lillian Violet Townsend applied for enrollment in the Saint Luke's School of Nursing. She had been born in England and was then 24 years of age. In her nursing school application she gave her religion as "Episcopalian," having attended the Church of England before she emigrated. She also named the then-rector of St. Mary's Church as a reference.

Upon completion of her nurse's training, Miss Townsend was employed as a surgical nurse at Saint Luke's at a salary of $50 per month, with the stipulation that she would "give her extra time to soliciting funds." Miss Townsend was elected the first president of the nurses' alumnae association. She resigned her nursing position for matrimonial purposes ... a later list of nursing school graduates indicated that she had become Mrs. Harry F. Mather.

• • • • •

The hospital needed to expand in order to accommodate more patients. The Reverend Cyrus Brady, rector of St. George's Episcopal Church, issued an appeal for funds in October, 1910. He solicited outright gifts and long-term, interest-free loans for Saint Luke's, "a small but admirable institution with a capacity of twenty-five beds, and with a nurses' home adjoining." The hospital, "housed in a made-over dwelling," was said to be "practically self-supporting" despite the fact that 25 percent of the patients were charity cases who paid little or nothing. According to Father Brady, almost every day many patients—charitable as well as those who were able to pay—were turned away for lack of room. More were refused than accepted, because of inadequate capacity. Superintendent Keely was described as a woman of unusual character, experience, and ability; and the nurses "under instruction" were said to be "drawn from an unusually high class of young womanhood."

The Brady appeal declared that a new hospital must be built at once. Said Father Brady: "Its record proves its usefulness, its inadequacy declares its needs."

Saint Luke's was identified as the one solitary diocesan institution in West Missouri and the only non-Catholic church hospital in Kansas City. Father Brady concluded:

> "For God's sake, for Christ's love, Christian people of Kansas City, give of your sweet charity your assistance to this noble Institution for ministering to the poor and suffering brethren in your very midst."

One of the rules governing the hospital was an unfortunate social commentary on that era in Jackson County, Missouri. It limited Saint Luke's patients to persons of the Caucasian or white race.

At the turn of the century, black residents of Kansas City had access to very limited health care facilities … at City Hospital, a white professional was in charge, and black physicians struggled to gain appointment to the medical staff. Such discrimination was not peculiar to Kansas City— blacks and foreign-born were almost completely absent from hospital staffs throughout the country. Then, in 1908, a new "General Hospital" was completed for the white community, and the old City Hospital— renamed "General Hospital #2"—began to provide services especially for blacks. In 1911, a few black physicians were elected to the staff of the latter hospital. The city also approved a Negro School of Nursing, to train nurses for General Hospital #2.

Another Saint Luke's rule of that era barred persons having a chronic or infectious disease from admission to the hospital.

Damage done to hospital property was charged to the patient's account. Disorderly conduct was cause for ejectment, and patients becoming uncontrollable—from disease or any other cause—were subject to removal by the superintendent. Profane or loud talk and any "unnecessary" disturbances continued to be forbidden, as was the use of tobacco in the wards and building. Unless upon admission patients deposited their money and valuables with the superintendent, the hospital assumed no responsibility for them. Visits between patients, and food and drink other than as prescribed by diet were allowed only if authorized by the superintendent. Patients were requested to comply with nurses' instructions and forbidden to give them money or gifts. Lights were extinguished at 9 p.m.

Patients paid fifty cents for a meal, and nurses were provided board at the patient's expense, which was $5 per week. There were additional charges for fruits, wine and liquor, electric fans and laundry, as well as for drugs and dressings, and for use of the new diagnostic X ray laboratory.

Scrupulous records were kept of all charity patients, and the same care was rendered to them as to those who paid. Their numbers were limited, however; only "designated" rooms or beds were available for their use, and the cost of their care was charged to a charity account.

Name plates on room doors identified the donors of those rooms; if a donated room was occupied when its contributor was admitted to the hospital, the occupant was quickly relocated. Rooms also were furnished by various church organizations, including the Girls Friendly Society of St. Paul's Church, the Women's Auxiliary of St. George's Church, the Men's Bible Class of St. George's Church, the Girls Friendly Society of Grace & Holy Trinity Church, the Business Women's Club of St. Paul's Church, and the Guild of St. Paul's Church.

• • • • •

Dr. O.S. Gilliland was a pioneer Saint Luke's physician of the day. He received his M.D. degree from the University of Kansas in June, 1910, after spending his first two years at the University Medical College. In his later years he praised faculty members of the old Medical College, including Dr. Jabez Jackson; he also lauded faculty members of the University of Kansas Medical School. He described them as "honored men of yesteryear" and stated that it was a privilege and an inspiration to have studied under them. He paid particular tribute to Saint Luke's Dr. Peter T. Bohan, describing him as one of the outstanding teachers of his day. Bohan had resided in the Midland Hotel at a time when Gilliland, working his way through medical school, was employed as night pharmacist at the hotel's drug store. Dr. Gilliland characterized a medical student of his era as "a young man or young woman long on optimism and enthusiasm, and short on finances, but with an abiding faith in himself and his chosen profession."

Dr. Gilliland later reminisced that he had practiced medicine in the horse and buggy days, the trolley car days, the Model T Ford days, the eight-cylinder car days, and the airplane days. "Who could ask for anything more?" His cash income from his fourth month of practice: $37.00. "Typhoid fever, malaria, and pneumonia were a good source of income for the general practitioner, as well as an occasional epidemic of smallpox or flu. Night calls were common, and about 80 percent of the babies were delivered in the home."

The street in front of Saint Luke's was paved with bricks, and hospital patients could hear the clip-clop of hooves as the horse-drawn milk wagon made its daily rounds. City ambulances were also horse-powered until 1911, when the Police Commissioner of Kansas City purchased two motorized ambulances. A cautious approach to horseless carriages seemed warranted because the experience of the local citizenry with automobiles had not been very satisfactory. A few years earlier, when there were only two such contraptions in all of Kansas City, their drivers managed to collide on 11th Street between Oak and Locust.

Bishop Atwill died on January 24, 1911, and was succeeded by Bishop Sidney C. Partridge, formerly Bishop of China. The new hospital head was described by nurse Meer Shane as "a dignified and wonderful person."

On May 28, 1913, Bishop Partridge broke ground at the rear of the hospital (11th and Euclid) for an addition. The addition was completed in 1914, increasing the hospital's capacity to fifty beds.

Provision was made for the care of sick and disabled seamen at the flat rate of $2 per day. Where these seafarers were expected to come from was not disclosed.

• • • • •

As late as 1897, there were no maternity hospitals in Kansas City, and women would wait for many years before it became safer to have a baby in a hospital than at home. (The dangers included contagion and puerperal—or "childbed"—fever.) However, in 1913 a doughty lifelong Episcopalian, Ursulla Burr, insisted on having her baby at Saint Luke's. She had moved to Kansas City from the East, where hospital births had become accepted. Saint Luke's provided no rooms for the delivery of babies, but at her urging the men's ward was vacated, and her baby was born there.

SEVEN
1914-1917

physician access and organization ... baby camp ...
Richard Cabot Club ... nurses' training

The hospital was under the benevolent dominion of the Episcopal Church in spiritual matters, but the church's religious ministrations were not offered to a patient unless he or his family so desired. Other religious denominations were given equal access.

The philanthropy initiated by the Sponable bequest was succeeded by other gifts. Thomas B. Tomb left $5,000 to the hospital, and the sum of $100 was bequeathed by Mrs. Louisa G. Musson. $1,500 was donated to the hospital under the will of Mrs. Olivia Thompson. Mrs. Ellen St. Clair gave the hospital a nearby vacant lot, a gift valued at $3,750. And Mr. Rufus Barton Green of St. Paul's parish left $922.21, which was placed in the Bishop Atwill Cot Fund. Donations of fruits, vegetables, and other necessities continued to flow from friends of Saint Luke's; all were entered in the hospital's records.

· · · · ·

The typical hospital medical staff organization in 1914 boasted a consulting staff composed of eminent, senior physicians. More important to the hospital, however, was its attending staff, which provided most of the patient care. In a teaching hospital there was also a house staff of young doctors in training who actually administered the treatment prescribed by the attending staff, in exchange for free room and board.

Saint Luke's initially permitted an open medical staff, allowing all competent physicians to practice there. However, a more selective approach was initiated in May, 1914, when an "approved" list of physicians and surgeons was compiled and those named were specially invited to make use of the hospital—its rooms, wards, and equipment. A letter of invitation to the selectees listed certain state-of-the-art additions to the hospital's facilities and noted that the nurses averaged one for every two patients. Hospital food was a concern even then, for the letter boasted that the hospital continued to enjoy a "reputation as to sufficient diet service." The invitation also offered assurance that the hospital would "as nearly as possible" comply with the requirements of the Clinical Congress of America.

Greater hospital control over staff membership was imposed in 1915, when Saint Luke's bylaws were changed to provide that medical staff members were to be nominated by the diocesan bishop and elected by the board of directors. The tenure of physicians was limited to three years unless their election to the staff was unanimous.

• • • • •

By 1915, an open air baby camp for underprivileged infants, founded by the Saint Luke's Hospital Club in 1905, was well entrenched. The camp was located originally at Fifth and Charlotte streets, in the center of the tenement district known as "Little Italy" and "the North End"—a part of the city occupied by many poor immigrants who lacked transportation and had to live near their jobs. It was the first enterprise of its kind in Kansas City, an outdoor clinic to care for infants during the heat of the summer. William Rockhill Nelson was credited with much of the support for the camp, soliciting contributions in the columns of his *Kansas City Star*. In 1906, another camp was opened by the Club—this one on the city's West Side. Later, both camps were consolidated at the West Side location, 21st and Jefferson streets.

The name of the Saint Luke's Hospital Club was subsequently changed to the "Richard Cabot Club," in honor of a Cambridge, Massachusetts, doctor. Dr. Cabot was a member of the Harvard medical faculty and a pioneer in medical social welfare. Club membership was described as large, enthusiastic, and nonsectarian. The name of the West Side clinic also was changed to the "Richard Cabot Clinic," although it was still associated with Saint Luke's. Lists of contributors to the camp included a number of prominent Kansas Citians as well as various Episcopal Sunday Schools and the "Saint Luke's Busy Bees."

In 1915, the baby camp had fifteen beds made of iron with white enamel coating, divided between two tents connected by a "modern" screen doorway. The attitude of the camp toward its clientele was decidedly paternalistic. When babies arrived at the camp, they were immediately bathed. Their old clothes were discarded, and sterilized new garments were provided. The babies' diet during their stay included goat's milk prescribed by the camp's attending physician, Dr. David Broderick.

The first prenatal instruction in the Kansas City area was offered by the same Dr. Broderick to expectant West Side mothers.

· · · · ·

By 1915, the School of Nursing was well established. Applicants for admission had to be between 21 and 32 years of age, and present evidence of good moral character, good health, and good education (at least one year of high school was required). Other prerequisites included good teeth, vaccination within a year prior to admission, books, uniforms, a long coat, scissors, a watch, and "noiseless shoes." Women of "superior education and refinement" were preferred.

Each applicant underwent a probationary period of two or three months, after which she was accepted or dismissed. Acceptance required her agreement to conform absolutely to all of the rules and regulations governing the hospital. She remained the object of careful scrutiny; during the next six months her record was carefully considered, and, if unsatisfactory, she was subject to dismissal by the superintendent. She could also be dismissed at any time for inefficiency, misconduct, or neglect of duty, as well as for failure to keep up with her studies.

Pupils were expected to attend Episcopal chapel services when their duties permitted. Make-up was prohibited, as were dates. The hospital furnished living quarters, and the nursing students were expected to reside there. The shifts were twelve hours in duration: 7 a.m. to 7 p.m. for day nurses, and 7 p.m. to 7 a.m. for night nurses.

The students' day began with breakfast at the hospital. Grace was said at all meals, and punctuality was strictly enforced. If students were tardy, they languished in the hall until an explanation was offered. The housekeeper presided over the dining table. And silence reigned; according to a graduate of that era: "It was all done very quietly. You could have heard a pin drop in the dining room."

In the second and third years, students were paid $5 per month and in case of illness were cared for at hospital expense. However all time lost, for any reason, had to be made up by the end of the term. Students were allowed one to two hours of free time daily as well as one afternoon each week and "when practicable" one-half day on Sundays. There were also three weeks' vacation each year.

A school publication described the work of a nurse as requiring intelligence, good temper, an orderly habit of mind, thorough trustworthiness, and a willing spirit. In addition, this paragon of virtue was to be endowed with a strong sense of duty and a willingness to conform to strict rules of discipline.

Diplomas were awarded only if students passed their examinations for state registration ... the school accordingly could boast that none of its graduates had ever failed to pass her state boards. Of the thirteen girls who entered the school in 1915, only four graduated. Mrs. Pearse took the graduating seniors to tea at the Hotel Muehlebach, where they were entertained by a string quartet.

Memories of Kansas City's frontier days were still vivid. Florence Parsons, a 1916 graduate who later became chief nurse on one of Saint Luke's floors, recounted a call on a sick neighbor:

> "One thing I remember, at the corner of Twelfth and Garfield there was an old lady who lived in there ... I had heard that she had been scalped by Indians ... I told Miss Keely that if we ever got a call to go down there, that I sure wanted to go ... I never knew whether it was true or not, but that was the tale they told. I did find out that she tied her head up in a handkerchief at night. But I didn't get to see how much hair she had, whether she had her whole scalp or not."

• • • • •

Space in the hospital was at a premium. In October, 1915, a room serving as a pharmacy was converted to a minor operating room, with the pharmacy's drug supply relocated under the watchful eye of Superintendent Keely. However, no significant quantity of drugs was kept on the hospital premises. During this period, most of the drugs supplied to patients were purchased from Samuel Robinson's Drug Store at Twelfth and Brooklyn streets. Orders were placed as needed by telephone, and the delivery boy/soda jerk would ride over on his bicycle with the supplies.

During the fiscal year ended October 31, 1915, the hospital cared for 909 patients, of whom 112 were treated without charge or at a discount. Free care amounted to 1,609 patient days. For the thirteen-month period from October 1, 1914, to October 31, 1915, hospital records showed a net financial gain of $8,376.55 reflecting income from various sources and numerous offsetting entries, including a "charity" entry of $3,022.01. A short list of life members paid $100 for membership, and an even shorter list of honorary members—Mr. Jacob L. Loose and Mr. Adam Thompson—each paid $500 for the honor.

Saint Luke's was hospitable. Patients were welcomed as guests and treated accordingly. After their departure, their rooms were sealed and fumigated with formaldehyde candles that burned for eight to ten hours; curtains were taken down and washed; and beds were turned down for the next patients.

There was concern in 1916, that the hospital's discriminatory "white patients only" rule posed a potential problem for Saint Luke's under its contracts to furnish hospital care for employees of the Navy Department and of railroads. However, there was some flexibility; when Rosie, the popular black cook, fell ill, she was hospitalized at Saint Luke's and two sympathetic nurses were assigned to her case.

At a December, 1916, meeting of the hospital board, Dr. John Hayden appeared and stated that a Mr. Thompson of Duluth had been his patient two years earlier, and that Thompson's father was a man of considerable means who had expressed his appreciation for the care given his son by offering to build a hospital for Dr. Hayden. In the ensuing discussion it was suggested that if the matter was pursued, it should be done with concrete plans in hand. Bishop Partridge also insisted that any such gift should be unconditional. There was then adopted a motion that Dr. Hayden communicate with Mr. Thompson, asking if he was ready to have plans for a new hospital submitted to him, providing for a 100-bed institution that would be fireproof and modern and situated on the present hospital grounds at Eleventh and Euclid. Nothing further came of this proposed gift ... apparently Mr. Thompson had second thoughts when confronted with reality.

• • • • •

A.C. Stowell succeeded John Harding in 1917 as lay head of the hospital.

A Saint Luke's memo in March, 1917, described the advantages of continued control over staff membership: development of the hospital to a "high plane of efficiency," distinguishing it from an "invalid home" or a "high class boarding house" for chronic cases; elimination of "slipshod methods" by the members of the medical staff, whose work would then "stand checking"; and further development of the School of Nursing.

The Saint Luke's medical staff table of organization was ambitious in 1917. There was a chief of service "A," with an associate, and a chief of service "B," also with an associate; there were chiefs of surgical services "A" and "B," each with an associate; there was a pathologist with a resident assistant; occulists "A" and "B" each had an associate, as did nose and throat "A" and "B;" and there also were to be a dentist, an orthopedist, a Roentgenology (X ray) practitioner, a superintendent of nurses, an associate superintendent who was also "teacher of student nurses," a manager, and a dietitian. There was also provision for a consulting staff in medicine, surgery, nose and throat, eye, and orthopaedics.

Staff officers were selected annually by their peers. Over the years, the term "chief of staff" was used interchangeably with "president" to identify the physician serving as head of the medical staff.

The hospital House Committee was made up of representatives from the board of directors, administration, nursing school, and medical staff. This committee supervised hospital management. However, the physicians clearly had assumed responsibility for the professional aspects of the hospital's activities. The policy of the hospital with respect to standards of excellence, therapeutic procedure, equipment, admission and care of patients, and patient records was determined by the medical staff alone. Similarly, the appointment of assistants to the staff was subject to staff approval, and the courtesies and privileges of hospital practice were extended to outside physicians only with staff approval.

All regular staff members could admit patients for treatment or diagnosis whenever the hospital could accommodate them. Free patients were cared for by the attending staff and assigned to particular "attending members" as their area of expertise dictated. The arrangements for such care and for attendance at the patients' clinics were subject to staff approval.

The United States' entry into World War I in 1917 necessitated some relaxation of control over staff membership due to doctor shortages.

Because several physicians were called away to the service, and others were likely to be, the policy was revised to permit practice at the hospital by any physician or surgeon approved by an admission committee of three staff members acting in concert with the superintendent of nurses.

That year a pharmacist and a business manager joined the hospital staff.

Woman doctors were a rarity in Kansas City. The Women's Medical College of Kansas City opened in 1895, and Dr. Alice Berry Graham and her sister, Dr. Katherine Berry Richardson, founded Children's Mercy Hospital in 1897. But until well into the 20th century most medical schools maintained quotas limiting the enrollment of women. Nevertheless, women began to enter the profession in increasing numbers. An employment application was received at Saint Luke's from a Dr. Ione Pinney of Abilene, Texas, who identified herself as "a churchwoman." Dr. Pinney had been in practice for a number of years and especially sought "hospital work." Saint Luke's replied that the only paid positions at the hospital, other than nurses in training and subordinate employees, were those of the superintendent and assistant superintendent.

EIGHT
1917-1918

World War I ... influenza ... American College of Surgeons

$\mathcal{A}$merica's entry into the First World War affected the hospital in many ways. Superintendent Keely joined other nurses in the service and was dispatched to France, taking with her fourteen student nurses from Saint Luke's. She became chief nurse at Base Hospital No. 28 in Limoges, staffed by several Saint Luke's physicians and surgeons. Other Saint Luke's RNs also served in France. Florence Parsons, now a brand-new RN, made the trip overseas aboard a troop ship. En route she contracted both measles and mumps from infected young soldiers. Recovering, she was stationed near battle-scarred Verdun in one of the busy general hospitals collected in an area called "Hospital Hill."

Nine other Saint Luke's nurses left the hospital to engage in "home service" during World War I.

Hospital directors also were called to the colors. Mr. Jay M. Lee, a director and Board Secretary, resigned to serve his country.

Because of World War I enlistments in the armed forces, Kansas City hospitals were understaffed in 1918, when a worldwide influenza epidemic struck. The disease killed more Americans than did the Germans, and Kansas City ranked in the top ten cities nationwide in flu-related deaths. Army draftees assigned for training to Kansas City's Sweeney Automobile and Tractor School died during the epidemic, some of them while patients at Saint Luke's Hospital. During the height of the contagion, Saint Luke's was converted to a military hospital, with a military doctor in charge for some three months. All but two of the Saint Luke's nurses fell ill with the disease and were placed on beds in the chapel. Several died. Two of the military patients had tuberculosis; their cots were placed on the hospital lawn to avoid contaminating others.

As would be the case later with poliomyelitis epidemics, little was known about influenza. Public health officials attempted to stop the contagion by asking people to stay home, by allowing only emergency operations, and even by banning kissing. Patients were isolated, attempts were made to reduce fever and control dehydration, aspirin was the chief medication, and prayers were offered that pneumonia would not ensue.

The war ended with the armistice on November 11, 1918, and Saint Luke's doctors who had served in the armed forces returned to private practice. Among them was Dr. O.S. Gilliland, who found it difficult to re-establish his practice after a prolonged absence. Typhoid fever and malaria were fast disappearing, and pneumonia was being successfully treated with serum.

· · · · ·

Upon returning after the War, Miss Keely organized rural nursing throughout Missouri and helped found the Missouri State Nursing Association. She had been replaced at Saint Luke's by Miss Clara Tulloss as superintendent, and Miss Cecelia Calpernia ("Callie") French later became principal of the training school.

Medical advances were accompanied by standards for improved hospital care instituted by the American College of Surgeons—among them a requirement that institutions concerned with treating the sick or injured submit to regular review. The standards were supported by the Jackson County Medical Society. The Saint Luke's board resolved that the hospital should comply "as far as possible" with the College's standards, and a letter advising of this policy was directed to the physicians and surgeons practicing at the hospital.

The same basic standards apply today, but now are implemented by numerous manuals and investigators. A Joint Commission (Joint Commission for the Accreditation of Hospitals or "JCAHO") administers a vast bureaucracy whose surveyors descend on the hospital periodically, necessitating preparation well in advance of their arrival and the devotion of two or three days to their visit by hospital administrators and physicians.

A request by the auxiliary that same year that it be represented by a voting member on the board of directors was rejected on the ground that the Board lacked the authority to grant the request.

The medical staff pressed the board for an "analytic laboratory"—the forerunner of the modern pathology lab. Dr. William K. Trimble, a pathology professor at the K.U. Medical School, was hired as the hospital's first pathologist. He equipped the lab at his own expense and recovered the cost through fees charged for lab work performed by him and his assistant. A $3.00 lab fee was assessed against each patient to cover analysis of blood, urine, secretions, tissue, etc. The arrangement promoted greater accuracy in diagnosis and reduced the hospital's costs.

A summary of the hospital's condition in 1918 noted that it was handicapped by inadequacies with respect to building, equipment, and funds. The ability to keep the doors open was attributed to a steadfast staff of physicians and a splendid, loyal nurses' training school. "With a capacity of fifty beds we have had at times over fifty patients. 996 patients treated, of whom 120 wholly or partially free." It was argued that a new hospital should be built or Saint Luke's would be relegated to second-class status. Hospital superintendent Clara Tulloss appealed to the board:

> "Let us build a hospital that will not only be a monument for the church but for Kansas City as well. We have made this our life work, make it your plaything."

There were working relationships with other hospitals. Nurses were sent to Children's Mercy Hospital to learn how to care for children. Nursing students also went to General Hospital, which was affiliated with the Saint Luke's school for "contagious work." The nursing school's curriculum required anatomical science and other academic courses, and nursing students attended Junior College for their first five months of classroom work.

NINE
1919-1923

A. W. Peet ... surgery ... Dr. Arthur Hertzler ...

preparations to build and move ...

medical education ... obstetrics

The hospital governing body's articles were amended in 1919 to change the parent organization's name from Church Charity Association to Saint Luke's Hospital. The board, which had been self-perpetuating, would now consist of nine persons elected by the Diocesan Convention in addition to the bishop of the diocese.

The annual meeting of members in March, 1919, empowered the board of directors to dispose of the existing hospital property, select a new site and erect a new hospital building, if in their judgment that course was necessary. The members deliberately avoided tying the board's hands with specific directions.

In August, 1919, Mr. F.C. Barber of New York City was employed to conduct a fund-raising campaign for the new hospital. Meanwhile, there had been efforts to determine the proper site for such a hospital. Some sentiment favored the existing site ... if it were chosen, a friend of Dr. Logan Clendenning would donate $50,000 for a clinic building to be erected on the Euclid Avenue alley corner.

• • • • •

On August 29, 1919, A.W. Peet was elected second vice president of the hospital. He would serve Saint Luke's in exemplary fashion for many years and through difficult times. Mr. Peet was aptly described as a "tower of strength" during the trying Depression years, when he contributed substantial personal funds to cover expenses, including, on occasion, the hospital payroll. Other members of the Peet family, as well as Peet Brothers Company and its successor Colgate-Palmolive-Peet Company, also were significant donors.

There were efforts to acquire nearby property because of a concern that it might be sold to "negroes." Dr. Pearse attempted to obtain it through a trade but was unsuccessful ... the tract was available only for cash.

Society was less litigious then, but it was prudent to insure Saint Luke's Hospital against liability on account of patients' personal injury or death. A liability insurance policy was purchased from the Fidelity & Casualty Co. of New York for $15,000 coverage—the premium was $3 per year per bed.

An estate bequeathed to Saint Luke's included one dozen dinner forks valued at $8. These were presented by the board to an old friend of the deceased, accompanied by "an appropriate letter of compliments" from the president.

There was "some misunderstanding in regard to who was the official X ray doctor"; to clarify things, Dr. E.H. Skinner was appointed to that position. The job carried with it the hazard of dealing with radioactive materials, a risk that was not fully appreciated at the time.

On September 25, 1919, the board hosted a dinner for the medical staff. The stated purpose was to draw the board and staff closer together. Another purpose: to hear from the doctors, personally, their attitude towards the new Saint Luke's Hospital plan. Dr. Arthur Hertzler, president of the staff, opened the discussion, and several others offered remarks. The doctors also seized the opportunity to voice complaints about the service, diet, and cleanliness of the hospital.

The medical staff recommended the immediate cancellation of a hospital contract to provide care for Army and Navy patients unless they were treated by members of the staff, and in September the hospital's president met with the director of the American Red Cross to implement that recommendation.

• • • • •

There was only one operating room at Saint Luke's. Artificial light was not as effective then as now, and a skylight in the center of the room's ceiling provided natural light for the operating table just beneath it. One side of the room contained sterilizer tables and instrument trays. Two stools and a small bench provided relief for the anesthesiologist. Outside the operating room were the sterilizer and sterile water, together with a sink in which the doctors could scrub up. A table held sterile solutions, such as bichloride alcohol, and sterile gloves.

A small, dark room adjacent to the operating room was used for eye, ear, nose and throat treatment.

A nearby doctors' dressing room contained a lavatory and storage space for the doctors' wooden, velvet-lined instrument cases. Each doctor furnished his own instruments; only in the event of an emergency would one doctor use those of another. The hospital supplied sterile gloves. While the surgeon was scrubbing, his instruments were boiled in the sterilizer and set up on the tables in the operating room, ready for his use. In later years the doctors donated their instruments to the hospital, where they were pooled and made available to everyone.

A blackboard outside the surgery door listed the daily operating schedule, naming doctors and patients.

The operating room was cleaned by nursing students, who scrubbed the ceiling, walls, and furnishings. A black man named "Pate" waxed the floor.

Great care was exercised for the comfort and protection of the surgical patients in 1919. Each was clothed in a cap and stockings. A hot water bottle was placed in his bed, and a cotton blanket covered him. Hospital gowns opened in the back, a fact that patients occasionally overlooked while traversing the hospital halls.

Postoperative patients remained in bed for several weeks. For many years it was the practice to place in a specimen bottle any parts of the patient's anatomy removed in the course of an operation—appendix, gall stones, or tonsils, for example—and exhibit them to skeptical patients as proof of their removal.

• • • • •

In 1919, the American College of Surgeons required hospitals wishing to receive its approval to organize their affiliated doctors into a "definite medical staff." The College was flexible: the staff could be open or closed, with as many active, associate and courtesy members as desired so long as they were competent and reputable, did not split fees, abided by formal bylaws, and held monthly meetings and reviews of clinical experiences. At a meeting in December, 1919, twenty-five doctors were chosen for a closed medical staff at Saint Luke's.

The staff included several specialists. A shift toward specialization in medicine began in the 1880s, and by 1912 the bylaws of the Jackson County Medical Society were revised to establish committees of specialists in internal medicine; surgery; gynecology; pediatrics; radiology; dermatology; genito-urinary; eye, ear, nose and throat; and pathology.

The president of the staff from 1917 to 1920 was Dr. Arthur Hertzler, later acclaimed nationally for his autobiography, *The Horse and Buggy Doctor*. Dr. Hertzler was very tall, with long arms and legs, a large nose, and a tie that "never looked quite right with his collar." He established a modest hospital in 1902 in Halstead, Kansas, where he received patients and operated on Sundays and Mondays. The remainder of the week he spent in Kansas City, teaching, operating, and writing. Dr. Hertzler did much of his writing while traveling on the Santa Fe train between Halstead and Kansas City. He joined the Saint Luke's medical staff in 1914, where he was a closed staff proponent. Although he had a specialty—thyroid and goiter surgery—paradoxically he derided specialization as a means of avoiding the greater demands of general practice. An expert pathologist, he was precise and swift at the operating table, where he sat on a stool and disdained the wearing of gloves (he did not want to impair the sensitivity of his fingers).

A medical staff stalwart in the Hertzler years was Dr. J.C. Minor, a proctologist. Today, a plaque in the hospital hallway commemorates a gift in honor of Dr. Minor and his wife, Marie. Minor practiced medicine in the grand manner. While making rounds he wore a beautiful black dressing gown and was described by one awed intern as "just about the most majestic person you ever saw." Dr. Minor owned a large, chauffeur-driven limousine. He would sit in the back in solitary splendor, his hands resting on the ivory head of his cane. When the car arrived at Saint Luke's, he would remain seated until the chauffeur stepped out and opened the door. Then he would emerge, remove his gloves and place them on the seat beside the cane, and proceed to the hospital's front door—ready to grapple with the medical problems of the day.

• • • • •

The hospital began raising money for a new building in 1919 and within a year had in hand $271,000 and a contract to buy four acres of what was once John Wornall's pasture land—the present site of Saint Luke's Hospital. The campaign produced an anonymous gift of $25,000 for a chapel. And a significant sum was collected from patrons of downtown show houses—$643 from the Gaiety Theater alone, which featured silent movies and vaudeville acts. Also, John Thompson of the Conservatory of Music promised to give a concert that would net $10,000; and additional funds would be generated from the sale of the old hospital building. A second fund drive yielded another $79,000, and construction of a new hospital was assured.

The firm of Keene and Simpson was selected as the architect, and the Long Construction Co. signed on to do the construction work. Ground was broken December 19, 1920. A.W. Peet served as chairman of the building committee. The building would lie to the south of 43rd street and be abutted by both Mill Creek Parkway and Wornall Road.

Mill Creek Parkway had been completed in 1913 and provided a boulevard connection from downtown by way of Penn Valley Park, Broadway, and Westport. Both the Parkway and Wornall Road led to nearby Brush Creek, along whose banks the Country Club Plaza was in the formative stages. Beyond Brush Creek, development of the prestigious Country Club district and affluent Mission Hills, Kansas, was underway, with easy access to the new hospital site. And across Mill Creek Park to the east was the Country Club Trolley Line of the Metropolitan Street Railway Company.

The selection of this site as the location for the new Saint Luke's Hospital contributed significantly to its subsequent success, as well as to the perception that it was a "silk stocking" institution.

• • • • •

The first prenatal instruction in the Kansas City area had been offered by Dr. David Broderick to expectant West Side mothers. By 1920, at a time when a relatively small number of women received instruction in prenatal care, Saint Luke's Hospital was operating a prenatal clinic.

In 1920, midwives still were delivering about 50 percent of the babies in Kansas City, and puerperal (childbed) fever took a heavy toll—the following year there would be thirty-six maternal deaths in Kansas City from this illness out of a total of 5,127 births. But the clinic operated by Saint Luke's Hospital did not experience a single death.

· · · · ·

Today Saint Luke's Hospital is a major teaching institution, affiliated with the medical school at the University of Missouri-Kansas City. The basis for accreditation of modern medical schools is a report by Abraham Flexner, funded by the Carnegie Foundation and published in 1910. The Flexner report recommended that the nation's strong medical schools be further strengthened, that a few from the middle ranks be improved, and that the rest be terminated. The result was the demise of many small medical colleges. Among the casualties was University Medical College, which closed its doors in 1913.

The responsibility for medical education was assumed by the surviving schools, separating academic medicine from private practice. The KU School of Medicine was one of the survivors.

Future doctors' training would conform to the standards and values of academic specialists. The lasting consequence was that a large number of schools became engaged in training specialists and an insufficient number concentrated on training general practitioners.

Upon graduation from medical school, doctors began to undertake additional training in hospitals, leading to further specialization. Internship was a necessary preliminary to the more specialized medical residency ... interns rotated through the emergency room (one month), pediatrics (two months), obstetrics/gynecology (two months), internal medicine (two months), and surgery (two months), with an additional elective month. In 1904, about 50 percent of the graduates received such advanced training; by 1912, the figure was 75-80 percent. The American Medical Association published its first listing of these hospital internships in 1914.

According to AMA records, Saint Luke's Hospital was approved "for furnishing acceptable internships for medical graduates" by 1920. During the period 1920-1923, while Saint Luke's was at the Euclid Street site, graduate medical education got its formal start at the hospital. The medical interns (sometimes spelled "internes") were young M.D.s in their first year of post-graduate medical education; the service exposed them to broad clinical experience and compensated them with free room and board.

In March, 1921, the Saint Luke's board wrote Governor Arthur Hyde, petitioning him to veto Senate Bills #433 and #342 liberalizing medical licensure, on the ground that they would make Missouri "a dumping ground for inefficient practitioners from other states." One of the objectionable provisions dealt with the qualifications of acceptable medical schools; the bill would require only that such institutions be "chartered" rather than "reputable." The board's letter stated that physicians licensed to practice in Missouri should come from "such high institutions as St. Louis University, Washington University, and the State University."

The board argued that while on the surface the proposed legislation appeared to be laudable as antidiscriminatory, the owners and managers of hospitals "must exercise the greatest discrimination in the character of the people we admit to practice in our wards and private rooms." One of the primary functions of hospitals was said to be "to protect their sick from incompetent practice," which power would be lost if the bills were to pass.

• • • • •

In November, 1921, it was noted that a Saint Luke's obstetrical department was added the previous month, and that there had been three cases thus far "with several more booked for the next few weeks." From the start these cases were a financial bonanza, bringing $10 extra for use of the delivery room in addition to the other charges paid by maternity patients "who always stayed two weeks." It was observed that "their care is easy as a rule, and their diets regular." Furnishing the new department involved only modest additional expenditures, mainly for baby cribs and an extra table for the delivery room. Future success was anticipated, for "we have been running almost full since adding this department ... ."

A report listed six "unimproved" cases dismissed from the hospital, representing a marvelous collection of ailments: fracture of radius (nonunion), insanity, hysterical insanity, pin in bronchus, thyroid or goiter, and smallpox. The report also noted that the nurse's training school had a fine academic record: "Out of the eight training schools which affiliate with Junior College for the first five months of nurse's theory—our pupils were the only ones who did not make a single failure."

A summary of 1921 noted that only 137 "government cases" were admitted during the year, whereas in 1920 there had been 330. The attrition had some financial impact because, "We are getting $3.00 per day on these cases in wards, where other patients pay only $2.50 per day." The decrease was attributed to the government "taking over" another unnamed area hospital.

A list classified 1921 admissions according to religion, with "unclassified" the most numerous, followed distantly by Methodist, Christian, and Roman Catholic, in that order. Among the remainder, Episcopalians were in the middle of the pack. The final religion named on the list: "Salvation Army."

An April 2, 1922, publication of Grace and Holy Trinity Church indicated that, of the funds contributed for the new hospital in 1920, only a small percentage was given by Episcopalians ... "There were more Roman Catholics and Jews contributing than Episcopalians."

The restrictions on medical staff membership were eroding. Another Grace and Holy Trinity periodical a week later answered a question about a "closed staff" as follows: "If you mean by a 'closed staff' a prohibition of any reputable physician or surgeon to practice at Saint Luke's Hospital, it emphatically has not a 'closed staff.' " Quality of care was not adversely affected; the hospital had "been given grade A by the American College of Surgeons," said to be "the highest award that can be given a hospital."

The nurses' caps were modified in 1922. Bestowed on freshmen in a capping ceremony after a probationary period, they featured three points symbolizing the "tools" of the nursing profession—head, heart, and hands.

A board meeting in December, 1922, adopted a resolution authorizing residence in the hospital by Ellen St. Clair, described as "a benefactress" of the hospital who had lost her home at the Montagne Hotel ... Mrs. St. Clair paid a stipulated sum to the hospital each month for her care. The rules prohibiting "chronic cases" were suspended in this instance.

At a January, 1923, meeting of the board, Dr. Trimble proposed that in the new hospital facility there be graduated laboratory fees, with Saint Luke's receiving a $3 fee for urinal and blood analysis from each patient upon entering the Hospital, and the laboratory physician receiving all other fees charged the patient as his compensation for services rendered. The latter services were later amplified as involving blood chemistry, serology, "and other highly technical and clinical work," which was itemized. It was anticipated that not all patients would remit payment to laboratory physicians without encouragement, for it was provided that the hospital would receive 20 percent of the physician's fees for its collection efforts.

Dr. Skinner presented a plan for X ray services, suggesting that the hospital own the equipment (to be purchased at a cost of $4,000) and that charges for services rendered be divided between the X ray physician and the hospital.

The medical staff committee on interns reported that three full-time men would be required at a cost to the hospital of $150 per month, including room, board, and laundry.

The list of physicians to comprise the medical staff of the new hospital facility also was approved, and rates were established respecting certain specialized care: rates for hospitalization of nose and throat cases were fixed at $12 per case for a period of twenty-four hours in ward beds, and for obstetric cases at $75 for ten days' single occupancy of west front rooms or $60 for double occupancy. Regular rates were to apply in each case after expiration of the specified period.

• • • • •

Aware that Saint Luke's would soon move from its Scott House location, a delegation representing the "Eastside Protective Association" paid a visit to the hospital, asking whether it was the intention of the board to sell the old hospital building to "colored" people. Their spokesman stated that the Association sought to impose racially restrictive covenants upon an area that included the hospital. Such restrictions would be stricken later by the United States Supreme Court but were valid and enforceable at the time. Specifically, the Missouri Supreme Court only a few years earlier had upheld a prohibition against sale of property to a black person for a twenty-five-year period. The Association asked the board to sign an agreement that would preclude for fifteen years the sale of the Saint Luke's Hospital property to blacks. The delegation was informed that the matter would be taken under consideration.

Others also expressed interest in the property for hospital use. One was an organization of Free Methodists, contemplating establishing "The Hogue Memorial Hospital." Another was a Jewish Committee consisting of Rabbi Blazer, Morris Biggus and Barney Stevens, with all communications to be addressed through Dr. Abraham Sophian. Nothing came of either of these inquiries. Meanwhile, the board resolved to decline the restrictive proposal from the Eastside organization ... not on moral grounds but because the property was a valuable asset and the board was unwilling to "tie its hands by restricting purchasers to the white race." The board urged the Association to find buyers "to take it for purposes they approve of." Nothing resulted from this invitation either, and the hospital's vice president was authorized to advertise the property in the newspapers and to place a "for sale" sign in the yard.

At a meeting in March, 1923, the board was informed that "Dr. Dibble, a Negro Episcopal Minister, wanted to take over the old hospital and operate it for colored people under the name of Saint Luke's Hospital for Colored People." Dr. Dibble was requested to reduce his proposition to writing, but nothing was submitted.

At another board meeting later that month, an offer was presented from Atlas Realty Company of $85,000 for the old hospital building, with "Wheatley Hospital at $25,000 to be considered in the deal." A committee was appointed to investigate the offer, with authority to immediately dispose of the property "at the best terms possible." No sale ensued.

Finally at an April 27, 1923, meeting of the board, word came of a proposal from the Vail Maternity Hospital for purchase of the old hospital building. The proposal was approved. This sale was consummated, and the Vail Hospital began operations shortly after completion of the new Saint Luke's building on Mill Creek Parkway. The maternity hospital operated for several years before the Swedish American Savings and Loan Association foreclosed on the property. In July, 1938, the old hospital building and the Euclid Avenue frontage were sold to St. Stephen's Baptist Church, a black congregation whose former structure at 910 Harrison had burned in a fire in February, 1938.

TEN
1923

new hospital ... John R. Smiley ... babies ...
Country Club Trolley Line ... Peter T. Bohan ... Christmas

T he new hospital building, a handsome, fireproof, brick-and-terra
cotta structure rising six stories from sloping pasture land, was
dedicated on Feb. 25, 1923. A special prayer service was conducted by
Bishop Sidney C. Partridge. Four motorcycle officers and six traffic
patrolmen were required to manage a crowd so great that automobile
traffic on Mill Creek Parkway came to a complete standstill.

Three days later, the Saint Luke's board of directors hosted a reception
for the medical staff.

On March 1, patients were transferred from the hospital's Eleventh and
Euclid location. Eighteen patients were conveyed by ambulance, with a
nursing student accompanying each patient. During the day, twenty-two
more were admitted. Six operations were performed, and two babies were
born ... all on the first day of occupancy.

The 150-bed facility was old-fashioned by today's standards, with roll-
up window shades and a coal-burning power plant. But it was state-of-
the-art at the time, featuring electrically operated dumb waiters and a
solarium on each floor—a source of considerable pride to board and
medical staff.

The hospital directors commissioned a portrait of Bishop Partridge to
be hung in the hospital lobby. Since then, incumbent bishops' portraits
have graced the Saint Luke's lobby.

That same year, the hospital's corporate articles and bylaws were amended by then-Chancellor William G. Holt of the Diocese of West Missouri. He inserted language formally establishing a closer relationship between the hospital and the Episcopal Church.

The first records of the new building's emergency room are dated March 1, 1923. Miss Ruby Shaw, R.N., head of the hospital's "central service," acted as head nurse of emergency service ... presiding over a steam sterilizer and a few instruments. At that time, and for many years thereafter, services in the ER were free of charge for all comers—patients were treated and then referred to their family doctor for any necessary further care.

There was a plan to help defray the cost of the new hospital by offering Second Mortgage Bonds in the amount of $150,000. The churches of the Diocese were called upon to underwrite and sell them in proportion to parish size. The vestry of St. George's Church agreed to sell $12,000 worth of the bonds, and Mr. Peet personally offered to underwrite them provided the other churches participated equitably. The vestry of St. Paul's agreed to take care of that parish's proportionate share.

The ladies of the hospital auxiliary used the lecture room one day a week for sewing.

Mr. Peet assumed responsibility for planting rye grass seed about the bare grounds of the new hospital building.

Room rates not previously established for the new facility were fixed, and the medical staff was advised of the charges. However, there was some flexibility ... use of higher-priced rooms at a reduced charge was authorized when all lower-priced beds were occupied; the patient was relocated as soon as a cheaper room became available. Meanwhile, the hospital was not squandering revenues on gourmet food—it was reported in June that the cost of meals averaged between seventeen and eighteen cents each.

• • • • •

Saint Luke's was built, and in the early years operated, by its board of directors. Their dedication, hard work and direct financial support, together with an increasingly influential medical staff, had created a totally new organization that was now at the epicenter of the city's health care system. However, the hospital's administrative and clinical complexity continued to grow, and on June 1, 1923, John R. Smiley was employed as Saint Luke's first professional administrator, with the title of "manager" (later "superintendent") and a salary of $4,000 per year.

• • • • •

That spring, Callie French and the nursing staff proposed a party for the graduating class of nurses at Mission Hills Country Club. The "festivities" were authorized by the board, provided the cost did not exceed $150.

By July, 1923, the baby business at Saint Luke's was booming. The thirty-bassinet nursery was frequently overwhelmed ... there had been thirteen births in March, eighteen in April, thirty-five in May, and twenty-nine in June. For the month of July, there were an average of ten babies per day in the hospital, and in the course of that month there were thirty-eight births. In August the board authorized, as part of a general reduction of room rates, a reduced flat rate for maternity cases "for the ten-day lying-in period," from $55 to $50. That month saw thirty-six births and an average of fifteen babies per day in the hospital.

The board also approved for the charitable Minute Circle Association the same rates as prevailed for the Richard Cabot Club, to wit, $4.50 for twenty-four-hour hospitalization for children's operative cases; for all other cases, $1.00 per day up to the amount stated on the admission card.

A contract for hospital services with the U.S. Veterans Bureau was renewed in August, 1923. That same month, the board authorized John Smiley to replace six white housemen drawing $40 per month plus room, board and laundry, with four colored housemen at $20 per week with no room or board. Smiley also was authorized to handle and sign for all narcotics and alcohol.

There was recognition of the growing professionalism of hospital administration when John Smiley was authorized to attend the annual meeting of the American Hospital Association in Milwaukee. However, the board continued to take its obligations very seriously. It did not abdicate responsibility in favor of a very competent professional administrator ... always a hallmark of the Saint Luke's directors.

A tennis court on hospital grounds was completed by September and put to use by the nurses and some patients.

Mrs. Clarke Salmon had paid the cost of furnishing a room at the hospital. After her death, her own day bed was placed in that room, and her wheelchair was given to the children's floor for use by the children.

At a meeting of the board in October, 1923, considerable time was devoted to discussion of the Country Club Trolley Line carrying passengers to and from the hospital. The board authorized the use of cinders produced by the hospital's coal-burning power plant to construct a walk through Mill Creek Park to the trolley tracks. This had the approval of the park board. Saint Luke's director Gordon Beaham was named a committee of one to call on the police commissioners for protection of disembarking passengers, because of "an experience of one of our nurses while coming from the car line to the hospital." He later advised that such protection would be handled by the Westport district of the police department.

The House and Grounds Committee spent $250 to build a waiting station at the trolley line, and the street railway company approved the new "Saint Luke's Hospital Station."

Dr. Peter T. Bohan was the hospital's largest admitter in October in terms of patient days; Dr. Harold P. Kuhn was second, although he actually had more patients, twenty-three. Dr. Van Eman had eighteen obstetrical cases … the obstetrical floor was maintaining an average of fifteen patients per day.

Prohibition was the law of the land, but Dr. Bohan and his sympathetic colleagues brought relief to suffering patients by prescribing whiskey for such complaints as bronchitis, insomnia, laryngitis and flu.

Costs were assessed against the hospital for the curbing and widening of Mill Creek Parkway. The directors tried to avoid the assessment but were advised by Judge Holt that the hospital would have to pay. The park board also was contemplating repaving the parkway surface; the board would exercise vigilance to insure that the hospital was not burdened with the entire cost of that project.

An article by student nurse Violet Smith described the 1923 Christmas festivities in the nursing school. All of the students gathered in the assembly hall at 6:30 p.m. on Christmas Eve and followed the superintendent into the dining room. Here, in addition to some small tables provided for faculty, there was a long table set for the students as well as small trees brilliantly decorated, wreaths, nut baskets, and favors. At the students' table there were place cards in the form of the various girls' heads, wearing the hospital cap and bearing a question which the nurse was required to answer—much to her embarrassment and the delight and amusement of her friends. There then followed a four-course dinner, and during the last course a vested boys' choir from one of the Episcopal churches sang carols from the hall. After dinner the students reassembled in a classroom where there was a large Christmas tree and where packages from home were presented. Then Santa entered with a pack of novelty gifts for each student nurse accompanied by a poem to be read aloud by the recipient. Many of the student nurses then attended a midnight service at Grace and Holy Trinity Church. The next morning—Christmas Day—all of the students sang carols in the hospital corridors.

ELEVEN
1924-1930

Dr. Logan Clendenning ... Peet generosity ...
hospital progress ... Dickson and Diveley ...
Dr. F.C. Helwig ... interns ...
Linda Hall Fund ... Robert Nelson Spencer

*T*he first three floors of a new nurses' residence were built in 1924. Such was the board's confidence in the future of the hospital that the contractors were authorized to proceed with construction before the financing was arranged.

Student nurses continued to live cloistered lives. Day girls worked from 7 a.m. to 7 p.m., with a half hour for dinner and for supper and three hours off duty (some of this free time was spent in classes); relief girls worked 7 p.m. to 9 p.m.; and night girls worked 9 p.m. to 7 a.m., with a half hour for midnight supper "if you could get it." Students were paid about 58 cents per hour. Unless on duty, all nursing students had to be in by 10 p.m., with lights out at 10:30. Everyone was expected at chapel daily, except Sunday, and at breakfast, where their appearance in uniform was inspected. They were allowed one all-night a month. There were "wonderful" school parties attended by every student not on duty, and the doctors also gave parties for them. Students were never permitted off campus in uniform except as a school body. They did attend night classes downtown at Junior College, rushing across Mill Creek Park after a 4 p.m. meal to the Saint Luke's Hospital Station to catch a north-bound Country Club streetcar. No smoking was permitted while in uniform.

Married students were barred from enrollment in the school, and marriage by a student was prohibited.

The summer well-baby camp was not equipped to care for sick infants, and in February the board approved a proposition by the Richard Cabot Club for a summer ward in the children's department of the hospital. It involved maintenance by the club of pediatric beds on the sixth floor, for which they paid $1 per day per patient, with a minimum of $350 and a maximum of $750. The club also furnished beds, linens, mattresses, diapers, clothing and medical attention by a pediatrician. The hospital furnished nursing care, supervision by the hospital children's superintendent, milk and other dietary items, laundry and incidentals. The total cost to the hospital was limited to the income from the Sponable bequest, $255 annually.

In a precursor of what the future held in store, there was a group contract for the hospital care of Kansas City Telephone Company employees, with the telephone company supplementing the employees' payments.

Each room in the hospital was equipped with a Bible, furnished by one Oscar Kreager. Dr. Hertzler donated four clocks for the operating room. Superintendent Smiley's request for a new typewriter was referred to the House and Grounds Committee.

It was reported at the April board meeting that no complaints on food had come to the hospital office during the month of March—a circumstance apparently worthy of note—and that in the course of that month 10,393 meals had been served at a cost of 23.1 cents per meal. At the same meeting, a letter from Dr. Logan Clendenning, then serving as president of the medical staff, was presented, outlining a plan for intern service at the hospital. The plan called for three internships per year at an expense of $25 a month per intern with a parchment certificate to be presented upon completion of service.

• • • • •

One of the more eccentric physicians on the local scene, Dr. Clendenning was a writer (author of the best-seller *Down the Alimentary Canal*) and instructor at the University of Kansas School of Medicine. According to the fall, 1995, issue of *Horizons Unlimited* (a publication of the Kansas University Endowment Association):

" … Dr. Clendenning often used his talents as a humorist and amateur actor to enhance his teaching. When he lectured on neurological disorders, for example, 'He really demonstrated neurological disorders,' said Susan Case, rare-books librarian for the Clendenning Library. In fact, 'It was so memorable that former students—now in their 80s—still vividly remember.' "

When the noise of air hammers used in constructing a new sewer line near his large home in a fashionable 55th Street neighborhood offended him, Dr. Clendenning proceeded to the construction site and destroyed the hammers and a compressor with a sledge hammer. He was jailed briefly on charges of disturbing the peace and destroying city property, and while incarcerated entertained fellow inmates with lengthy quotations from William Shakespeare.

Dr. Clendenning wrote a syndicated column in which he once maintained that American football should be prohibited in all secondary schools for boys under age fourteen; it was his contention that the bones of such boys were not sufficiently formed for the contact sport.

• • • • •

The continuing dedication of the Peet family to Saint Luke's was demonstrated in a variety of practical ways. The hospital lawn in 1924 was cut by a horse-drawn mower loaned by Mr. Peet. And it was noted at the June board meeting that a Mr. K.A. McVey, superintendent at Peet Brothers, had spent much time and labor in surveying reports and figures regarding electric current used at the hospital. In January, 1925, Mr. Peet advised the board of a "splendid" gift of $1,000 from his father, William Peet. And in December, 1925, Mr. Peet expressed the wish to be Santa to the nurses; their yearbook—*The Luke-O-Cyte* (a leukocyte is a white blood cell)—commented that although he didn't dress the part he was "Santa" to the nurses throughout the year.

Peet Brothers Company contributed $5,000 in 1925 toward the installation and maintenance of a new hospital ward and later that year made a gift to the hospital of $5,000 in hospital Second Mortgage Bonds; Mr. and Mrs. Peet contributed $2,000 in such bonds at the same time. Minutes for October, 1926, reflect a $2,500 gift from Peet Brothers Company and $2,000 from Mr. and Mrs. A.W. Peet. In March, 1927, it was noted that a Bryce McMillen, an employee of Peet Brothers, had given very efficient voluntary service to the hospital for the past four years. At a June, 1927, meeting the board gave a standing vote of thanks to Mr. and Mrs. Peet for a gift of $4,206. The Peets' generosity continued in 1928 and 1929, frequently in the form of gifts of hospital Second Mortgage Bonds. And Peet Brothers kept the nurses supplied with their popular Palmolive soap.

The hospital ministered to a variety of patients. During a Shriners' convention from June 3 to 5, six Shriners were hospitalized and emergency treatment was given free of charge to conventioning members of that convivial organization.

In July, a staff recommendation was presented for a cardiac clinic in the outpatient department, with free service for those patients certified by a social agency to be needy and worthy. A cardiograph machine was purchased, which was operated by the nurses; there were no specially trained technicians at the time.

There were fifty-three births during the month of July and an average of twenty babies in the hospital per day.

At the October, 1924, board meeting, the purchase of a cystoscopic table was approved. Dr. Nelse F. Ockerblod, a genito-urinary specialist, stated that the table would pay for itself in six months and also that there would be "added prestige" to the hospital. His arguments were persuasive, for Smiley was instructed to have the table shipped by express.

The concluding passage in the October minutes summarized the hospital's comfortable condition at the time:

> "It was the opinion of the board that Superintendent Smiley's report for the month was fine and the hospital going along nicely."

In the board meeting of December 8, 1924, there was a motion "that the House and Grounds Committee provide a radio machine to the Nurses for Christmas."

Robert Nelson Spencer, the rector of Grace and Holy Trinity Church and chaplain at Saint Luke's, praised the hospital in his January, 1925, church bulletin. In describing various services and ministries at Saint Luke's, Spencer found it strange that there were not more Episcopal patients in an Episcopal hospital. (He had done his part to strengthen the church's presence by baptizing two nurses.) He described Saint Luke's as "the hospital of the Beloved Physician," and proclaimed it to be a hospital that any diocese in America might well covet "if to covet were not to break the Tenth Commandment."

The previous year's arrangement with the Richard Cabot Club for a sick infants' ward in the summer months was renewed on virtually the same terms, subject to approval of the Charities Committee of the Chamber of Commerce of Kansas City, Missouri.

Dr. Harold P. Kuhn was chosen Commanding Officer, Saint Luke's Hospital Unit Reserve Corps, U.S. Army. An army major had requested that such a unit be formed at the hospital.

· · · · ·

In May, Dr. Frank D. Dickson was invited to bring his thriving orthopaedic practice to Saint Luke's. Dr. Dickson, an Easterner, had been affiliated with the University of Pennsylvania when asked to attend Kansas Senator Frank Capper's polio-stricken daughter in Topeka, Kansas. He was attracted to the area and soon settled in Kansas City, the city's first orthopaedic surgeon.

An architect submitted an estimate of $10,500 as the cost of remodeling the hospital's sixth floor for use by Dr. Dickson. Dickson later directed a letter to Mr. Peet regarding the number of "guests" he might have in the hospital should he make arrangements with Saint Luke's. The Board authorized the expenditure of about $25,000 for improvements to the sixth floor, and a room on the fifth floor was to be converted into an operating room for Dr. Dickson. The board refused, however, Dickson's request for other privileges not enjoyed by the remainder of Saint Luke's admitting physicians.

Dr. Dickson joined the Saint Luke's staff. Later he would serve both as president of the American Orthopaedic Association and president of the American Academy of Orthopaedic Surgeons—one of only two physicians ever to hold both offices.

· · · · ·

The Richard Cabot Club was informed that they would no longer be able to use the sixth floor for the annual summer baby camp because of its occupancy by Dr. Dickson's patients. This generated protests from an influential constituency, and a compromise was effected: the board approved continued use by the club of the Southeast corner room of the sixth floor and access to the sun parlor on the floor's Northeast corner. Charity care in the form of discounted rates was offered throughout the sixth floor.

That same year the club's well-baby camp, which in 1916 had been moved to Scout Hill in Penn Valley Park, began to use Saint Luke's Hospital. Here nursing service was provided as part of the regular nurses' training at the Saint Luke's School of Nursing.

There continued to be reduced hospital charges for the clergy, including the wife of a missionary to the Philippine Islands. A request from the rector of an Episcopal church in Atchison, Kansas, for special dispensation also was approved by the board. It was becoming difficult to keep track of the free and reduced charges being offered, and, adopting a suggestion by Bishop Partridge, the Finance Committee prepared a schedule listing the priests of the diocese and their families, members of the board, graduate nurses, student nurses, doctors, employees, and "any others."

The increasing importance of the business aspects of Saint Luke's activities was reflected by efforts to collect hospital bills from solvent patients. The cooperation of physicians in this regard also was solicited ... deadbeat patients were to be avoided.

Payment was received from the Chicago, Rock Island and Pacific Railway Company for the hospital bill of two men who had been travelers in an automobile that was struck by a train. The remittance was accompanied by a letter from the railroad advising that the company did not ordinarily assume bills for travelers on the highway. The hospital was not impressed: it replied that in the future the hospital would continue to hold the railroad accountable for the bills of any patients sent to Saint Luke's by the Railroad's surgeons.

Superintendent Smiley and Callie French were given salary raises of $300 per year effective January 1, 1926. In March, the Finance Committee was directed to investigate the cost of adding north and south wings to the hospital. Mr. Peet, the hospital's principal benefactor, was prudently added to that committee.

In November, 1926, the Chamber of Commerce asked Saint Luke's to assist in bringing a meeting of the American Hospital Association to Kansas City, which the hospital agreed to do. It developed, however, that Saint Luke's did not belong to the AHA, and application was made that same month for membership.

Saint Luke's doctors continued to support the Richard Cabot Clinic. Dr. Don Carlos Peete later remarked that he first saw patients at the clinic following his graduation from the KU School of Medicine in 1926, and served the West Side there every Thursday morning for the next eighteen years. Like his colleague Dr. Ralph Ringo Coffey, he was first introduced to Saint Luke's Hospital through his work at the clinic.

Dr. Coffey had served as a second lieutenant in the infantry in World War I and then set about becoming a surgeon. In the course of Coffey's surgical training at Saint Luke's, he undertook the duties of hospital orderly or general handyman for the Saint Luke's surgeons ... part of his education was to stand by to assist, move patients to surgery, answer a few night calls and perform emergency work; he labeled it "dog-robbing," an old army term.

•••••

In January, 1927, A.W. Peet was elected first vice president, succeeding George B. Richards as the lay head of the hospital.

The auxiliary regularly served refreshments at the nursing school's graduation exercises, conducted on the hospital lawn before a large gathering of relatives and friends. The auxiliary's annual meeting in 1927 was held on Saint Luke's Day, a practice that continues today. All of the auxiliary's money, raised or donated, went into the Chapel Fund that year. The bank balance reflected in the treasurer's annual report was $772.45.

In 1927, Dr. Frank D. Dickson was joined by Dr. Rex Diveley, and the Dickson-Diveley Orthopaedic Clinic was founded.

•••••

In November, 1927, the board responded to medical-staff urging by authorizing the employment of a full-time pathologist and the establishment of an adequate laboratory. There was recognized the importance of autopsies in order to be absolutely certain of the cause of a patient's death. The physician who did not have his diagnoses checked in this fashion "might form careless habits." Also, continued progress in medicine generally was said to depend upon autopsies.

In December, 1927, Dr. Ferdinand Christian Helwig, pathologist at the University of Kansas Medical Center, offered his services part-time until June 1 for $4,000 and full-time thereafter for $7,000 per year. The application was supported by every member of the medical staff. The appointment of Ferd Helwig was approved and marked a significant milestone in the progress of Saint Luke's. He was the city's first specially trained pathologist and was described by Dr. Peter Bohan as having "brains to burn." In time he would raise the standards of all of the departments in the hospital. Another colleague characterized him as "the supreme court for all medical decisions made at Saint Luke's."

• • • • •

In February, 1928, construction was authorized of two stories and a basement of a new South Wing to the hospital at an estimated cost of $200,000. Two additional floors were roughed in but left without partitions. The work proceeded quickly, and the building was dedicated the following November. It added 100 beds, bringing the bed capacity to 250.

• • • • •

Fifty-page hospital booklets were distributed in August, 1928. The first few pages included a history of the hospital. There were forty physicians on the executive staff and ninety on the general staff, and the hospital was training eighty-five nurses and six interns. In 1927, 4,634 patients had been admitted, some fifty patients a week were treated in the outpatient ward, and 1,464 partial-pay patients were served, with an average payment by such patient of $3.05 per day and an average total cost of $5.75. The net cost to the hospital of this charity work, $2.70 per day, amounted to $39,536.10 for the year. Then as now, cost-shifting resulted, with the burden falling on the private patients who paid full charges.

The booklet disclosed donations, including a handsome bequest by Herbert Whitehead Mackirdy, former British Vice Consul, of $40,000 to care for deserving poor children. And Charles W. Armour had left $5,000 to the general revenue fund of the hospital.

The religious census for the previous four-year period did not reflect much change among the various denominations during that span, except for the lone Spiritualist listed in 1924, and the number of those who professed no religion, which grew from 1,124 in 1924 to 1,787 in 1927.

The booklet featured a section on the nursing school. It noted that all of the drudgery of former years had been eliminated from the school's courses—cleaning and scrubbing were now handled by maids. The student was expected to do only the things necessary for proper patient care. The section listed some of the advantages accruing to the nursing profession, including preparation for home-making and motherhood … nursing was said to be "absolutely a woman's sphere and work." There was also the statement that remuneration "should, of course, be considered as only secondary in this sort of work." Callie French, now superintendent of nurses, wrote this section and stated:

> "The idealistic high type girl is the desirable applicant, for there is no place where such an individual is more necessary than in a hospital."

The paragon of virtue continued to be in demand.

A reprint from *The Modern Hospital*, dated June, 1928, was in effect a defense of hospitals against common criticisms of the day—some of which have a familiar ring. Hospitals were charging too much or were badly managed and inefficient. Several pages of the booklet were devoted to refuting these complaints.

The children's ward on the sixth floor was described, noting that usually there were twelve to fifteen patients, ranging in age from two to fourteen. Some were recuperating from infantile paralysis. The children came from many states.

Dr. Helwig authored a section on pathology, noting that in addition to a large number of purely clinical procedures, his department performed tissue and postmortem work. The clinical work was described as very beneficial to the hospital as a check and a record, and was often of immeasurable assistance to the surgeon … particularly in regard to malignant tumors. Postmortems were said to be an excellent index as to the quality of work being done by the men on the hospital staff. It was the final quality-control procedure—otherwise doctors simply buried their mistakes. Hospitals were judged on the frequency of such examinations. There was also a teaching function served.

Twenty-four rules governing interns were listed near the end of the booklet. At least three interns were on duty at all times, and all gained experience in the departments of surgery, ob/gyn, pediatrics, urology, radiology and orthopaedics. For them, interning in a good community hospital such as Saint Luke's was preferable to a university hospital experience. According to one of the physicians trained at that time:

> "The house staff looked with some disfavor on university-affiliated hospi-

tals as being sort of slave institutions, where we continued in servitude from our student days. Anybody who was going into general practice would gravitate to the community hospitals."

• • • • •

Interns also rotated through the department of ear, nose, and throat, where tonsilectomies, thought to be beneficial to many children, were a common medical procedure.

A *Kansas City Star* article contained a recollection by a former Saint Luke's nurse, Kathryn Hurd, of a six-year-old boy named "Tommy" who was admitted to the hospital for a tonsillectomy, to be performed the following morning. Ms. Hurd reassured him about the operation, but when the time came to go to the operating room he balked. The nurse then told him that if he would get on the gurney he'd be rewarded with ice cream. Tommy thought that he was being offered an alternative to the operation, not an incentive for undergoing it, and climbed on the roller bed. The article does not disclose how he was persuaded to submit to ether—the anesthetic of the time. Later, in the recovery room, when the nurse asked Tommy if he wanted his ice cream, she was told to "go to hell."

Interns' pay was $25.00 per month, plus room and board, three pairs of white trousers, and three white jackets. Interns were not supposed to date nurses, but they did—meeting them away from the hospital and parting from them afterward at a nearby street corner. More than one marriage resulted from these clandestine romances.

If the nurses attracted suitors from the hospital staff, it was not due to seductive uniforms. Dress was severe and subject to daily inspection by the assistant superintendent of nursing. According to Thelma Walsh, R.N., such inspection was rigorous:

> "You were particularly suspect if you didn't have a petticoat on. We had big full dresses with aprons on them and you couldn't have seen through them for anything in the world, but she would pull up your dress to be sure that you had a petticoat on."

Business-like black oxfords were furnished by the hospital. New pairs were kept in the linen room, and nurses in need of replacements simply went there and got them.

The hospital's new chapel, located on the first floor in space formerly occupied by the cafeteria, was dedicated by Bishop Partridge on Christmas Eve, 1928. The auxiliary had furnished the pews, kneeling benches, lighting fixtures, altar rail, organ, Oriental runner for the aisle, and kneeling cushions.

Bargain 1929 prices are reflected in a bill for hospital services in connection with the birth of a baby boy. The bill for delivery and an eleven-day stay: $76.30. This did not include the charge by the doctor but did cover the mother's room ($44), anesthesia, delivery room ($10), lab, drugs, dressings, circumcision ($2), and nursing bottles, caps and nipples.

The ladies from the Richard Cabot Club again demonstrated their clout when three of them appeared at the February, 1929, board meeting to protest increased charges for the club's obstetrical cases. The board capitulated, making an adjustment with respect to cases already booked. There was another appearance by club representatives at the August meeting on the same subject; the board passed the buck to the Executive Committee "with power to act." At the November, 1929, meeting of the board, the Executive Committee reported that children's rates for the club would remain at $1 per day, that the obstetrical rate would continue at $35, and that ward beds for adult operative cases would be at a minimum charge of $5.50 for the first day and $2.50 for each day thereafter.

A gift of $300 was received from the graduates of Yale University to furnish a room in the new South Wing. A plaque mounted on the door of the room read:

> "The Yale Room—This room is furnished by Graduates of Yale University in memory of Walter Camp and William Hutchinson of the class of 1880. Champions in Foot-Ball and Base-Ball."

A proposal for a convalescent home for patients of Saint Luke's Hospital was referred to the House and Grounds Committee for investigation and report.

• • • • •

Among the highlights of 1930 was a magnificent gift by Mrs. Linda S. Hall, wife of Herbert F. Hall, president of the Hall-Baker Grain Company. Her contribution of money and property, valued at $250,000, (the result of solicitation by A.W. Peet), was the first large endowment for the hospital and was heralded as the largest gift for a specific purpose ever

made to any Kansas City hospital. The specific purpose of the philanthropy was "the furnishing of medical treatment, care, food, attention
and nursing in Saint Luke's Hospital in Kansas City to such children and
women as may be found by the directors, in the exercise of their discre-
tion, to be unable to pay for such medical treatment, preference being
given to children under the age of fifteen years who are patients in the
hospital." A *Star* article reported:

> "Mr. and Mrs. Hall live in a handsome Georgian house, one of the finest
> in Kansas City, in the center of a wooded tract of fifteen acres at 5109
> Cherry Street.
> "Just a mile to the northwest, across Brush Creek valley, is Saint Luke's
> Hospital, topped by a sixth-floor roof garden, where science is doing its
> utmost to bring health and vigor to little children. There, too, is centered
> the orthopaedic work directed by Dr. Frank D. Dickson and Dr. Rex L.
> Diveley, the correction of deformities that otherwise would be lifelong
> handicaps."

Dr. Dickson stated with satisfaction that the Hall Fund's income would
maintain twenty beds, relieving General Hospital and Children's Mercy
Hospital of congestion and enabling them to divert their funds to other
medical uses. Newspaper coverage pointed to the gift as recognition of
the fact that medical institutions were not businesses but places of refuge
which carried debts because of the lack of adequate support:

> "Most hospitals really are not self-supporting at all, and could not function
> even at the rates now charged without supplementary financial aid."

An appropriate, eloquent resolution of appreciation for the gift was
engraved and personally presented to Mrs. Hall at her home by Mr. Peet.
In ensuing years, numerous charity cases would be charged against the
Linda S. Hall Gift Trust Fund.

· · · · ·

Bishop Partridge died in the summer of 1930. At its August meeting,
the board adopted a resolution expressing sorrow at his death and appreciation for his service to the Hospital. Later the new Bishop, Robert
Nelson Spencer, was notified "that he automatically becomes President of
the Board of Directors of Saint Luke's Hospital."

Bishop Spencer was succeeded by Charles Tyner as hospital chaplain.
Father Tyner was also full-time rector of St. George's Church. Fortunately

he was energetic, described by one of the nurses as "always bouncing around and giving spiritual advice to patients."

At the December, 1930, meeting, after a general discussion of what was termed "the food situation" at Saint Luke's, the Building and Grounds Committee was directed to make a special study of the hospital's food and its service to patients. The problem was ongoing ... at the July 11, 1932, meeting, the board would move that the same committee "make an investigation of the service of food," with Mr. Peet being added to the committee.

A $100 gift from Ursulla Burr, now president of the auxiliary, initiated a general endowment fund effort for the hospital. This was followed early in 1931 by a publication entitled *Building for the Centuries,* intended to encourage gifts to the endowment fund. A foreword by Bishop Spencer introduced the history of the hospital, its status as an educational institution (only the school of nursing was discussed), the daily cost of operation (average cost per patient day of $6.55 versus ward beds, which were free or for which patients were charged $1 to $2.50 a day), the hospital's characteristics as a non-profit corporation, opportunity for the future, and benefits derived from charitable gifts. An Endowment Resolution later was adopted, establishing the fund and providing for its investment and use. There would be continuing efforts to enhance the fund.

TWELVE
1931-1936

The Great Depression

*T*he Great Depression of the 1930s did not spare Saint Luke's. The annual report of the hospital in the 1932 *Convention Journal of the Diocese* stated that for the year 1931 the hospital was "forced to join all other activities of this Community in reporting a decided decrease in the amount of work done for the year." Paying patients who in ordinary times would have been hospitalized remained at home for less-expensive treatment.

Dr. Peter Bohan pre-empted the entire South Wing of the first floor, twenty-eight beds. It was convenient for Dr. Bohan to have all of his patients concentrated in this location, but there was some resentment on the part of his colleagues on the medical staff. However, he helped keep Saint Luke's afloat by filling twenty to thirty percent of the hospital's beds.

Dr. Bohan devoted hours to reviewing his patients' charts, puffing on cigarettes screwed into a quill holder while sitting at an old porcelainized table at the nurses' station. Often a patient's problem proved to be a simple one, disclosed by Bohan's painstaking interrogation.

Doctors Dickson and Diveley were also vital to Saint Luke's survival, doing all of their work in the sixth-floor area assigned them.

Patients entered the hospital only if they were quite ill and required greater care. As a result, the hospital, while still very busy, was called upon to render more service for less pay, and at the year's end had a $5,000 deficit from operations. The board was forced to reduce salaries, lay off employees, and close the South Wing of the third floor.

In April, 1931, a goiter clinic was conducted at the hospital. Many of the doctors in attendance were attracted to the hospital gowns used at Saint Luke's, asking for the patterns and where they could have them made up. The gowns were described as "keenly efficient," a quality attributed to several years of study.

The city's General Hospital could not handle all of the indigent cases, and in December the Executive Committee was authorized to act "in the matter of receiving patients from General Hospital to Saint Luke's Hospital in cases of emergency, with suitable safeguards."

Baseball's Babe Ruth explained that he had made more money than President Herbert Hoover in 1931 because "I had a better year."

1932 proved to be worse than 1931, with the demand for free service increasing fourfold. Consequently the need for an endowment fund at the hospital was apparent, and an Endowment Committee joined the Executive, Finance, and Building and Grounds committees as a standing committee of the board. However, despite financial problems, the hospital in 1932 furnished hospitalization to men, women and children unable to pay in the sum of $60,860.68.

In May, 1932, Dr. Herman E. Pearse discontinued active practice and transferred from the general staff to the honorary staff.

In November, 1932, the board mourned the death of director H.T. Poindexter. Mr. Poindexter was the long-time chairman of the Building and Grounds Committee and left a generous bequest to the hospital in his will.

The churches of the diocese collected funds at Thanksgiving time for the care at Saint Luke's of indigent men. And Mr. Peet paid hospital bills sent to him for both indigent men and indigent women. The Depression Grinch almost stole Christmas in 1932; at the board's December meeting that year it was voted that "on account of the condition of our finances ... the amount of $20 only be expended for Christmas decorations this year."

The 1933 *Convention Journal* indicated that 1933 would be a better year financially for the hospital ... for the month of April there had actually been a net profit of approximately $700. The *Journal* also reassured communicants of the diocese with respect to the quality of the medical staff:

> "There is not the remotest chance that any but the most skilled of the profession will obtain an appointment on our staff. Not only are the members carefully selected by the Executive Committee of our medical staff, but all must be approved by our board of directors."

That year the Ways and Means Committee of the auxiliary decided to concentrate on one annual benefit, a Holiday Ball, to be held in the PlaMor Ballroom.

All of the mortgage bonds of the hospital were extended, and the treasurer, C.S. Alves, wrote the manager of the bond department of the Mississippi Valley Trust Company in St. Louis expressing appreciation for its cooperation in this regard.

The 1934 *Convention Journal* noted that the hospital's total mortgage indebtness was $271,000. That same *Journal* stated that Saint Luke's had "by rigid economy, careful supervision and management" been able to pay its expenses and maintain its standards "notwithstanding the severe financial depression that has had such an injurious effect upon the whole country."

• • • • •

The auxiliary established a circulating library at the hospital with twenty-five used books purchased from the Women's City Club. An appeal for additional books, published in each parish bulletin, produced results, and the hospital carpenter fashioned a book cart that could hold sixty volumes. The cart visited each room weekly, with an average of 270 books loaned monthly the first year.

After the hospital lost its chief housekeeper, a problem developed with cockroaches; the ladies of the auxiliary attacked the infestation with vigor and success.

At its April, 1934, meeting, the board authorized the submission of Saint Luke's regular rates to the federal government for the care of disabled soldiers and transients. At the same meeting the board noted the demise of A.W. Peet's father, William Peet, and adopted a resolution which began:

> "BE IT RESOLVED, by the Board of Directors of Saint Luke's Hospital of Kansas City, in regular meeting assembled, that we record with infinite pleasure the sterling worth of a man of high ideals, generous impulses, and Christian life, our friend and benefactor Mr. William Peet, late of Beverly Hills, California, and with his family and friends we sincerely mourn his passing, but we are comforted in the thought that his life, pure and unblemished as we know it to have been, has obtained for him the great reward promised by our Heavenly Father to all who have done His will."

The gift from Linda Hall included real estate at Twelfth and Troost.

Prohibition had been repealed in 1933, and at its June, 1934, meeting the board was confronted with an opportunity to lease part of this property for use as a nightclub. The board initially declined, but finding a tenant proved difficult, and in July the board recanted and approved the nightclub tenancy.

In October the board was advised that Saint Luke's nursing school alumnae requested an end to "twenty-hour duty" for nurses. The medical staff supported this request, which was referred to the board's Executive Committee. At the same meeting Mr. Peet advised the board that Superintendent Smiley's automobile, used for hospital purposes for a number of years, was in very bad condition and offered to purchase a car for the hospital to be used by Mr. Smiley and others. After discussion this generous proposal was accepted.

The auxiliary's gift shop had its modest genesis in November, 1934, when the president of that organization requested the privilege of "placing a sales cabinet in the hall of the hospital."

The 1935 *Convention Journal* carried an excerpt from the report of an American Hospital Association survey, reflecting that Saint Luke's was by no means an inner-city hospital:

> "Its distance from the downtown section of the city operates against the establishment and maintenance of an outpatient department which would be very useful and in time a profitable adjunct to the hospital. This not so much from the standpoint of income as from the benefits the institution would derive from the closer contact of the people of Kansas City, particularly the poorer and middle-classes and in the building-up of the personal interest of the Kansas City public welfare work in which Saint Luke's Hospital might well engage. The board of trustees is composed of representative citizens who are interested not only in the successful operation of Saint Luke's Hospital from a public welfare standpoint, but for its permanency as a leading institution of its kind in Kansas City."

• • • • •

The *Journal* report also reflected the impact of the continuing Depression, commenting: "In spite of the reduction of the number of nurses and the necessary lowering of salaries, the quality of nursing service in the hospital has not been impaired." The article stated that "through continued economy" the hospital in 1934 had been able to meet its "running expenses" and show an increased amount of business over 1933. Although unable to reduce indebtedness, Saint Luke's was able to carry its current load without increasing debt, characterized as "a splendid accomplishment."

The hospital was urged to broaden its base of financial support. "Every revenue-producing patient coming to the hospital cuts the unit cost of care, and of course, adds to the hospital income. The overhead of operation remains practically the same … ." Diocesan support of Saint Luke's also was urged, through contributions and through communicants' use of its facilities.

Times were tough for physicians as well, especially beginners. Dr. Mervin Rumold later would remark that when he started practicing in 1935 he sat in his office for thirty-two days before a soul walked through the door.

Mervin Rumold's medical-school roommate was Maxwell G. Berry, later recognized as one of Kansas City's leading physicians. Max Berry moved in on a cold night when a penny-pinching landlord was conserving fuel, and Merv Rumold was afraid that his new roommate would want to open a window at bedtime. There occurred this exchange:

> Rumold: "Max, what's your idea about fresh air?"
> Berry: "Merv, it belongs outside."

After that, according to Mervin Rumold, they "got along just fine."

At the February, 1935, board meeting Mr. Peet commented that in light of Saint Luke's "poor financial showing" in 1934, immediate steps should be taken to reduce fixed charges such as bond interest. In reviewing the list of holders of the hospital's Second Mortgage Bonds, he had found the names of people with an interest in Saint Luke's welfare, and he felt sure many of these bondholders would be willing to donate their bonds. Minutes of later meetings reflect the surrender by various hospital supporters of their Second Mortgage Bonds.

Dr. Ralph Wilson, a very busy obstetrician, advised that "the old faithfuls" continued to bring patients into Saint Luke's, doing their best to fill hospital rooms.

• • • • •

In March a new schedule of discounts was adopted for various patient categories, including physicians and their families, nursing school graduates in good standing in the alumnae association, Episcopal clergymen and dependents, board members and dependents, and employees.

An attempt to rezone property at 45th and Main for a bakery was successfully opposed ... it entailed a change from retail to industrial classification and would open the door for other industrial uses in the area.

The IRS ruled that the hospital was exempt from federal income tax and that contributions to Saint Luke's were deductible by the donors, for federal income tax purposes.

In April, new rates adopted for the fourth (obstetrical) floor included $50 "special concession, Payable In Advance" rates available only to eligible patients upon determination by Superintendent Smiley prior to admission.

Much of the May board meeting was devoted to a proposal submitted by the "Harry M. Evans Children's Home Finding Society," operating the Kansas City Cradle. Mr. and Mrs. William J. Brace and Mr. Hal Brace appeared before the board to present plans for the home's future. This institution, established in 1915 at 520 Woodland, was now situated next door to the hospital. It had functioned for twenty years as a home-finding society for illegitimate infants up to two years old. More than 2,000 sets of parents throughout the country had adopted Cradle babies. However, the home found itself unable meet the current demand ... sixteen babies were presently in the home, and thirty-two babies had been turned away in April because of lack of accommodations. Under the proposal the Cradle would be operated by Saint Luke's, and the name of the institution would be changed—both "Saint Luke's Cradle" and "Children's Hospital" were under consideration. The directors' reaction was favorable, but nothing further transpired for ten years.

In June Mr. Peet reported that the interns' quarters had been relocated on the fifth floor of the hospital, where two rooms also were set aside for the care of alcoholic patients brought to the hospital in "an intoxicated condition." According to the minutes, these patients would be required to employ male nurses for their care while inebriated; the practicalities of this requirement were not challenged.

In July the hospital took over the management of the X ray Department and subsequently authorized a contract with Dr. Fred Kuhlman to handle X ray services.

There were continuing financial pressures: the Missouri Savings Bank asked the hospital to retire its Second Mortgage Bonds held by the bank; Mr. Peet reported efforts to persuade two other banks to reduce interest rates on outstanding loans.

In October there was received a welcome check for $226.75 from the contestants in a "Jelly Contest" conducted by *Household Magazine,* the funds to be used to purchase "a suitable article" for the crippled children at Saint Luke's Hospital. Senator Frank Capper's "Capper Publications" of Topeka, Kansas, was the magazine's publisher. The contest offered a prize for the best glass of jelly submitted, an invitation which produced hundreds of entries from every state in the Union. After the winner was determined the jelly was sold, producing the $226.75.

The "Senator Capper Fund" sent children to Saint Luke's Hospital from all over the State of Kansas—many of them afflicted with cerebral palsy. Also, under provisions of the Social Security Act relating to crippled children under age 15, Children's Mercy Hospital and Saint Luke's were designated to care for children from Missouri's rural areas, to be reimbursed at the "all-inclusive" rate of $3 per day. At the May meeting the board implemented this when it approved a contract with the Board of Curators of the University of Missouri, providing for the care of crippled children at Saint Luke's under the supervision of doctors Dickson and Diveley for the period April 1 to June 30, 1936. The two doctors furnished their own services "gratis."

Dr. Helwig's efforts extended beyond pathology. In 1936, a program of medical-technology education at Saint Luke's under his direction was one of the original ninety-six in that specialty approved by the AMA Council on Medical Education. And in April 1936, Dr. Helwig was charged with administration of the X ray Department. He also presented educational programs at staff meetings; indeed, according to one admiring colleague, "he was the staff meeting."

In June, "a boy by the name of Evans on the Andrew Drumm Farm" was approved for full hospitalization, with the account to be charged to the Carrie J. Loose Fund. The Andrew Drumm Institute was located near Independence and had been established under provisions in the will of Major Andrew Drumm, a wealthy cattle baron. When Major Drumm's widow died in October, 1937, she left a bequest of $5,000 to Saint Luke's.

In September E.F. Swinney requested payment in full of a $32,000 note owing the First National Bank, and the hospital complied. However, after payment to the bank, Mr. Swinney presented the hospital with his personal check for $4,000.

A new bookkeeping machine, a mobile X ray unit, and a cardiograph machine were acquired with funds donated by Mr. and Mrs. A.W. Peet.

In October and November, the Peets surrendered a total of $10,000 in bonds in exchange for a $5,000 payment from the hospital.

In December the Finance Committee "with Mr. A.W. Peet" was authorized to call or refund First and Second Mortgage Bonds of Saint Luke's Hospital. In January, 1937, the board adopted a resolution providing for refinancing, with $200,000 borrowed in exchange for First Mortgage Bonds and $150,000 borrowed in exchange for Second Mortgage Bonds. This refinancing, which permitted the retirement of the outstanding bonds, was facilitated by Mr. Peet's personal endorsement of the note at the First National Bank.

Economically the worst was over. The 1937 *Convention Journal* would state: "Saint Luke's has weathered the years of the depression and is now functioning normally in its great work."

THIRTEEN
1937-1941

group hospitalization ... David Beals ... X rays ...
Gray Ladies ... cat gut and milk

$\mathcal{E}$mergency-room care remained under the supervision of the hospital's central-supply operations until 1937, when the increased volume of emergency cases—an average of five or six patients daily—led to the creation of a separate Emergency Department. Mrs. Mary Thomas, formerly the night supervisor, was placed in charge. Shortly thereafter the emergency service opened an ear, nose, and throat room for the doctors on staff.

In 1937, parts of the fourth and fifth floors were air conditioned, including all operating rooms, delivery rooms, nursery, most work areas, one labor room and the doctors' locker room. This also permitted the removal of radiators in those areas, which would now be heated by circulating air. The improvement received considerable attention in the press inasmuch as central air conditioning was a recent innovation.

After completion of their one-year internship, young doctors pursued advanced training through residency programs. Internal-medicine residents were heavily involved in patient care, with primary responsibility for the maintenance of medical records. These were in some disarray in early 1937. A regular records meeting was proposed, to be held each Friday at 5 p.m., to insure that the records of all discharged patients were up to date. The records were to include the final diagnosis. If the resident was uncertain as to that diagnosis, he was still held accountable and was to consult the physician on the case as to his opinion. The physician was to sign the completed history or have his associate sign it for him and add his own initials. If the physician's name was lacking, the resident was to sign as his proxy. If the resident failed in these duties, he was subject to discipline … the superintendent was authorized to withhold the monthly stipend or even the diploma of the offender until the records were completed. These measures achieved the desired result; Dr. Dickson advised the board in April that the records "showed great improvement and marked success."

Dr. Helwig and others made several suggestions relating to the house staff. One dealt with the need to provide incoming interns with literature clarifying the duties of interns and provide resident physicians with a nomenclature book. Another stated that a "dangerously ill" list should be provided to the residents by 7 p.m. daily. Also, the cooperation of the nurses' training school was "earnestly requested" in efforts to improve records, utilize the interns to best advantage, and achieve an effective working relationship among the medical staff, interns, and nurses staff. The executive committee of the medical staff requested that each attending physician ask the operator to give notice of his arrival in the hospital "so that he may avail himself, as far as possible, of the services of his interns."

The doctors suggested that relationships of the hospital with members of the public would materially benefit from a closer contact between the superintendent of nurses and the patients, and recommended a personal visit with each private-room patient and to each ward, at least once a week.

Superintendent Smiley stated in October, 1937, that "at the present time the hospital was running at total capacity."

There had been a dispute with the city and the county over the amount of taxes assessed against the Linda Hall Fund's property at 12th and Troost, the site of the earlier nightclub operation. This was settled in January, 1938, by payment of 25 percent of the amount originally claimed by the taxing authorities. The property at this time continued to be devoted to profit-making activities … at the September, 1938, meeting one of the directors "announced that the results from the 12th and Troost Avenue property have shown a splendid increase during 1938." This success would be short-lived, however.

The persistent generosity of Mr. Peet was recognized by the board at its January, 1938, meeting when there was a motion that a "rising vote of thanks be extended by the board to Mr. A.W. Peet for his untiring efforts, generosity and loyalty to Saint Luke's hospital." In response, "the board arose in a body to cast their unanimous vote." Those were more courtly times.

• • • • •

The Depression underscored for hospitals across the country the financial hazards of their humanitarian mission. The American Hospital Association took an active role in seeking a solution. This led to AHA endorsement of hospital insurance in 1933. Insurance would assist hospitals' budgeting process, a difficult procedure complicated by the uncertainty of payment of bills by patients.

Group hospitalization was a concept dating back to 1929, when some Texas hospitals, experiencing low occupancy and financial problems, supported a new organization called "Blue Cross"—initially on the premise that there was little to lose and possibly much to be gained from its novel insurance program. Blue Cross originated with a group of Dallas school teachers who, unable to pay emergency hospital bills, determined that collectively they could solve their problem. They persuaded Baylor Hospital to provide twenty-one days' hospital care for $3 per semester. Other groups and hospitals followed suit. Although payment to hospitals was originally a flat per diem amount, other methods had since evolved—in some cases, full charges as billed by the hospital. Blue Cross and the hospitals were partners in this group-insurance venture, with the hospitals assuming an obligation to provide the subscriber with the services called for by his Blue Cross contract.

The group plan spread across the country. In cities having more than one hospital, Blue Cross included nearly every area hospital, and the patient was entitled to choose which hospital would treat him. The first such group of hospitals was located in Sacramento, California.

A committee of the Saint Luke's board studied two "all-inclusive" hospitalization plans, intended to meet the demands of people unable to pay their full hospital bill at the time of entrance. Both plans provided for payment of doctors and hospital in one lump sum.

One of these was the Blue Cross plan used by hospitals elsewhere in the United States, which enjoyed the support of the Jackson County Medical Society as well as the approval of the Missouri State Medical Society, the Chamber of Commerce, the Council of Social Agencies and the Hospital Council of Kansas City. However, the plan did not have the support of

A.W. Peet—a formidable obstacle. Mr. Peet believed that participation by Saint Luke's would "put the hospital in the insurance business," which he considered objectionable. He also disapproved of a feature that would limit hospital payments to the plan's available funds.

Plan proponents responded that the hospital would not be in the insurance business but would only continue to render hospital service. And the limitation on payment was the same as provided in the fifty cities with comparable group-insurance plans, none of which had found it to be a problem.

Proponents also argued that the middle and lower classes would be able to budget and prepay the plan's $9 per year premium—"less than the cost of the daily newspaper." Without such a plan, many people remained at home rather than accept charity hospital care, thereby prolonging illness, increasing their economic loss, and risking their lives. Adoption of the plan would enable doctors "to obtain some fee from the beginning" and increase the occupancy and income of hospitals.

Supporters also had to refute the damaging rumor that the plan's patients would not be free to choose their hospital or physician.

Saint Luke's leadership was not persuaded. Supporters of the plan did not want to go forward without Saint Luke's participation; the plan would be much more difficult to sell. Consequently, no plan was implemented in Kansas City for a time. Then, on May 13, 1938, "Group Hospital Service of Jackson County" was formed, to offer the Blue Cross plan. It was apparent that the plan was going forward, with or without Saint Luke's. Business Men's Assurance Co. reportedly was considering underwriting insurance to protect the plan's participants in the event of a severe epidemic.

The Saint Luke's board at its May, 1938, meeting got on the bandwagon. They approved the plan and agreed to participate, provided that all contracts and specific arrangements were satisfactory to the Executive Committee. Despite the hospital's initial reluctance, it would see Group Hospital Service become a major source of patients and revenue in the years to come.

The president of the medical staff predicted that the plan "would be very difficult to sell"—his crystal ball was murky, however; group hospital insurance was in Kansas City to stay. By September, 3,894 people had enrolled in the plan, with "many prominent firms being supporters of Group Hospital Service, Inc."

Aided significantly by the Jackson County Medical Society, the non-profit Group Hospital Service had an immediate impact on Saint Luke's occupancy. A December 25, 1938, article noted:

> "The hospital is already beginning to feel the pressure of the group hospital-ization movement, now growing at the rate of several thousand a month, and when this program gets fully under way, a shortage of beds is expected … "

Equitable Life Assurance Society and Business Men's Assurance Co. presented rival group insurance proposals for Saint Luke's employees. However, in January, 1939, the board opted for the Group Hospital Service Plan for hospital employees, with financial aid for lower-paid employees in the form of part-payment of the premium cost.

At that same meeting Mr. Peet stated that for the first five months' operation of Group Hospital Service, the hospital had charged off $454 … discounts were already being allowed. He recommended that a committee of the board "study the method of handling these cases." The Executive Committee was directed to "make a thorough study of the method of bookkeeping on Group Hospital Service cases" and report to the board.

By February, 1939, there had been a rapid increase in contract holders in Group Hospital Service, with 25,000 members now in Kansas City. This was not without its problems, apart from the discounting. Superintendent Smiley "outlined some of the dangers of organized groups of unemployed who are desirous of becoming members of Group Hospital Service." The executive director of GHS believed that if a letter were written to the President of the GHS Board on the subject "it would assist in keeping out these undesirable groups."

There was also a problem with accommodations: most of the insured patients did not want the $4.50 double rooms which their contracts provided but insisted on $5.50 private rooms, paying the difference themselves. This forced uninsured patients to accept higher-priced accommodations. The Executive Committee was directed to "make a study of the hospital problems created by the Group Hospital Service cases."

In March, 1939, Smiley reported that GHS continued to grow, at a rate of 1,500 to 2,000 contract holders per month. GHS was paying the hospital once a month, and Mr. Peet suggested that this should be accelerated to twice a month in view of the volume. There also continued to be problems over the demand for $5.50 private rooms. During February the average amount received by the contracting hospitals per patient was $7.07.

• • • • •

While group hospital plan developments were transpiring, other events of note also took place.

There were articles in the newspaper noting the death of the 81-year-old director, Henry D. Ashley.

At the September, 1938, meeting, the board expressed its appreciation to Mayor Bryce B. Smith and the members of the park board for resurfacing the driveway in front of the hospital.

Financing for completion of the third and fourth floors of the South Wing also was discussed at the September meeting. A campaign to raise the necessary funds was contemplated, and it was proposed that a fund-raising firm be employed for this purpose. But Mr. Peet objected to such a stratagem, stating that in the first hospital fund-raising campaign an outside agency had been employed and "it created so much criticism that an indignation meeting was held at his home which resulted in the dismissal of the agency." It was then determined that the possibility of a government loan should be investigated as well as other sources of available construction funds.

A loan from the "Nelson Art Gallery Fund" was approved in October; the hospital's officers were authorized to borrow $75,000 from the Nelson Trustees upon such terms as they deemed advisable, the proceeds to be used to complete and furnish the third and fourth floors. The financing had not been finalized by the end of the year but nevertheless a December 25, 1938, article in the *Kansas City Star* noted:

> "Anticipation of future demand, particularly that developed by group hospitalization, has prompted the trustees of Saint Luke's Hospital at 44th street and Mill Creek Parkway to proceed with the unfinished floors in the south wing."

• • • • •

David Beals, who would later succeed A.W. Peet as lay head of the hospital, was elected a director, and, at the October board meeting, "Mr. Peet welcomed him with open arms."

The purchase and installation of new X ray equipment was authorized in October, necessitating considerable remodeling. The hospital's X ray operation and related diagnostic activities brought in more income than any other department despite the fact that they functioned with the poorest equipment in the city.

X ray patients encountered a "rather awkward" problem, according to director Gordon Beaham: "When Barium Enemas or intravenous treatments are given patients, there is no toilet connection in the X ray Department, and it is necessary to go down the hall to the bath." To avoid such mad dashes, toilet facilities were "added to the new arrangement."

It was suggested that, when a patient entered the hospital for a serious operation, he be requested to sign a form or waiver "clearing the hospital of any responsibility." The rationale: it was the doctors and not the hospital who brought the patients into Saint Luke's, and the patients assumed any risk of injury by accepting their physicians' advice before entering. "The hospital should not be held responsible for the results." This was especially true of charity patients: "Charity patients are accepting hospitalization, and no doubt the services of the doctor or surgeon, for nothing and should have no come-back." Judge Holt was asked "to draw up a form."

Beginning in October, 1938, a "See for Yourself Committee" of two directors was appointed, on a rotating basis, to go through the hospital, taking meals at the hospital and visiting with supervisors, nurses, and patients, and then reporting their findings to the board.

Franklin D. Roosevelt was well into his second term as President, and national health programs were under consideration. However, although FDR endorsed the principle of compulsory national health insurance, he did not submit legislation to accomplish this—his first priority was economic recovery, and a costly national health program would not advance that goal.

A federal minimum-wage law was enacted in 1938. At twenty-five cents per hour, it posed no immediate problem for Saint Luke's, but subsequent increases in the mandated minimum would require significant payroll expenditures.

The storage of the hospital's voluminous patient records was burdensome, and the House and Grounds Committee looked into the transfer of those records to 16 millimeter film. Mr. Peet asked how long it was necessary to keep these files, wanting to avoid the burden of transferring older records. It was determined that case histories, charts and other patient records should be recorded on film and the negatives carefully indexed and preserved. Original records were then to be destroyed after five years, unless involved in pending litigation.

In February, 1939, the gift committee of the auxiliary sought to expand its merchandise sales through the use of the east end of office space in the general lobby for a display of items. A myopic board determined that "it was not advisable to use the lobby for a gift shop."

In March, 1939, there was a conversation with Mr. F.H. Hall regarding difficulties the hospital was experiencing in finding suitable investments for the Linda S. Hall Trust Fund. The terms of the gift required investment of the fund in specified kinds of bonds and mortgages. However, recitation of investment problems fell on deaf ears; Mr. Hall "refused to talk about it as he said that was the reason they had given the money away so they would not be bothered with investing it."

Group Hospital Service matters continued to occupy the board's time. Smiley's April report noted that in March there had been forty-two insured patients in the hospital. There was further discounting: $1,954 had been paid for their care, and the hospital charged off $348.66 for the month. There were now 25,477 members of the local Plan, including dependents.

In June it was reported that the hospital had refused to admit the patients of ten doctors on the staff because of lack of space; there was suspicion that GHS patients were being brought to the hospital to the exclusion of medical-staff patients, but no corrective measures were taken.

The third and fourth floors of the South Wing opened in August, adding ninety beds. A few rooms were equipped with bulky window air conditioners.

In October, a committee was appointed to investigate the possibility of offering the hospital's facilities to more boys from the Drumm Farm, most of whom were presently being sent to Children's Mercy or General Hospital. This later occurred, and there were repeated instances thereafter when Drumm Farm boys received free care.

In previous months there had been doubts expressed about continuation of the annual ball, and one of the directors spoke of a fashion show staged annually by a Chicago hospital auxiliary; it was moved that this possible alternative be brought to the attention of the Saint Luke's

Auxiliary. However, no fashion show was organized, and the following year there was a post-Easter "Cotton Ball" on March 30, which enjoyed a great deal of newspaper publicity.

The Board approved a motion to offer the hospital's facilities to "any deserving children who might need hospitalization during the Christmas holidays, as a gesture of good will to the community." This practice was continued in subsequent years, primarily in the form of free tonsilectomies.

· · · · ·

January, 1940, was the busiest month ever at Saint Luke's, with an average of 204 patients per day. Part of the activity could be attributed to the length of stay of insured patients:

> "Often patients were able to leave the hospital but on account of the fact they were privileged to remain for a certain additional period, they generally took advantage of it."

It was reported in January, 1940, that there were 36,423 GHS members, prompting Mr. Peet to renew his call for twice a month remittances. He was advised by Mr. Beals, a member of the GHS board, that given the large volume of GHS business and the necessity of reviewing each bill, this was impossible. At the same meeting, the president of the medical staff reported that physicians favored the plan because it helped patients to obtain hospitalization, and consequently the doctor was paid without waiting for the hospital bill to be settled.

· · · · ·

The hospital by-laws were amended in January to create the title of First and Executive Vice President, an office to which A.W. Peet was promptly elected. This officer was the de facto president of the hospital, with the bishop actually functioning as board chairman.

· · · · ·

A recurrent nursing shortage prompted the American Red Cross to form and train an organization to provide limited patient care—called "Gray Ladies" because of their gray uniforms and veils. In November, 1939, the Gray Ladies organization was accepted for volunteer work at Saint Luke's if the medical staff and the auxiliary approved, with membership preference favoring Episcopal women. Initially, the medical staff was "lukewarm" about acceptance, but further investigation by the doctors led to approval, and the Gray Ladies served faithfully for many years at the hospital. The Red Cross ultimately discontinued the organization, but a handful of alumnae remain as volunteers at Saint Luke's.

February, 1940, was even busier than January—214 patients per day. In March the same director who had come back from Chicago with the fashion show proposal had been in the Windy City again and returned to report that a hospital auxiliary there had installed a small gift shop and soda fountain, and expressed the belief that this would be an attractive feature for Saint Luke's to consider.

A resolution was adopted commemorating the death of Dr. Harold P. Kuhn. As a memorial to Dr. Kuhn, who had served as medical-staff president and enjoyed one of the busiest surgical practices at Saint Luke's, there was established the "Harold P. Kuhn Fellowship for Medical and Surgical Research."

A new policy resulted from a police department request for $50 to help sponsor a horse show. Mr. Peet "moved to discourage such practice," and the request was refused. Without passing judgment on the merits of a particular enterprise, the board has continued to recognize that those who donate funds to Saint Luke's have their own philanthropic interests and do not contribute to the hospital in order that it might in turn give to other causes.

John Smiley chaired a committee formed by various hospitals to study the GHS financial performance. Losses sustained to date were a concern. Maternity cases were a drain on the insurer, but hospital employees, comprising just 2 percent of the plan members, were the only group showing continuous loss. An employee "group" was not defined, and Smiley's committee recommended that the contract be offered only to hospital employees "proper" and their dependents. Also, their length of hospital stays should be limited, with "further restrictions on type of disease." And GHS should pay out to each hospital group only an amount equal to the amount received from that group. The board endorsed these recommendations, but only four hospitals (Saint Luke's, St. Mary's, Independence Sanitarium, and Providence) implemented them. Consequently, Kansas City's hospital employees continued to be losers for GHS.

Plans were authorized for a new building, to house interns on the second floor and provide class and recreation rooms for nurses on the first floor. In May, 1940, measures were taken to prevent mingling … the plans were revised to provide two entrances instead of one. This would permit "an entrance on Wornall Road which would enable the interns to park their cars there and enter the building without going to the far side and having to enter through the part which will belong to the nurses, thus avoiding the intimacy of the nurses and the interns in the same part of the building." Construction got underway in September, and the building was completed the next year.

World war was raging in Europe in May, 1940, and Smiley reported that "due to the recent upset of market conditions caused by the war situation, all firms had been contacted for supplies for the purpose of protecting the hospital on both securing supplies and prices."

There was extended discussion of the cost of rubber gloves and cat gut used in the operating rooms. The surgeons had supplied these but now objected to the expense, saying that many of their cases were charity cases for which they received no fee and that after the gloves were discarded because of cuts or tears, they were patched and given to the interns and nurses. The total cost of these two items for one month averaged $350. It was determined that the hospital should absorb this expense.

• • • • •

Another discussion topic was the source of milk for the hospital. It was the opinion of Saint Luke's doctors that the hospital should serve pasteurized milk, whereas presently the hospital served only raw milk. There was no milk-control ordinance, and many opposed pasteurization on the ground that the process destroyed calcium and protein. Consequently some 150 local dairies still sold raw milk.

Mr. Peet proposed turning his farm into a dairy farm and equipping it to furnish the hospital with the highest-quality pasteurized milk. He planned to ask the Turner Brothers of Belton ("well educated, from a nice family and of good stock") to join him in this enterprise. There was a general discussion of the kind of herd and the amount of investment that would be required, water supply, location, and other details. The board then accepted Mr. Peet's proposition.

• • • • •

A complaint was filed about the care of one patient. After a conciliatory visit from Messrs. Peet and Wallace Goff, another board officer, the patient was "somewhat appeased." Part of the problem was determined to be "patient relations" … patients were influenced by the hospital people they met and the general atmosphere of a hospital. They should leave the hospital with the feeling that everything possible had been done for them. At the same time it was recognized that "a sick man was hard to please." A closer relationship between the board and the medical staff would be helpful. Closer contact with patients also was suggested, and not only by the nurses and doctors … the office staff "left impressions" as well, especially those who worked at the front desk and those who handled the telephone. Better communication among employees was urged, through the use of memos. A publication later encouraged kindness and courtesy on the part of those employees dealing with the public.

Antitrust-law prohibitions against price-fixing were not a hospital concern in those days, as a report at the September, 1940, board meeting demonstrated. Mr. Peet referred to a conversation with a Mr. Ennis from Research Hospital regarding Saint Luke's ward bed rates:

> "Mr. Ennis contended that Saint Luke's and Menorah Hospitals maintained $3.00 ward bed rates. Mr. Peet stated that we were not the only hospital, besides Menorah, charging $3.00 ward rates, since St. Mary's, Trinity, and some Kansas City, Kansas, hospitals charged these same rates. Mr. Ennis had stated that the insurance companies were well able to pay $4.00 for ward beds; also that they had decided to raise hospitalization rates on school teachers … doubling the rate … making it $1.50 a month, and, even then, they didn't break even."

It was determined that there should be no change of Saint Luke's rates. In November, doctors complained of slow elevator service, a minor but exasperating problem, and also urged that relatives and visitors be kept out of the operating and delivery rooms.

• • • • •

Medical staff efforts to obtain a Saint Luke's surgical residency were successful, and Dr. Eugene Parsons became Saint Luke's first surgical resident. Part of his time was devoted to medical research, and it was determined that funds from the Dr. Harold P. Kuhn fund would be used to finance research activities appropriate for a surgery resident "and, if possible, the results of such investigation be published in one of the national scientific medical journals."

GHS membership continued to expand rapidly, and all was in conformity with the GHS yearly budget, except for the number of people hospitalized, which was very high. Superintendent Smiley and Mr. Peet attended a conference at the office of prominent attorney Arthur Mag to discuss GHS problems. GHS hoped to inaugurate an educational program to overcome mistaken ideas regarding GHS and its progress, and representatives of the organization intended to visit the various hospitals and provide information in this regard. As a consequence, the December 20, 1940, meeting of the board was attended by GHS representatives. Their remarks were summarized as follows:

> "Mr. Earl R. Sweet, Executive Director of Group Hospital Service, Inc., gave us some very interesting information about the hospitalization plan from the administrative standpoint. We next heard from Mr. F.K. Helsby, Assistant Director of Group Hospital Service, Inc. He stated that the hospitalization plan was a national movement, there being sixty-five such plans in effect at this time. The third representative from Group Hospital Service, Inc., was Dr. Ira H. Lockwood, one of the trustees. He spoke of the needed cooperation of the Physicians with the Group Hospital Plan in dismissing their patients as soon as they were well enough to leave the hospital."

At the January, 1941, board meeting, the House and Grounds Committee recommended "that we have two Coca-Cola containers located in Saint Luke's Hospital," and that there be a gift shop in the lobby to be used by the auxiliary. Both were approved. Smiley urged that Saint Luke's join the other hospitals in the Kansas City area in preparing and publishing a set of rules to control visiting; the Public Relations Committee was authorized to prepare such a plan.

Patients sometimes requested certain rooms that were not available at the time of admission, and it was proposed that if the request was for a $5.50 room and only a $7.50 room was available, the patient be offered a $6.50 rate for the higher-priced room until the $5.50 room became available. Also, higher-priced private corner rooms in the South Wing were to serve as double rooms in case of emergency rather than turn people away from the hospital.

In September the auxiliary opened a coffee shop furnished with a large gift case. Success was immediate, according to the auxiliary's annual report:

"There is a widespread expression of pleasure and gratitude over the service we are now able to render to the families and friends of the patients in Saint Luke's."

The clouds of war were hanging over the country, and none of the auxiliary "felt very much in the mood for a ball this year." Consequently, they raised additional funds by expanding their membership.

• • • • •

The benefit to hospitals of GHS did not escape physicians, and the president of the medical staff reported that "the Jackson County Medical Society is working on a plan to prepay doctors' fees in surgical, obstetrical and orthopaedic cases to be sold in conjunction with the Group Hospital Service contracts." In October, Surgical Plan, Inc., was put into effect. This was the genesis of Blue Shield in Kansas City, although initially it was limited to people with low incomes.

• • • • •

To help cope with the greater patient volume resulting from group hospital insurance, Callie French, superintendent of nurses, "offered two practical suggestions:" 1) allow nurses' aides to provide some nursing care; and 2) place a girl at each chart desk on all floors to handle phone calls and clerical work.

Miss French had been both director of nurses and director of nursing education since 1920, having replaced Miss Tulloss in those roles. Now the responsibility for nursing activities was divided, with Miss French continuing as director of the School of Nursing but relinquishing her supervisory duties relating to patient care. Miss Helen B. Valentine was appointed Superintendent of Nursing Service; as such she would be responsible for seeing that the patients received proper nursing care and responsible also for all the other employed personnel in the nursing department.

The nurses' training school was enlarged on September 15 by adding twenty-five girls; the sun rooms in the nurses' home were converted into sleeping quarters for the additional students.

Miss Valentine suggested that one reason for the difficulty in securing adequate nursing care for patients was that the hospital underpaid its nurses. Subsequent salary increases to supervisors living outside the Nurses' Home improved conditions from a supervisory standpoint, and the hospital experienced less difficulty in securing nurses and nurses' aides.

In December, 1941, the board approved the employment of Dr. Louis Scarpellino as Director of the X ray Department. And the board again decided to "accept children for hospitalization as a part of our Christmas celebration," and also to "carry out our usual decorations to cost approximately $50.00."

FOURTEEN
1941-1945

World War II ... Max Berry ... crippled children ...
Arnold Arms ... discrimination ... Roger C. Slaughter ...
congestion ... Kansas City Cradle

*A*merica entered World War II with the bombing of Pearl Harbor on December 7, 1941. This would have a profound impact on the hospital for the next several years.

Several members of the medical staff were granted leaves of absence "for the duration of the war." These included Rex Diveley and Ferd Helwig. This was a repeat performance for Dr. Helwig, who had served as a very young Army first lieutenant in World War I. He predicted victory in World War II when, looking out a hospital window at the stream of traffic on Mill Creek Parkway, he declared: "There is your answer to the outcome of this war ... No other nation on earth can produce armament as fast as we can!"

Dr. Helwig arranged for Dr. Morris Jones to take over his work in pathology and for Dr. Scarpellino (recently employed to manage the X ray Department) to supervise the laboratory employees as chief of radiology.

The day after Pearl Harbor, Maxwell Berry—now a Saint Luke's internist—went down to the General Post Office and volunteered for the Army Medical Corps. Dr. Berry would serve as Chief of Medical Services for the Army's 133rd General Hospital and as a consultant in tropical medicine; he would be awarded the Bronze Star medal.

Fifty-nine of Saint Luke's 132 physicians ultimately served in the armed forces. A number of them were assigned to the 77th Evacuation Hospital whose head nurse, Ms. Bessie Walker, had been a Saint Luke's R.N.

The arrangement with the University of Missouri for the care of crippled children had been in effect for several years, with only very small rate increases. The contract expired at the end of 1941, and Mr. Peet agreed with the University's Dean Conley that Saint Luke's would henceforth accept only emergency cases (Dr. Conley was to decide whether an "emergency" existed in a given case), but would continue to care for those crippled children already in the hospital. This arrangement was subject to change on thirty days' notice; meanwhile, the hospital conducted studies to support its request for increased compensation. The financial strain was somewhat relieved when an agreement was reached for additional billing for outpatient work that would generate $4.10 per patient day; on this basis the contract was renewed to June 30.

The *Diocesan Journal* for 1942 reported that the war would affect the hospital just as it would affect all other industries and that the hospital would have an important part to play in preparation for civilian defense. It would be called upon to furnish emergency beds in case of a major disaster and to send teams of doctors, nurses and orderlies to disaster scenes to render first aid. The hospital immediately lost several nurses to the armed forces and expected to lose more very soon.

The availability of nursing students proved to be a godsend. In February, 1942, the nursing "situation" was alleviated by putting to work thirty-eight freshman students who had been in the classroom since the previous September.

To partially offset the nurse drain, the School of Nursing was enlarged by another twenty-five students. A February class of twenty-five new students was accepted, and they would be ready to assist in June. This would enable the hospital to meet the shortage anticipated from more and more nurses being called into Army and Navy service.

The progress of GHS continued to be "very good." The growth of hospital insurance everywhere was stimulated when the national War Labor Board determined that fringe benefits up to 5 percent of wages could be permitted without having inflationary effects; employers increased group health benefits to attract and retain workers.

The level of occupancy by plan members led to a constant shortage of hospital beds … a national phenomenon. Mr. Beals observed that "the final hope was that the 'Blue Cross' Plan would admit its members to any hospital in the United States … however, this would be up to the member hospitals."

Contributing to the persistent overcrowding at Saint Luke's were the soft-hearted night admitting clerks, known to be more accommodating than the day shift. Recognizing this, doctors sometimes sent patients to the hospital in the dead of night after they had been advised in the daytime that no room was available.

Mrs. Herbert Peet was commissioned to paint the portrait of her father-in-law, A.W. Peet, for a fee of $200. When completed, the painting was installed on the south wall of the board room. Mr. Goff, second vice president, was asked to say a few words at the installation ceremony; he praised Mr. Peet's leadership. Mr. Peet made an appropriate, gracious response, thanking the bishop and the board and expressing his pride in what the hospital had become.

Brigadier General William Rumbaugh of Camp Crowder, Neosho, Missouri, was scheduled to be the commencement speaker for the School of Nursing, and the auxiliary organized a reception for him. However, he was ordered to Washington by the War Department and was replaced as speaker by the chaplain of Camp Crowder. There was no mention of a reception for the chaplain.

The hospital's cost studies bore fruit when the Crippled Children's Service of the State of Missouri proposed a rate increase to $4.00 per patient day. The board approved that proposal and authorized renewal of the contract with the University of Missouri beginning July 1, 1942.

Callie French was in ill health, and in September she resigned as superintendent of nurses. She moved to Albuquerque, New Mexico, and was succeeded by Miss Valentine as superintendent.

• • • • •

A Scroll of Honor was approved by the board bearing the names of doctors, nurses, and other hospital personnel called into "Active Service for our Country," to be placed in the elevator lobby. The Scroll, entitled "The Roll of Honor Board," was ordered and carried an inscription written by Bishop Spencer.

A board resolution recognized the distinguished services rendered the hospital by Ferdinand Christian Helwig, M.D., expressed pride in his patriotism in "volunteering his services to our country" and expressed "the earnest hope that his services elsewhere being terminated, he may return to the hospital to carry on the work which has been to the hospital one of its outstanding services to humanity."

By September, there were twenty-eight doctors, thirty nurses and ten hospital employees in the armed forces of the United States.

They turned up all around the globe. When Dr. Ralph Ringo Coffey—back in the army as a medical officer—suffered a broken neck on a French reconnaissance mission, Colonel Rex Diveley (Chief of Orthopaedic Surgery for the European Theater) made the repairs.

The armed forces used a skin-grafting device patented by Saint Luke's Dr. Earl Padgett as the "Padgett Dermatone." Dr. Padgett was compared by Dr. Mervin Rumold to a bantam rooster, with energy galore but little tolerance for the slow-witted. Much of his minor surgery was performed using local anesthetic, described by Rumold as "vocal anesthetic" as Padgett constantly ordered his wide-awake patients to "keep still."

· · · · ·

The hospital's obstetrical department, particularly the nursery, was overflowing … a condition reportedly prevailing throughout the city. To help alleviate the crowding at Saint Luke's, attending obstetricians were instructed to send all maternity cases home "at the end of a ten-day period, except those with definite complications." The president of the medical staff suggested that a room next to the doctors' sleeping room on the fourth floor be assigned as a "loafing and sleeping room" for obstetricians. Meanwhile the Margaret Chapman Guild of Grace and Holy Trinity Church contributed eighty-three pairs of baby mittens to the hospital.

The 12th Street property was now a liability—a fire had caused a significant loss in January, and the building was put up for sale at a price of $30,000. Mr. Bettinger of the Bettinger Trunk Co., the current tenant of the property, offered to pay $15,000 for it. The board indicated that it would disapprove of any price below $25,000.

· · · · ·

Meanwhile the war's impact continued to be felt in many ways.

The United States Surgeon General allotted $3,000 for use in training twelve additional student nurses, who enrolled in September.

Compensation increases effective October 1, 1942, for hospital employees were limited by a presidential order freezing salaries above $5,000 per year.

Despite the hospital's location in the middle of the country, there was also raised—and dismissed—the question of whether war damage insurance should be purchased on hospital property.

Government authorities attending an AHA meeting advised that there would soon be a shortage of food and containers, particularly cans, and of farm labor. Care and conservation of all food supplies was stressed, but the hospital dietitian stated that the hospital had on hand a year's supply of most major canned goods.

· · · · ·

The Fund for Indigent Men was still receiving contributions in November, 1942.

In December, each employee and each student nurse received a gift of $5. Christmas decorations were less elaborate than in most prior years. The Shrine Chanters sang carols the Monday night before Christmas, the Student Nurses' Glee Club caroled in the corridors on Tuesday night, and the Grace & Holy Trinity Boys' Choir sang carols on Christmas Eve. Passengers in automobiles on Mill Creek Parkway were cheered by lights in every hospital window, creating an effect similar to old Williamsburg. Once again the hospital took children for free service "in order that they may enjoy the Christmas Eve activities in our Children's Ward."

Judge Holt stated at the December board meeting that he and Senator Cooper had turned the matter of adjustment of taxes on hospital property over to Mr. Matz, "who had done a bully job of it." It appeared that taxes on hospital grounds would be reduced from $5,000 to about $28. There was no suggestion that hospital property should be tax exempt, but the tax burden was certainly minimal and seemed to the board to be hardly worth challenging.

Saint Luke's was unable to expend all of the income from the Linda Hall Fund because there were no beds available for charity cases. Moreover, there was "not a big demand for charity." Group hospitalization revenues contributed substantially to this comfortable financial condition. Hospital counsel, asked to comment on the embarrassment of riches, verbosely advised that because the fund's earnings were "greater than the demand therefor at the present time furnishes no valid reason for complaint … it is a prudent matter to have at all times earnings of that fund on hand more than sufficient for present needs, so as to be able to hospitalize women and children in Saint Luke's Hospital in the event of demands for their hospitalization becoming greater than at the present time." More succinctly put: it was acceptable to accumulate for a rainy day.

In January, 1943, a "North Wing Building and Equipment Fund" was established for the purpose of building a North Wing to the hospital. The nucleus was a $10,000 gift from Mr. E.F. Swinney, payment against a $50,000 bequest that he had established for the hospital's benefit. The general feeling of the directors at the time was that they "would rather run their hospital without government aid" … recognition that with such aid came government intrusion. But the board's laissez faire philosophy would not prevent subsequent acceptance of federal funds for hospital construction.

The auxiliary's continuing interest in the comfort of the hospital's nurses was demonstrated by a gift of a Victor Combination Radio for the Nurses' Home (cost: $186.15).

The war decimated employee ranks at Saint Luke's. At its February, 1943, meeting the board was advised that securing nonprofessional help was a growing problem, exacerbated by a recent government order requiring all available men and women to register for war plants and by the departure of several key men for the armed forces.

A bill pending in Congress classified osteopaths as physicians and surgeons and provided that they should be permitted to practice in any tax-supported hospital. A biased board directed hospital counsel and Mr. Peet to "take such steps as they deem necessary to defeat this bill."

The president of the medical staff suggested that hospital admissions be limited to patients of the Saint Luke's medical staff because of crowded conditions in the hospital. In March the board approved preference for Saint Luke's staff members in the admission of patients, excepting, however, members of the board and their families, members of the auxiliary, the Episcopal clergy, and "special friends of the hospital" whose physicians might be attached to another hospital. Doctors were cooperating by dismissing patients earlier than they ordinarily would. Because of prevailing, overcrowding a request for assistance in treating the county's emergency hospital patients was rejected.

A rationing program went into effect on March 1, 1943. A ration bank account was established with the First National Bank of Kansas City, Missouri, agent for the Office of Price Administration.

Food rationing became a major problem immediately. The Office of Price Administration established regulations fixing Saint Luke's allotment at 36 percent of the amount used during the month of December, 1942 … unfortunately a very low month in terms of patient numbers. The same formula applied throughout the area, and the resulting food shortage was a common complaint in all of the city's hospitals. The local rationing board agreed to grant hospitals additional allotments of rationed foods upon application setting forth their requirements. Meanwhile Saint Luke's meat supplier advised that it would continue to furnish the hospital with "everything possible for our needs."

The House and Grounds Committee stated that the time was "opportune" to assemble property in the area to permit future development of the hospital. The "whole matter of acquiring additional ground" was referred to the Executive Committee.

The Executive Committee felt it would improve the hospital's "labor situation" if it owned additional quarters in which to house lower-paid employees; and it was decided to "get a price" on the Muder property across the street and purchase it if possible. However, Saint Luke's interest in acquiring the property was not to be disclosed. There was a report on other efforts to acquire properties near the hospital, again "keeping the name of the hospital out of the discussions."

Employment at the hospital was stabilized by the government's classification of hospitals as essential war industries. It was now necessary to hire all employees through the U.S. Employment Office, a cumbersome process, but once employed they could not leave without establishing that the new job was more essential to the war effort than their hospital work. And they would need a certificate of availability from the hospital, stating that they could be spared for employment by another war industry.

A schedule of proposed payroll increases, authorized by the board, was submitted to the War Labor Board and received its approval.

Doctors on the hospital staff raided the hospital for nurses for their private offices. The president of the medical staff expressed no remorse over his colleagues' piracy, arguing that they did not encourage such defections but that nurses preferred the regular hours in the doctors' offices to hospital schedules, and also that the hospital's nurses were underpaid. He suggested that the solution lay in increased student enrollment in the nursing school.

In May, John Smiley advised that the training of an adequate number of nurses was a national problem in which the federal government was taking a very active interest. Government representatives suggested that, to increase the capacity of Saint Luke's School of Nursing, the senior class be housed outside the Nurses' Home for their final six months' training and their places filled with additional students. Smiley recommended that additional housing facilities be secured in the neighborhood.

Other employment problems continued, with the hospital's laundry now being in the worst straits. It was almost impossible to get or keep help in the housekeeping department. Employees in the kitchen and housekeeping departments were said to be far less efficient than those of a year ago, since many had been available only because of physical handicaps which prevented them from doing war work.

The Missouri Furniture Co. offered $20,000 for the 12th and Troost property, a price that would net the hospital $19,000 after the broker's commission. The board had lowered its expectations, and the sale was approved. When the sale was consummated, the proceeds were invested in a United States Government Bond.

• • • • •

Internist Arnold Arms, M.D., was admitted to medical staff membership in May, 1943, a significant event not recognized as such at the time. He was to become a hospital stalwart. Arms was attracted by the caliber of the people and the presence of the Church at Saint Luke's. Later he reminisced:

> "Although the staff was small, it was great, and above all of them towered the presence of the Reverend Bishop Spencer, who spent very much of his time in Saint Luke's Hospital in his capacity as Bishop of the Episcopal Diocese."

• • • • •

The Federal Works Agency was investigating the need for more hospital beds in the Kansas City area, and in June asked Saint Luke's for data. In the course of their investigation, FWA officials disclosed that government aid for the construction of the North Wing might be available under the Lanham Act if the area was indeed short of beds and if Saint Luke's served war workers. If the hospital could raise one-quarter of the funds needed, the application for a federal grant under the act would be given very serious consideration in Washington. The Executive Committee was directed to formulate plans and apply for the grant. The committee subsequently authorized Mr. Peet and Superintendent Smiley to negotiate with government officials.

However, a question arose concerning Saint Luke's policy against admitting blacks as inpatients. It appeared that this might prevent government funding for the North Wing as well as government aid for nurses' training and acceptance of patients from the armed forces. One of the directors expressed his "grave doubt as to the effect on Saint Luke's Hospital" if black patients were admitted.

A memo from another hospital director reflected the times in Kansas City and the State of Missouri. The state Constitution then—and indeed for ten years thereafter—mandated segregation in the public schools. "Caucasian birth" was a requirement for membership in the Jackson County Medical Society. Also, there was considerable discrimination in Kansas City's public accommodations and housing. Even the nation's blood supply was segregated, as were the armed forces and the war plants.

The memo warned that a literal interpretation was likely to be enforced by the Fair Practices Board, "which is headed by a darkey who has no other duty or thought except to enforce the constitutional rights of the colored people." The memo went on to state:

> "I have lived among darkeys all my life and usually our household servants have been colored.
>
> "I do not believe that this plan is practical or workable and I further believe that if it is enforced, it will lead to bloodshed and set the colored race back rather than improve their position.
>
> "In no place that I can think of is the contact of patients and employees more intimate than in a hospital. I cannot conceive of your white nurses giving darkey patients a bath. I cannot conceive of ward beds being occupied by both black and white in comfort and happiness and I cannot conceive of your nurses training school embracing both races in harmony.
>
> "It is my well considered judgment that this will multiply your operating problems ten-fold and create many unsolvable situations both embarrassing and detrimental to this institution which it has taken so many years to build.
>
> "It is my judgment that if these policies are agreed to and placed in effect,

it will result in the hospital being ostracized by the major part of our most profitable clients."

"I believe that I am moved to make these statements solely because of my interest in the hospital and not because of any racial prejudices."

The board at its September meeting unanimously resolved "that the hospital not admit Negro patients for inpatient care." However the effort to obtain a federal grant proceeded.

A racial issue also was raised by the Bolton-Bailey Bill, establishing a U.S. Cadet Nurse Corps and providing payment to the Corps' nursing students as well as payment to the hospital for maintenance and tuition fees. The hospital took forty of these girls into its September class, all of whom joined the Corps. Fifty-eight of the nurses in training also joined. The cadet nurses were readily distinguishable in their smart, military-style uniforms.

The bill provided that "there shall be no discrimination in the administration of the benefits and appropriations made under the respective provisions of this act, on account of race, creed or color." John Smiley wrote the surgeon general asking for an opinion on the admission of black girls. His request was referred to the Federal Security Agency of the U.S. Public Health Service. A reply, signed by the director of the division of nurse education, cited a legal opinion previously rendered to the Surgeon General. That opinion declared that the non-discrimination requirement would be complied with "if in the administration of the Act, no plan is disapproved or payment denied to any institution on account of the race, creed or color of its students, teachers or other personnel." There was no affirmative duty to take black girls, but discrimination against institutions that did accept blacks was prohibited. It was also pointed out that "each school sets its own admission requirements." The letter concluded: "It is hoped that this gives you the answer you desire."

With this in hand, legal counsel for the hospital had no difficulty in determining that Saint Luke's could, without violating the Act, decline to accept black students. The board unanimously resolved "not to admit negro students to the nursing school."

• • • • •

In September, a request was rejected that Saint Luke's accept an undetermined number of Veterans Administration patients for the years 1944,

1945, and 1946, because of the hospital's crowded condition. And cases referred from the Children's Bureau involving maternity care for the wives of servicemen were to be accepted only when the hospital had space, even though the government paid both the doctor and the hospital. (The Saint Luke's maternity department was averaging more than 100 deliveries per month.) Also rejected due to lack of space were requests from the medical department of the Naval Air Base in Gardner to accept patients from the Navy's Kansas City clinic, and from the V.A. in Excelsior Springs to take patients from the armed forces who suffered illness or injury, particularly WACs, WAVEs, and nurses.

The greatest problem continued to be lack of personnel; consequently, salary increases for all departments were approved. Meanwhile the hospital continued to operate at capacity with fewer employees, and "the strain is beginning to tell on our department heads." One department had a turnover of 600 percent during the year, which greatly impeded efficiency.

The U.S. Public Health Office and the Federal Works Agency endorsed construction of a Nurses' Home but were hesitant to recommend construction of a North Wing for the hospital proper pending a decision as to availability of beds at General Hospital for private patients. The War Production Board indicated its opposition unless all beds in Kansas City were 90 percent occupied, a very high standard. Then, in November it was reported that FWA representatives wanted Saint Luke's to contribute 40 percent of the cost of the new buildings, rather than 20 percent. Prospects for a new wing dimmed.

At the November meeting the Board was told that the Office of Defense Transportation would not permit dairies to make daily deliveries, and the hospital would have to provide a milk box with additional cold storage space. John Smiley also reported on a meeting of the Missouri Hospital Association concerning the effect of the war and government-sponsored programs on hospitals. Volunteer nurses' aides (Gray Ladies) sponsored by the Red Cross were doing a good job throughout the state. And the government program for payment of obstetrical bills for service wives was explained. (Saint Luke's was now accepting these cases and received the same compensation for them as the hospital's ten-day rate for private patients. To be eligible the husband had to be an enlisted man with the rank of sergeant or less.)

The steadily growing importance of GHS's Blue Cross Plan in Kansas

City was noted; all hospitals were urged to give their full support to this plan and also to the companion surgical plan. Surgical Plan, Inc., was now "Blue Shield," with the same focus on physician coverage. Some 400 physicians contributed significant working capital, and for the next forty years doctors would spend untold uncompensated hours on various boards and committees of "the Blues."

Efforts were made to extend these programs to rural areas. Meanwhile, GHS increased its payments to Saint Luke's for dependents by fifty cents per day in exchange for elimination of certain hospital charges.

The hospital continued to run at capacity in December, with a large number of influenza cases adding to the burden.

•••••

The Wagner-Murray-Dingell Bill, introduced in 1943, proposed an expansion of Social Security to include hospital and medical care. It called for a payroll tax on employers and employees to finance the health care coverage. This was perceived as socialized medicine.

The specter of socialized medicine haunted the medical establishment, which was sensitive to any encroachment in the medical field by governmental agencies. The success of GHS did much to curtail the movement in Kansas City. The State Board of Health also used its considerable influence to prevent "further socialization" of the practice of medicine. These efforts, and their counterparts elsewhere in the country, were effective; despite repeated attempts over a period of several years, the bill went nowhere.

•••••

The North Wing project was not forgotten. It was suggested that a fund-raising effort should get underway and that meanwhile board members should contact senators and congressmen home for Christmas ... one congressman in particular:

> "It was the general feeling that Mr. Roger C. Slaughter would be the man to follow the thing through for us."

On December 30, 1943, several members of the board met with Congressman Slaughter at the Kansas City Club to discuss an application for federal funds for the construction of the new Nurses' Home and

North Wing. Mr. Slaughter indicated his willingness to assist in any way possible and became heavily involved.

• • • • •

At the January, 1944, meeting, John Smiley listed three important factors affecting the operation of the hospital: the changing attitude of the medical staff, the insistence on the part of patients for accommodations, and the effect of the first two conditions on hospital personnel. When the president of the medical staff presented his report, he stated that the hospital was blessed with physicians unequaled in the area, due in part to the staff's morale and cooperation. However, he acknowledged that "of late the staff has not been as cooperative as it might have been." He then presented a written set of proposals concerning the medical staff for the Board's acceptance or rejection. These included: close cooperation among doctors; the perfection of the procedures for room reservations in the interest of fairness to doctors and patients; and an inquiry of the medical staff as to whether they would care to have a member of the board of directors attend staff meetings. The proposals were approved.

The medical staff in February recommended (1) that patients be admitted to the hospital only when such admission passed through and was accepted by the admitting clerk of the hospital, and (2) that two beds in the hospital be kept available for emergency cases at all times. They also expressed the hope that closer cooperation between the medical staff and the board "will in the future be effected."

One medical-staff problem was poor attendance at meetings, leading the staff president to complain to his colleagues that "for several months, attendance at staff meetings has been rapidly approaching the vanishing point." He proposed that the staff bylaws be amended to reduce the quorum requirements, but he was unable to muster sufficient doctors to formally adopt the amendment. A general staff letter resulted:

> "It should be obvious to everyone that nothing can be done until you attend meetings in sufficient volume to permit the transaction of business. The only alternative is to continue the sport of hollering, in which pastime the hazard and inconvenience of doing something is entirely eliminated. Members of your Executive Committee have had much experience with this sport and if it continues popular would like to be considered for admission to one of your teams."

• • • • •

Board committees recommended that Keene & Simpson, architects, be retained to prepare plans for a complete medical center at Saint Luke's, working in conjunction with a nationally known hospital consultant. They further recommended that efforts to obtain a government construction grant continue, that there be an organized effort to raise any balance needed, and that a booklet be prepared "giving the entire story of these proposals." The recommendations were approved.

There were now 158 nursing students. Sixteen were housed at recently purchased property at 4410 Wornall "under the care of Mrs. Avery."

The Muder property was fully occupied by employees, and as soon as two other houses purchased by the hospital could be renovated and furnished they also were rented to hospital employees.

It appeared in March that the Nurses' Home project would produce Lanham Act funds. Mr. Beals was satisfied that there would be no difficulty under the Lanham Act with respect to "the race problem." A consultant would assist the architects with construction plans at a fee of $100 per day. The North Wing approval was still in limbo.

In March the medical staff was given control over all physicians practicing medicine in the hospital, through the promulgation of rules and regulations approved by the board. The staff also was authorized to make changes from time to time in medical services as they deemed advisable and necessary, subject to certain controls vested in the superintendent and board. And the doctors were to be consulted regarding modifications in the buildings maintained for the care of patients. However, the staff recognized "the complete and supreme authority of the board of directors of the hospital in the management of the institution" with the right "to modify or eliminate any change in the medical care of patients that may from time to time be directed by the Executive Staff under the authority requested in the above proposals."

In April, 1944, the staff president "reported that the situation with the room clerks and doctors is now very tranquil and he thinks the future holds nothing but promise." Nevertheless, the hospital remained crowded, with beds at a premium. To alleviate the problem, a plea was directed to patients:

> "During ordinary times you have been welcomed, even encouraged, to spend as much of your convalescent period in the hospital as possible, but during these trying times we ask that you leave the hospital as soon as your physical condition allows."

Applications for medical staff appointment also were put on hold, with applicants told:

> "Due to the extreme shortage of beds for patients at Saint Luke's Hospital … the Executive Staff and Board of Trustees of the Hospital have decided for the present war emergency there will no additional members appointed to the staff at Saint Luke's Hospital."

The emergency room was busy as well, and the medical staff suggested larger and more adequate ER facilities. They also suggested that emergency cases be examined in ER by the resident there, before admission to the hospital.

In May, Helen B. Valentine resigned as Superintendent of Nurses because of ill health and was succeeded by Miss Virginia Harrison, who was described as "an Episcopal girl and a graduate of Saint Luke's Hospital in St. Louis … with considerable experience in the nursing field."

At the suggestion of the medical staff, a room was set aside until the start of school in the fall "for just tonsil patients."

In June, Mr. Beals pronounced himself "a bit discouraged with the situation regarding the War Production Board and the delay that our already approved Nurses' Home will probably have." He stated that "even though we raised our own funds we will be referred back to the War Production Board for approval, and since our plans call for critical materials and the government wants only the cheapest construction, I am very doubtful of the approval of our project by this agency."

Three months later, Mr. Peet told the Executive Committee that plans should be made for raising funds to supplement or replace government aid for the North Wing. It was determined that professionals should be hired for this purpose. Meanwhile, government red tape slowed the approved Nurses' Home project, with the hospital's application returned twice for changes.

In October, 1944, the hospital received an offer of a combined loan ($123,000) and grant ($393,360) from the Federal Works Agency (FWA) … leaving a balance of $123,640 to be raised by the hospital for the construction of a new Nurses' Home and conversion of the existing nurses' residence into a convalescent building. The proposed North Wing was not to be funded. The board adopted a resolution accepting the offer.

The Muder house, on the site of the proposed new Nurses' Home, was relocated on other Hospital land. The house was vacated by its employee occupants, who joined other employees housed in three nearby houses owned by the hospital.

The war news indicated that the tide had turned in favor of the United States and its allies. Dick Powell, movie star, spent a week in Saint Luke's Hospital after contracting a severe cold while making appearances for the U.S.O.

· · · · ·

The medical staff proposed to honor Herman Pearse at a dinner but Dr. Pearse declined, writing from his Bonner Springs, Kansas, residence:

> "The weight of my years is commencing to throw shadows that warn me that I should not let my footsteps lead far from my home and my resting place."

Dr. Pearse died that fall.

· · · · ·

In November, the board authorized the employment of a campaign director to raise a fund of at least $750,000 for building and equipping the North Wing.

In December, the building campaign was announced to the press and received favorable coverage … aided by the fact that Roy A. Roberts, Editor of the *Kansas City Star,* was a member of the Executive Committee for the campaign organization, representing St. Andrew's parish.

The campaign commenced officially in January, 1945, accompanied by a booklet stating the case for the effort. In a foreword to the publication, Bishop Spencer referred to the hospital's patron Saint Luke as "Tenderest of all Christian writers of nineteen hundred years ago," and pointed out that Luke was a doctor of medicine … "the best doctor that they had in his day." He prophesied that Kansas City, Missouri, would be the site of a medical school as well as laboratories "which hold the light for the modern doctor and surgeon."

A section authored by A.W. Peet recounted a brief history of the hospital, followed by a section on its financial condition by David Beals, hospital treasurer. Among other points made in the booklet: due to lack of capacity, the hospital in recent months had denied beds to an average of five patients daily. One reason for this was the "remarkable growth of group hospitalization plans and the sale of hospitalization insurance since 1939." More than 130,000 people now had such insurance. "It has made adequate and needed hospitalization accessible to thousands who formerly did without." Other causes: population growth and the need of industry to reduce absenteeism. One-third of Saint Luke's patients came from the territory outside of greater Kansas City, a pattern that would continue—Saint Luke's had truly become a referral hospital.

The booklet featured an architect's drawing—labeled a "vision of Saint Luke's destiny"—depicting the "Great Medical Center" which the hospital would ultimately become. The completed campus would include a separate women's and children's building and a separate research laboratory. A psychiatric building also was contemplated.

· · · · ·

At a special meeting of the board on January 9, 1945, bids were opened on the Nurses' Home project and the contract was awarded to Swenson Construction Co., the low bidder. Work was begun the next day—January 10, 1945. When completed, the nurses' residence would have accommodations for 200 nursing students, as well as classrooms, laboratories, office, auditorium, and library.

At the regular January board meeting, various cases were charged to the Linda S. Hall Fund, the Fund for Indigent Men, and the William Harvey Chapman Memorial Fund. A concise report of these cases would be prepared in aid of the building campaign, since "some people have the idea we don't do much charity."

In March, window bars and a combination safe were installed in the drug room at the insistence of the United States Narcotics Department.

Although the war would end in victory later in the year, food supplies at the hospital continued to be a problem, with a scarcity of chickens, meats, butter, and other items.

Local boys continued to die far from home. A room in the hospital was furnished "in memory of Richard Lee Shelton killed in action on Leyte December 13, 1944."

In May, the board addressed a profit dilemma: "The matter of profits shown in the first three months of this year, particularly the large amount in January, was discussed with a view to correcting, if possible, any thought that this profit was excessive." However, there would be need of these funds ... the hospital's largest employee group, the nursing department, requested immediate salary increases.

In June, Mr. Peet was approached by William J. Brace, who renewed his earlier proposal that Saint Luke's "take over" the Kansas City Cradle next door to the hospital. Judge Ray Cowan of the Juvenile Court of Jackson County had been discussing with Mr. Brace the possibility of enlarging the mission of the institution to include hospitalizing children three to six years old ... creating a place where polio, rheumatic fever and heart patients could be cared for especially. Kansas City lacked facilities for this specialized child care. Further, the hospital's chief of pediatric services had been consulted about the use of the Cradle for pediatric training for nurses. The proposal was approved, and Saint Luke's assumed responsibility for operation of the Cradle as the Children's Hospital.

Harry S Truman, a Baptist, had become president of the United States following the death of Franklin D. Roosevelt on April 12, 1945. At a board meeting in September it was suggested that Mrs. Truman (a communicant of Trinity Episcopal Church in Independence) be made honorary president of the Women's Auxiliary of Saint Luke's Hospital of Kansas City. "This met with the approval of the members of the board, and Mr. Peet suggested that the idea be passed on to the auxiliary for their action." Nothing further occurred ... either the proposal was not well received by the auxiliary, or the invitation was not accepted by the first lady.

The war ended with V J Day on September 2, 1945.

FIFTEEN
1945-1948

veterans ... polio ... H.O. Peet ... convalescent care ...
Crittenton ... Hill-Burton and expansion

*I*n September, 1945, physicians who had served in the armed forces were starting to reappear at Saint Luke's. The president of the medical staff proposed that for three months patients of these returning veterans be given priority access to hospital rooms. Returning servicemen also were exempted from paying medical-staff dues; when the medical director of the Major Clinic paid his 1946 dues, this note accompanied his check:

> "I am adding a little to the regular amount to help make up the deficit due to the fact that our men who are or have been in the service are not expected to pay dues."

The collegial note was signed "Cordially and Fraternally."

A party for the returning doctors also was suggested.

Among the returnees was the estimable Ferd Helwig, who was promptly re-employed at $12,000 per year although he declined a formal written contract. Addressing the board at its November meeting, Dr. Helwig said that many of the nation's hospitals were "in terrible shape" and that the Saint Luke's board and administration deserved tremendous credit for the way their hospital had been maintained.

· · · · ·

Dr. Helen Kingsbury Coffin also came to Saint Luke's in 1945. She was an anesthesiologist—a new specialty then. As Dr. Coffin and her surgical colleagues went about their work in the operating room, they were observed by medical students occupying stands against the surgery walls. Operating tables were elevated manually. Drop ether was still the anesthetic of choice for tonsillectomies, but cyclopropane had come into use for other surgical procedures. Cyclopropane was volatile, and there were one or two minor explosions in the operating room, but no injuries. The later introduction of gas machines that put patients to sleep with a mixture of oxygen and gas was an improvement.

Due almost entirely to Congressman Slaughter's continuing efforts, the board was advised in November, 1945, that a government North Wing construction grant was approved. However, David Beals reported in December that the building fund campaign was lagging ... "probably due to the fact that there has been a definite change in the thinking of people due to the termination of the war." Meanwhile, the new Nurses' Home was completed at the end of December, just across the street to the west of the hospital.

Three children received free tonsillectomies for Christmas.

The wave of physician returnees necessitated a renewed moratorium on medical staff additions. In February, 1946, the medical staff secretary wrote the hospital board as follows:

> "The staff feels that we are unable to take care of our many present members and until such time as more bed space is available we do not wish to make any additions to the Staff."

Virginia Harrison resigned as superintendent of nurses and director of nursing education; Miss Valentine returned in an interim capacity until June 1, when Miss Alicia Sayre would assume both positions.

The FWA approved plans for conversion of the former nurses' residence into a convalescent building, and, in February, 1946, the contract for this work was awarded to Inter State Construction Co.

National Life of Vermont agreed to finance the North Wing construction. However, it would involve incurring a debt of $625,000, and one prominent director—Judge Holt—opposed the project. Nevertheless, the Long Construction Co. was authorized to proceed with construction commencing July 1, 1946. A contract was approved on a cost-plus basis rather than for a fixed fee. Construction actually got underway before any formal written agreement was signed.

• • • • •

The board lost its congressional ally, Roger Slaughter. Mr. Slaughter, a Missouri Democrat, had been a member of the House Rules Committee, which stalled the Fair Employment Practices bill championed by President Truman. Angered by this, Truman decided not to support his fellow Democrat for re-election and enlisted the aid of political crony Jim Pendergast. Pendergast, heir to the late Thomas J. Pendergast's powerful political machine, consequently backed another candidate, Enos Axtell, in the Democratic primary held the first week of August. Roy Roberts' Republican *Kansas City Star* was outraged. After Axtell won the primary, there was suggestion of vote fraud, but it didn't do Slaughter any good—he was out of office ("purged"), and Saint Luke's would get no special treatment in Washington.

Hospitals in the area were unhappy with inadequate compensation provided by the Blue Cross plan (GHS was now uniformly referred to as "Blue Cross') and began to marshall data concerning hospital operating costs. Meanwhile, at the board's October, 1946, meeting, Smiley advised that Blue Cross had granted Saint Luke's a temporary increase of $1—to $7.50 per day per patient—retroactive to the previous July. A review of Saint Luke's financial data had indicated a loss of $600-$800 per month on Blue Cross patients, but in August—with the additional $1 rate in effect—the charge-off was only $51.

The hospitals produced data demonstrating that the $1 increase should be made permanent, and this was accepted. Hospital operating costs would be reviewed every six months and payments adjusted if inadequate.

By October, 1946, some 168,000 Kansas Citians were covered by the Blue Cross plan. The corresponding Blue Shield Surgical Care plan—a newer enterprise—covered 95,616 people.

The convalescent building conversion work also was progressing, and Florence Parsons was named to serve as its supervisor upon completion.

Saint Luke's room rates were raised to match those prevailing elsewhere. David Beals stated "that it was his feeling as treasurer that Saint Luke's should make the same charge for the same type of accommodations as is made in other hospitals in the Kansas City area."

• • • • •

The ravages of poliomyelitis were keeping the Children's Hospital busy. An inflammation of the brain and spinal cord, polio's most common victims were children between the ages of one and nine … hence the name "infantile paralysis." John Smiley in October reported that sixteen beds were occupied by polio cases in addition to sixteen other pediatric cases on the second floor. In the first year of its operation, the Children's Hospital cared for more than 800 children, whereas the previous year only eighty had been placed in the Cradle facility for adoption. William Brace was pleased with the utilization. And, the new hospital produced $40,000 in revenue in twelve months.

When the contract for care of crippled children was renewed with the University of Missouri's Board of Curators, the rate was increased to $7.17 per inpatient day and $2.71 per outpatient visit. Many of the crippled children were polio victims.

Saint Luke's was one of three primary polio treatment centers in Kansas City, and there were a great many disabled children in the hospital. On behalf of the Jackson County Chapter of the National Foundation for Infantile Paralysis, Mr. James J. Rick forwarded a check to the hospital for $10,000. In the transmittal letter Mr. Rick said:

> "Frankly … I do not know what would have happened in Kansas City and vicinity if Saint Luke's Hospital had not taken care of polio victims this year. Kansas City has had almost 200 resident cases of polio and our Kansas City, Missouri, hospitals have cared for more than 450 patients. This is more than three times as many cases as we have ever had here and they all received excellent care and without any excitement or inconvenience. I have received many letters from national authorities commending Kansas City on the fine way the situation was handled, particularly for the fact that we were prepared before polio struck. Certainly your fine hospital is entitled to a great amount of this credit."

The contribution bought special apparatus for treating polio patients and equiping the hospital's swimming pool for paralysis therapy.

William Brace and James Rick attended the November board meeting, where Brace "spoke briefly on the wonderful work being done in the Children's Hospital." Rick again expressed his appreciation for the care given to victims of poliomyelitis. The magnitude of the polio epidemic was indicated by the statistics he recited: 520 cases in Jackson County, for whom the local chapter of the National Foundation had brought forty-one nurses and eight physiotherapists to Kansas City. Mr. Rick's remarks were followed by those of Melvin H. Dunn, assistant superintendent of Saint Luke's, who reported that since July 17, 100 children had been

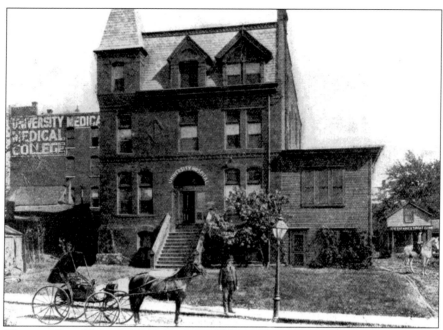

The progenitor of Saint Luke's Hospital was All Saints Hospital, which was established by charter of the Church Charity Association of Kansas City on October 3, 1882. Construction began at 1005 Campbell Street on a 50-bed hospital in 1883, and the facility, shown above, was opened on May 10, 1885. The hospital building has since been razed.

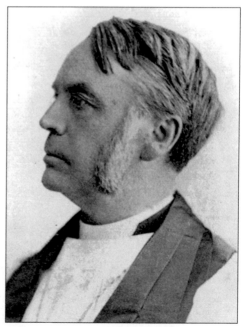

The Right Reverend Edward Atwill was appointed the first Bishop of the Diocese of West Missouri in 1890, and as such inherited a struggling All Saints Hospital, which closed its doors in 1893. However, he witnessed the resurrection of the hospital in 1902, when Saint Luke's Hospital was established.

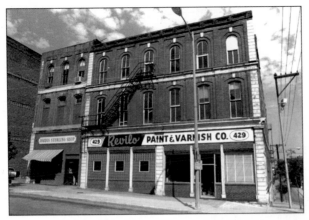

Saint Luke's Hospital's
first home was located on
the northeast corner of
Fifth and Delaware streets,
in a building that
formerly housed the
Western Surgical Institute
of Dr. d'Estang Dickerson.

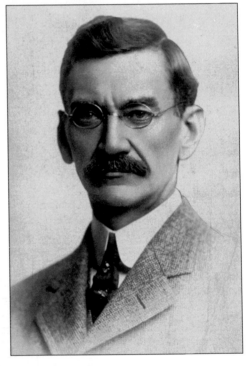

Dr. Herman Pearse, right,
was a communicant of St. Paul's
Episcopal Church. With the help of
pastor Percy Eversden, he opened
Saint Luke's Hospital in 1902.
Pearse mortgaged his home in 1906
to purchase new quarters for the
hospital at 11th & Euclid streets.
Pearse's home, below, still stands at
4515 Wornall Road, a block south
of the current Saint Luke's campus.

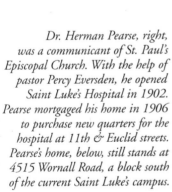

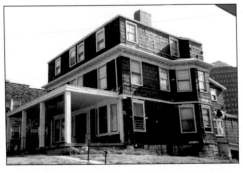

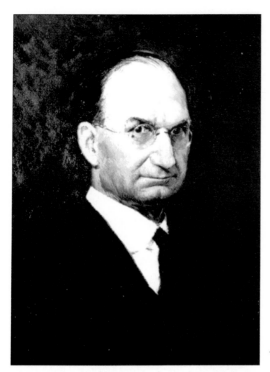

Dr. Arthur Hertzler, one of the colorful characters from Saint Luke's early days, later became nationally acclaimed for his autobiography, "The Horse and Buggy Doctor."

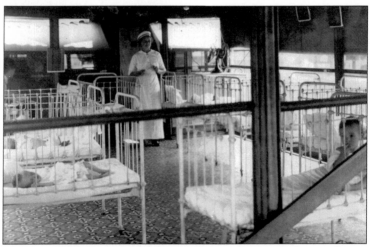

The Saint Luke's Hospital Club began sponsoring "open air baby camps" in 1905 to provide medical care for underprivileged infants in the city's tenement district, known as "Little Italy." A second camp was opened on the city's West Side in 1906. The group subsequently changed its name to the Richard Cabot Club in honor of Dr. Richard Cabot, a member of the Harvard University Medical School faculty and a pioneer in medical social welfare.

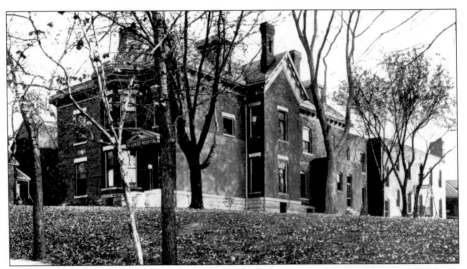

With Dr. Pearse's help, Saint Luke's moved into the Scott House in 1906. This photo shows the 1914 addition to the back of the hospital, which increased capacity to 50 beds.

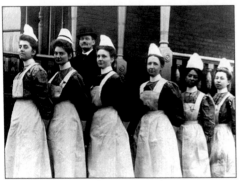

Saint Luke's established a diploma school of nursing in 1905, offering a three-year course of study. The school's 1906 class, shown with Dr. Pearse, included the first graduate, Virginia Pate.

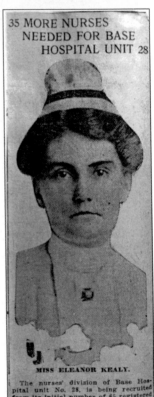

35 MORE NURSES NEEDED FOR BASE HOSPITAL UNIT 28

MISS ELEANOR KEALY.

The nurses' division of Base Hospital unit No. 28, is being recruited from its initial number of 65 registered nurses to its full strength of 100 members. Miss Eleanor Kealy, in charge of the division, is holding the nurses in readiness to leave on 24 hours' notice, although it is not expected that the call will come before spring.

The government has not only increased the pay of the nurses who go into foreign service, but it is now providing uniforms and all wearing apparel.

Miss Lou Eleanor Keely served as superintendent of nurses from 1903 to 1916. A strict disciplinarian, she was noted for setting a high standard of conduct for Saint Luke's nurses. After serving her country during World War I, she returned to Kansas City and helped found the Missouri State Nursing Association.

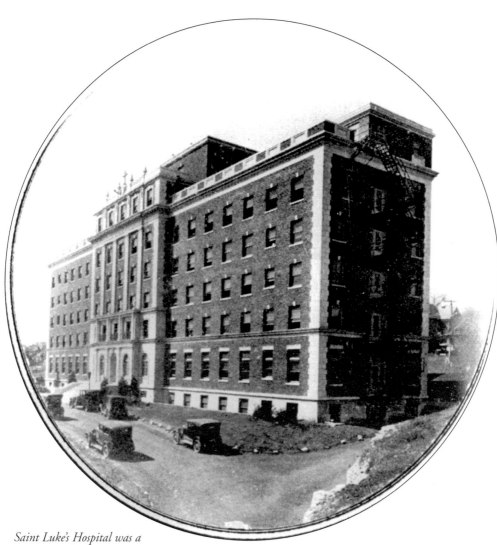

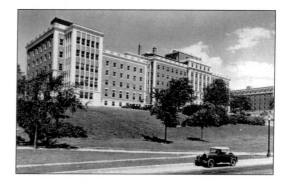

*Saint Luke's Hospital was a
state-of-the-art facility when it
opened with 150 beds in 1923.
Hospital directors soon found
it necessary to expand and
authorized construction
of a south wing, shown
right, adding 100 beds
to the hospital.*

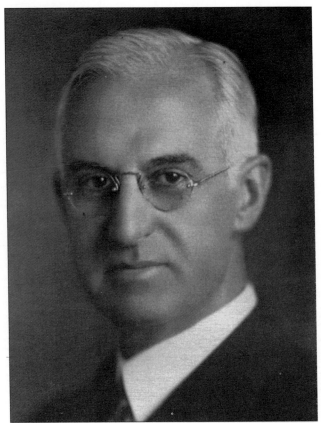

The Peet name has been affiliated with Saint Luke's virtually from its start. A.W. Peet, the lay leader of the hospital from 1927 to 1952, willed life into the institution during the Great Depression, donating products and services through his company, Colgate-Peet-Palmolive, providing personal funds to meet hospital payroll, and purchasing, then donating, hospital bonds.

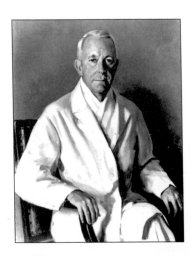

Dr. Frank Dickson, Kansas City's first orthopaedic surgeon, joined the Saint Luke's staff in 1925, after the hospital spent $25,000 to remodel the sixth floor for his use and create an operating room for him on the fifth floor. Dickson, an Easterner, had come to the area to care for Kansas Senator Frank Capper's polio-stricken daughter.

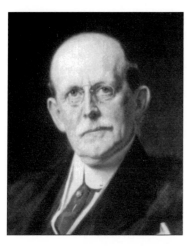

Many Kansas City luminaries were involved in the early Saint Luke's Hospital. Jacob L. Loose, the namesake of Loose Park, donated $500 in 1915 to become an "honorary member" of the hospital.

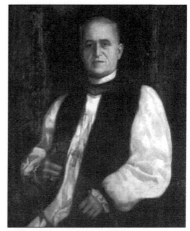

The Right Reverend Sidney C. Partridge succeeded Edward Atwill as Bishop of the Diocese of West Missouri in 1911. Partridge oversaw the dramatic expansion of Saint Luke's Hospital during the next 19 years.

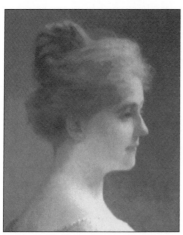

Linda S. Hall's $250,000 donation in 1930 was the first large endowment for Saint Luke's. It was heralded at the time as the largest single contribution ever made to a Kansas City hospital.

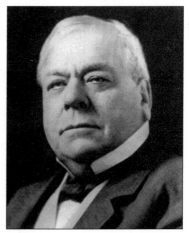

William Rockhill Nelson, the powerful publisher of The Kansas City Star, was an ally of the fledgling Saint Luke's Hospital, and he is credited with much of the support for the Rich Cabot Club's outdoor baby camps.

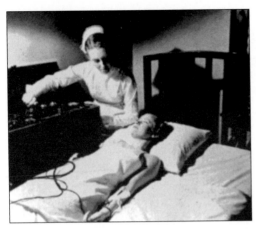

Medical science was evolving rapidly during the 1930s and 1940s, and Saint Luke's kept abreast of the new technology. Advances included the electrocardiograph ...

... the iron lung ...

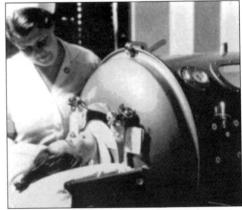

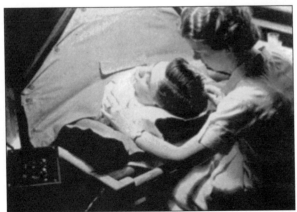

... and the hyperexia cabinet.

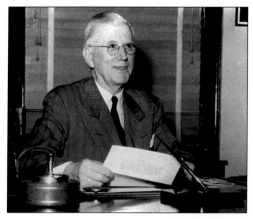

John R. Smiley was the first professional administrator of Saint Luke's, joining the hospital in 1923 at a salary of $4,000 a year. He served the hospital until his retirement in 1953.

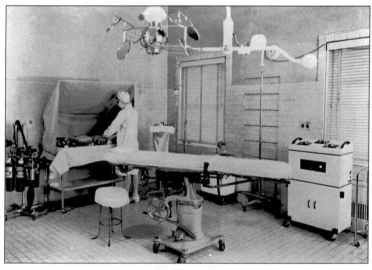

An operating room at Saint Luke's Hospital, circa 1944.

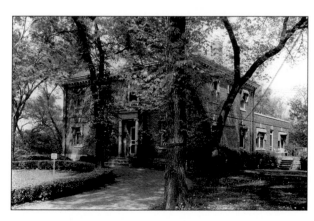

Saint Luke's took a larger role in providing pediatric care when it assumed control of Kansas City Cradle, a children's hospital, in 1945.

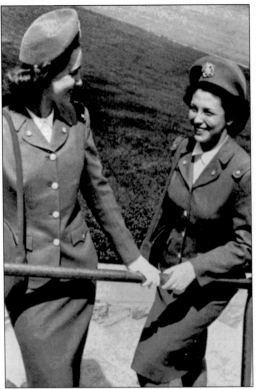

Cadet nurses lent a regimental air to the corridors
of Saint Luke's Hospital during the 1940s.

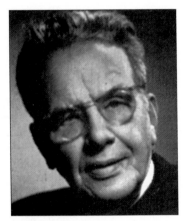

Robert Nelson Spencer, who
served as chaplain of Saint Luke's
Hospital during the 1920s,
guided the institution from
1930 to 1950 as Bishop of the
Diocese of West Missouri.

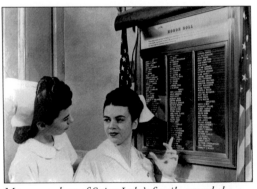

Many members of Saint Luke's family served the
country during World War II. Their sacrifice was
commemorated through the Scroll of Honor in the
Saint Luke's Hospital lobby.

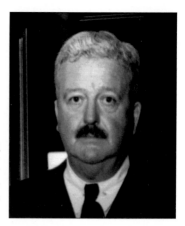

*Dr. Logan Clendenning,
president of the medical staff,
introduced the concept of training
young doctors at Saint Luke's
when he presented plans for the
hospital's first interns in 1924.*

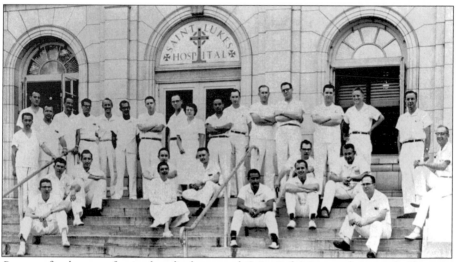

*Because of a shortage of trained medical personnel, Saint Luke's interns, know as the "house
staff," were invaluable in providing high quality patient care during the 1950s.*

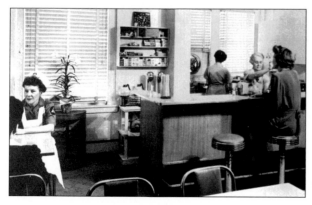

*The Coffee Shop,
operated by the Saint
Luke's Auxiliary, opened
in 1941 and quickly
became the favorite
gathering place for
visitors and staff alike.*

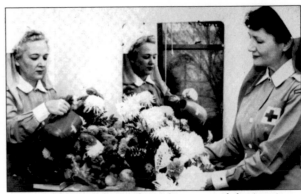

A nursing shortage during the 1940s prompted the American Red Cross to form and train the "Gray Ladies," so called because of their distinctive uniforms and veils. These volunteer women provided limited patient care at Saint Luke's Hospital for many years.

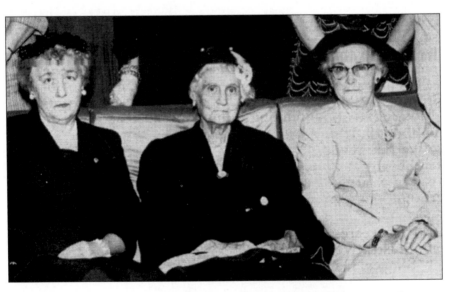

The women of the Saint Luke's Hospital Auxiliary volunteered with less notoriety but no less significance than their husbands, whose contributions are noted in board minutes and newspaper articles. In 1954, the hospital recognized many of these faithful volunteers, including, from left, Mrs. Carl D. Matz for 20 years of service; Mrs. A.W. Peet for 40 years of service; and Mrs. F.B. Walbridge for 35 years of service.

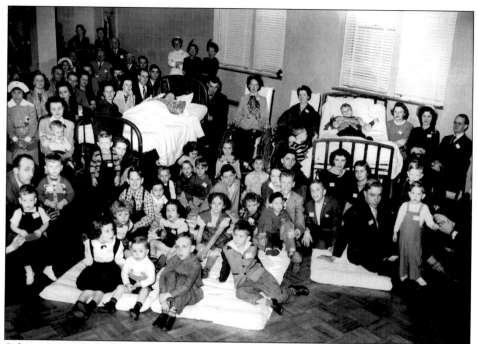

Polio patients who had been treated at Saint Luke's Hospital during the 1950s convened in happier times for a party in 1958. The polio vaccine had all but eliminated the disease by this time, but for many victims, physical disability provided a constant reminder of the terrible epidemic.

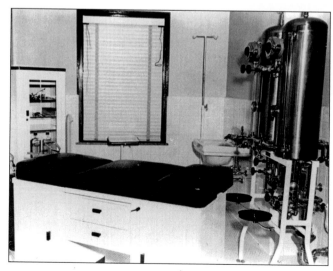

Tanks holding sterile water were a prominent feature in the emergency rooms at Saint Luke's Hospital in the early 1950s.

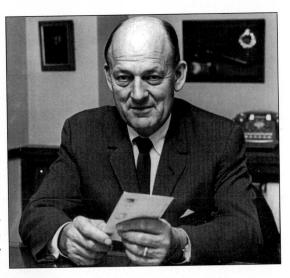

Many capable physicians, who contributed greatly to the prominence of Saint Luke's, joined the staff in the 1940s and 1950s. Dr. Maxwell Berry, served as chief of medical services for the Army's 133rd General Hospital during World War II and received the Bronze Star. He later helped develop the hospital's novel Code Blue cart used for CPR.

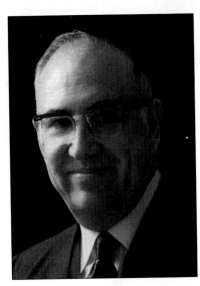

Dr. Arnold Arms, an internist, came to Saint Luke's in 1943 by way of Argentina, where he was born to missionary parents. A loyal supporter of Saint Luke's, Dr. Arms' opinions were highly respected both by hospital administrators and other physicians.

Dr. Mark Dodge, a Mayo trained endocrinologist, was admitted to the medical staff in 1951, joining Dr. Arms' internal medicine practice. Dodge became an influential proponent of Saint Luke's efforts to expand medical education programs and provide charity care.

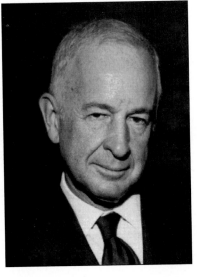

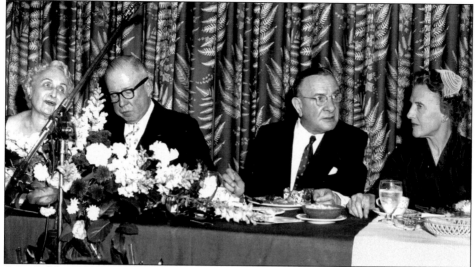

Saint Luke's commemorated Dr. Ferdinand C. Helwig's 30th anniversary of service with a dinner in 1958. Dr. Helwig, third from the left, was considered by his colleagues to be "the Supreme Court for all medical decisions at Saint Luke's Hospital," and he served as the first president of the Saint Luke's Foundation for Medical Education and Research, from 1963-1967. He is pictured with his wife, Helen, and Mr. and Mrs. David T. Beals Jr.

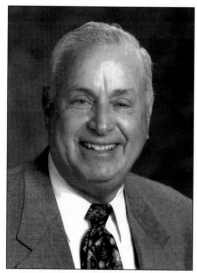

Pediatrician R. Don Blim came to Saint Luke's not because of the facilities—he found them "woefully inadequate"—but because of the caliber of the medical staff. Toward the end of his career, Dr. Blim became the hospital's director of medical affairs.

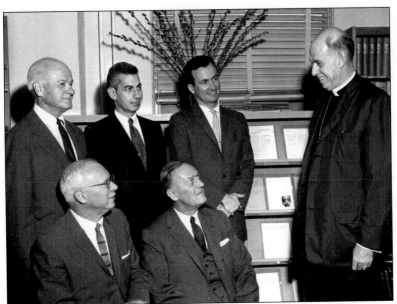

Bishop Edward R. Welles, right, welcomes new hospital board members in 1961.
Seated, from left, are Donald W. Bush and Paulen Burke. Standing, from left,
are David Mackie, Keith P. Bondurant, and Edward T. Matheny Jr., a future lay
head of the hospital. In 1974, as a Jackson County Circuit Judge, Bondurant
shocked Saint Luke's leadership by revoking the hospital's tax-exempt status. His
decision later was overturned on appeal.

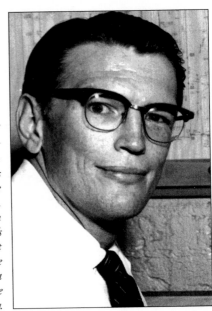

Dr. J. Tenbrook "Tim"
King developed the first
cardiac catheterization
lab at Saint Luke's
when he joined the
hospital staff in 1960.
Such was the premium
on space at Saint Luke's
during this period that
Dr. King's first office
was the anteroom of a
public toilet off the
main lobby.

admitted to the Children's Hospital as polio patients. Forty-five of these were discharged to go home, forty-eight had to have further hospitalization and treatment, and seven died.

Orthopaedic resident surgeon Dr. Asa C. Jones described the care required for polio patients in general and for Ann Louise Anset, age nine, in particular. Ann Louise was introduced "to demonstrate by her appearance the winning fight medical men are waging," and her mother expressed "her deep appreciation for the wonderful care Ann Louise received while a patient in the Children's Hospital." Bishop Spencer gave Ann Louise a china flower vase containing "baby ivy." With the help of bubble gum, Ann had made a complete recovery (a later article noted that "the child overcame residual paralysis in the throat and limbs by chewing bubble gum to strengthen the throat").

• • • • •

Senator Cooper nominated Herbert O. Peet to fill a vacancy on the board, stating that "he was moved to make this nomination, not only on Mr. Herbert O. Peet's own high qualifications but also from the impulses of his heart towards his distinguished father, Mr. A.W. Peet … " The motion was approved ceremoniously by a rising vote of all members of the board.

Director C.A. Searle, age eighty-one, resigned. Senator Cooper, himself no stripling, tried to talk him out of it, arguing "that Saint Luke's needed him." But Mr. Searle was adamant, and his resignation was accepted with regret.

In December, 1946, rates were fixed for the convalescent building, now commonly referred to as "the Annex," at 25 percent less than similar accommodations in the main hospital. When the remodeled building was opened to patients, the accompanying publicity identified it as a "pavilion for ambulatory patients" … an early commitment by Saint Luke's to less-expensive ambulatory care, with a significant facility dedicated to that use. "Only ambulatory patients from Saint Luke's who no longer require intensive treatment will be admitted to the new unit." There was no connecting corridor between the convalescent facility and the main hospital building, and for a time ambulatory patients requiring hospital treatment bumped over the short distance between buildings in a Chevrolet sedan.

Treasurer David Beals noted that the hospital's books showed it to be clear of debt "for the first time in a long time," although accrued accounts by reason of the building project had not as yet been entered. The November 30 financial statement reflected an average number of patients per day of 296, crammed into a hospital that was "supposed to have a maximum capacity of about 240 patients." Many patients waited weeks, even months, for hospital admission; 1946 saw an increase over the previous year of 14,549 patient days—an average daily increase of forty patients.

According to Mr. Beals, much refurbishing was needed at the busy hospital. All of the rooms needed new furnishings and everything looked badly worn.

Two children received tonsillectomy "Christmas presents"—Richard Cabot Club patients Peggy and Larry Evans, ages ten and five, respectively. The costs were charged to the Linda Hall Fund.

• • • • •

Alicia Sayre and Helen Valentine proposed revised personnel policies for nurses, in response to "an alarming number of resignations." Valentine stated that the policy revisions "were not lightly or inadvisedly presented." Nursing was a service profession, she said, but the nurses were overworked individuals who required time for social life, should have economic security, and needed to feel that they were appreciated.

To alleviate the nursing shortage, John Smiley offered an extraordinary proposal. He suggested that English-speaking graduates from recognized German schools of nursing might be interested in contracting to provide nursing services for a specified period of time at Saint Luke's. He argued that "such action would contribute materially to the program of indoctrinating these people with American ideals and our conception of the Democratic Way of life." Smiley was authorized to write to General Lucious D. Clay, Headquarters E.U.C.O.M., Berlin, Germany, for advice and assistance. General Clay later responded, proposing that Saint Luke's accept graduate German nurses for further training and offering to use a competitive examination in the selection of these girls … with the assurance that "they would be the best possible material available." However, no German nurses ever appeared at Saint Luke's.

The United States Public Health Service recommended that practical nurses or nurses' aides be trained for bedside care. They would be paid less than registered nurses, who favored the idea of such nursing assistance. Miss Valentine commented favorably on the nurses' aides, advising that Saint Luke's had aides' positions open for women eighteen to fifty years of age, in good physical health, with at least two years' high school education. New aides attended a series of lectures and "actual demonstrations" in the new convalescent building, and would receive meals, uniforms, laundering of uniforms, and a salary—the latter to be increased at six-month intervals as warranted.

The nursing program included affiliations for pediatrics at Children's Mercy Hospital, for tuberculosis at Leeds Hospital, and for psychiatry at St. Louis State Hospital.

Fifteen-year-old Ike Skelton (later Congressman Skelton) of Lexington, Missouri, a patient in Saint Luke's Hospital, received a "get well" letter from President Harry S Truman.

Work advanced on the North Wing. The wing's foundation and first-floor slab were completed by April, 1947. Work was then halted while the contractor recalculated costs under the cost-plus contract. Strikes by the construction trade unions led to significant cost increases for area building projects. Revised estimates for completing the North Wing were much more than the original plan called for—and consequently the board stopped construction until such time as adequate funds were available.

The bed crunch occasionally provoked desperate measures. In April the medical-staff secretary wrote to chastise a physician for sending a patient in labor to the delivery room despite being advised by the hospital room clerk "that there was no available bed and requested by her that you admit her elsewhere." The offending doctor was told that he had been guilty of a "breach of conduct" which "must not happen again."

There was also a great deal of discussion about whether the convalescent building would be successful "on the basis on which it has been operating." It was suggested that there should be another month's trial "to try and make it work, as originally planned." In May, Superintendent Smiley reported that the building was "fairly well patronized," but Dr. Rex L. Diveley, now president of the medical staff, argued that it should provide care for seriously ill patients and for those awaiting surgery in the main hospital building. Dr. Diveley's views prevailed; the need for beds for acutely ill patients was so great that two converted floors in the convalescent building promptly filled to capacity.

The board in June approved a proposal by the Cerebral Palsy Nursery School, headed by Mary Shaw Branton, for space in the basement of the Children's Hospital. A *Kansas City Star* article reported on the operation of the school, a facility where ten children "born with two strikes against them" were now making progress. There were a physical therapist, an occupational therapist, a once-a-week speech teacher, and two mothers of pupils all working with the children at the time of the reporter's visit. Dr. Robert E. Bruner, father of a handicapped child, served as the medical consultant. There was a tuition charge of $200 per child, and Saint Luke's provided space, heat, and light without charge.

· · · · ·

In September, the Finance Committee recommended against resumption of work on the North Wing after the property was put into condition to withstand the elements. Not only had the cost of completion now escalated to $1,035,844, but further increases were expected. However, John Smiley offered some hope for the North Wing's future when he reported the passage of the Hill-Burton Bill providing $85,000,000 nationally for hospital construction. The federal government had determined that more hospitals were needed to guarantee access to everyone.

Saint Luke's might be eligible for assistance under the new law. A survey found need in the Kansas City area for 425 additional beds for white patients. Within ten years, another 400 beds for white patients would be needed. The same survey determined that "the colored patients had the needed facilities."

Harvard sociologist Paul Starr, in his monumental *The Social Transformation of American Medicine* (Basic Books, Inc., New York, 1982), suggests:

> "In the long run, the Hill-Burton program probably retarded integration in the industry, since it provided money that enabled smaller and uneconomical hospitals to keep operating."

However there was no doubt that in Saint Luke's case, the money, if available, would be a godsend, making possible badly needed expansion.

· · · · ·

The nursing shortage continued in October and was not expected to be alleviated until January 1, 1948, when a new class of student nurses, having sufficiently completed their theory and clinical work, could be "put on the floors for five or six hours a day." The convalescent building, where patients numbered fifty-five to sixty per day, was being staffed largely with nurses' aides and "was running into difficulties for the reason we could not give the patients all the nursing care needed."

A November 30 newspaper article reported dissolution of the Kansas City Cradle organization, noting that its building and equipment had been used by adjacent Saint Luke's Hospital since July, 1945, as a children's hospital. Deeds conveying the property formally to Saint Luke's were executed. The property had a value of approximately $40,000 and was being operated as "Saint Luke's Children's Hospital."

In December Smiley reported the purchase by the Florence Crittenton Home of a corner lot at 43rd and Wornall Road, just north of the Children's Hospital, where they would erect a residence for unwed mothers. Thus the original mission of the Cradle was assumed by Crittenton. Smiley also recommended that "we take two children from the Richard Cabot Club for tonsillectomy operations again this year."

A *Kansas City Star* article for January 6, 1948, discussed rate increases at area hospitals. The increases were attributed to higher nurses' salaries, multiplying labor wage scales, skyrocketing food prices, a particularly heavy jump in equipment costs and advanced fuel prices. It was noted that hospitals subsisted on narrow, nonprofit budgets and operated on a twenty-four-hour-per-day schedule. They required three shifts of nurses and two or three labor shifts. Men had to be in the boiler rooms at all times, and manual labor was needed throughout the day.

● ● ● ● ●

The price of drugs was becoming significant as well. Penicillin attained general use following World War II, and now sulfa drugs had reached the market—called "wonder drugs" because of the medical miracles they wrought. Aureomycin capsules, dubbed "capsules of gold" by the hospital's cost-conscious pharmacists, soon followed.

Cortisone was another pharmaceutical marvel. When cortisone was first developed, Merck delivered limited quantities to Saint Luke's Hospital in insured wooden boxes. The contents were allocated among deserving patients by a committee of physicians. (There was precedent for this approach—when penicillin originally became available in limited quantities in 1944, the medical staff president appointed a similar committee, announcing: "The Executive Committee of the executive staff feels that control of the dispensation of the penicillin supply which is to be allotted to Saint Luke's Hospital should be vested in a penicillin committee so that the product will be used only in conditions for which it is beneficial.")

Saint Luke's pharmacists also filled prescriptions of tonsil powders for ENT doctors—medication no longer in use.

At the board's January, 1948, meeting, John Smiley reported that it cost about one-third less to care for patients in the convalescent building because of the extensive use of nurses' aides and because patients came "downstairs" for meals.

In January, A.W. Peet and his wife each contributed $2,500 to the building fund. There was the rising vote of thanks by the board that greeted many of their philanthropic acts.

In May, thirteen graduates of the nursing school found employment elsewhere, but John Smiley expressed the hope "that we can get along at least during the summer with the help of high school girls acting as nurses aides, plus the fact that our student nurses will be out of school, giving some additional time … " Also, John Smiley's salary was increased to $12,000.

In June, Chief of Staff Dr. Paul Gempel reported a significant boost for medical education and quality of care at Saint Luke's: his colleagues had voted an assessment of $50 per executive staff member and $25 per general staff member, as well as a monthly charge per physician of $5, to establish and maintain a medical library. The hospital would provide a home for the library.

• • • • •

A July article in *The Midwest Hospital Courier* by John Smiley noted that pending expansion plans for the nation's hospital facilities would add more than 100,000 beds at a cost of approximately $1,125,000,000. Financing for this unprecedented growth was provided by the Hill-Burton program.

The need for expansion was said by Smiley to be imperative, owing to five factors: 1) the busy doctor who found it necessary to concentrate all of his patients in one place so that he might better treat them, and where the newer drugs could be administered and newer procedures followed; 2) the great population increase in urban centers without corresponding expansion of hospital facilities; 3) crowded housing making it necessary to care for the ill outside the home; 4) the rapid increase of prepaid hospital insurance plans "and our own Blue Cross and Surgical Care"; and 5) a wider and more favorable acceptance by the public generally of hospital service. Still, many of the hospitals soliciting federal construction funds were doomed to disappointment.

Meanwhile, to help remedy overcrowding in the nation's hospitals, Smiley advocated a more rapid turnover of patients. This was said to be primarily the function of the doctor, who should be encouraged to move patients "as rapidly as feasible." The use of early ambulation also was to be encouraged, based on the experience in Army and Navy Hospitals, where as a result of this practice patients were processed in one-half to one-third of the time formerly required for their care.

Also consideration should be given to a convalescent unit in all major hospitals. It had been established that the cost of this type of care was 25 to 30 percent less than in the main hospital units. Smiley's experience with Saint Luke's convalescent building (now becoming known as "the Annex") doubtless contributed to his conviction.

Smiley advocated the construction of doctors' office buildings adjacent to hospitals to encourage the closer cooperation between the doctor and the hospital "for which we should all strive." The "one-stop-service-station" for patients was urged.

Finally, Smiley advocated study of hospital construction planning, looking to ways to reduce personnel needs through adoption of mechanical improvements and other measures.

This was a remarkably foresighted and statesmanlike article.

John Smiley also played a leading role in the search for a solution to a widespread problem: proper identification of patients in hospitals' multiple-bed accommodations. Patients in a ward or semi-private room sometimes received medication or treatment intended for another occupant of the room. One hospital responding to Smiley's survey cited a blood transfusion given to the wrong patient, which almost killed him. In another instance, both patients in a multiple-bed room were scheduled for surgery; the wrong patient was taken to the operating room and an operation completed before the error was discovered. The solution which evolved was simple: the plastic bracelet familiar to all hospital patients.

• • • • •

A July 30, 1948, *Kansas City Star* story reported that a Chinese doctor—Lin Tung-Kuang—had begun a one-year internship in general medicine at Saint Luke's, aided by two Chinese girls working for the summer at the hospital. A different priority of care was noted by the Chinese: in China the older persons primarily received treatment and veneration, whereas in America nearly everyone was more solicitous of children.

The government Cadet Nurse program was discontinued at the hospital in 1948. A September report by the superintendent of nurses stressed the value of nursing students to the hospital. Graduate nurses were in short supply, and every effort would be made to increase the number of students and thereby aid "in handling the nursing problem."

A member of the board's two-man visitation team praised a group of youngsters in the Nurses' Home who were caring for babies of nurses working in the hospital.

Hill-Burton money would be allocated among the states, which in turn were to estimate regional hospital needs and distribute funds to applicant hospitals. John Smiley was instructed in September to obtain application forms from the State Division of Health. By the October meeting he had obtained the forms and advised the Board of the availability of Hill-Burton funds for teaching hospitals in particular. The latter were to have plans and funds ready to the point that a contract could be let by June 15, 1949. They were invited to submit applications with the understanding that they would be considered in the order received.

Smiley reported at the October meeting that two black graduate nurses had been employed for service in the Annex ... "they are working out very well."

• • • • •

The November, 1948, issue of *Hospitals* magazine contained an article lauding the gift and coffee shop maintained by the auxiliary at Saint Luke's. The coffee shop was opened in September, 1941, to raise funds for the auxiliary and to serve the hospital's patrons. The gift shop was added later and was immediately successful. The profits went to the hospital in the form of equipment and furnishings.

SIXTEEN
1949-1952

Dickson-Diveley Clinic ... North Wing ... chaplain ...
Edward Randolph Welles ... Dr. Mark Dodge

At the January 21, 1949, meeting of the board, John Smiley reported that he had been investigating whether Saint Luke's nurses were underpaid. In any event, the nurses believed that they were being overworked, but he anticipated relief the following December, when some forty student nurses would be starting to work two or three hours per day. Alicia Sayre, director of nurses, predicted that this would be a great help; in some instances it would reduce the number of registered nurses needed.

The February 18 board meeting fell on Bishop Spencer's seventy-second birthday, celebrated with a surprise party featuring a cake trimmed in red and white. There were also treats for the children's ward in his honor.

Construction was underway of a new clinic building at 4312 Mill Creek Parkway, with Dr. Rex L. Diveley and Dr. Frank D. Dickson as the principals, and another associate, Dr. Richard H. Kiene, as a third participant. Upon completion, the clinic building, financed by the George S. Diveley Foundation, was leased to Saint Luke's for ten years and then given to the hospital.

A March 31 article in the *Star* reported that Saint Luke's was solving its intern shortage by accepting young Chinese doctors who wanted to learn American medical methods. The year's experience with Dr. Lin Tung-Kuang had been mutually beneficial, and so Saint Luke's agreed to take two more young men from the medical college of China's National Central

University. Dr. Lin became a medical resident at Saint Luke's for a three-year period when his internship was completed. The experiment with foreign residents soon was extended to a Brazilian and a Mexican doctor.

• • • • •

Contributions to the Building and Equipment Fund were reported, and the Finance Committee met several times to consider resumption of the North Wing construction. One of the meetings evidenced the collegiality then existing among hospitals; it was attended by representatives of Menorah, Kansas University Medical Center, Blue Cross and others. The Menorah and KU representatives encouraged the hospital to proceed with the wing, citing community need. The Blue Cross representative, with a wary eye on the price tag, declined to express any opinion. Meanwhile, William Brace stated that he would oppose any expansion of the Children's Hospital until a connecting wing was built, so that children could be transported to the main hospital through corridors rather than out of doors, as was the procedure at the time.

The most pressing problem of the hospital was "imbalance": additional rooms had been added over the years with no corresponding increase in kitchen, laundry, or other service facilities. The new wing would address this; it would only add 100 beds but would provide service capacity for a 450-500 bed hospital.

To finance the new construction, the hospital approved a plan anticipating receipt of Hill-Burton funds for one-third the cost, a loan commitment for one-third, and a campaign for one-third. It was proposed that the board be enlarged to provide the manpower for the campaign. A list of suggestions for additional directors was compiled by referring to the rosters of the various parishes of the diocese. Twelve additional men were then elected.

The board subsequently authorized completion of the North Wing utilizing the finance plan previously approved. One possible stumbling block was the application form for federal funds, which required the acceptance of patients "regardless of race, creed, or color." However, the law provided that this nondiscrimination provision was satisfied if separate but equal facilities were available in the area. John Smiley advised that the 1947 survey of Kansas City had determined that there were sufficient available beds for colored people and that KU's expansion program would provide two more floors in "their negro section" with sixty-five additional beds. Consequently, "we can say in the application to the government that additional facilities have been provided and there is no occasion for Saint Luke's to accept colored patients." (The separate but equal provision of Hill-Burton, relied upon in this instance, was determined by the U.S. Supreme Court to be unconstitutional in 1963, but that did not affect the Saint Luke's project, by then long since completed.)

The application subsequently filed adopted this approach.

Smiley also advised that the hospital would have to elaborate on the specific use to be made of the beds being provided. He stated that the number of beds allocated to chronic cases and mental patients could be enlarged. Rheumatic fever was prevalent, and a nearby convalescent center cared for children with acute rheumatic fever and the rheumatic heart disease which often resulted. Smiley stated that there was a very strong desire to do some work in rheumatic fever since there were 700 to 800 afflicted Kansas City children not being cared for, and that further provision also was needed for infantile paralysis cases that remained in the hospital for weeks or even months and hence were considered to be chronic. The bed allocation for the new wing also would include twenty beds for chronic heart disease cases as well as twenty beds for "mildly nervous mental cases."

David Beals met with the sympathetic director of the U.S. Public Health Service, who informed him that unallocated Hill-Burton funds for fiscal 1949 would be "returned" if not used and that such reversion of the funds would be "too bad." He was given valuable advice as to how to proceed.

However, when the application for construction funds was filed with the Hospital Survey and Planning Agency in Jefferson City, it appeared that all of the Missouri allotment for the fiscal year had been tentatively committed. In May it was confirmed by the Division of Health in Jefferson City that there was nothing further to be accomplished on the federal grant application until after July 1, 1949.

• • • • •

The new medical library opened in May; interns and residents were grateful for the resource.

The board approved affiliation with Missouri Valley College, permitting candidates for a B.S. in Nursing at the College to receive their practical training at Saint Luke's.

In June the board approved a program for training hospital administrators—a two-year rotating internship that would expose trainees to all of the key departments of the hospital.

An Episcopal priest, the Reverend Thomas Bridges, was hired as Saint Luke's resident chaplain—the city's first. The auxiliary paid his stipend of $3,600 per year, while the diocese made his annual retirement-fund contribution of $500, and the hospital provided his apartment and meals. Father Bridges, a graduate of Harvard and of Cambridge's Episcopal Theological Seminary, had spent the previous eight years as chaplain of Massachusetts General Hospital. On the eve of his assumption of duties at Saint Luke's, he stated that the counseling of family members was as much his task as counseling the patient.

Seventy-two-year-old Bishop Spencer retired, and an appreciative resolution was adopted by the board.

In August, during a recurrence of the polio epidemic, patients in the "contaminated area" of the polio ward of Saint Luke's Children's Hospital made a radio broadcast. This was later relayed nationally by radio station KCKN and the story told in more than 900 newspapers. It also was published in the *Journal of the American Hospital Association* and a series of pictures of the broadcast were entered in a competition at MU's School of Journalism.

Two deaths occurred that year in the polio ward. A later reunion was attended by forty-seven of fifty-four patients treated during the epidemic. In 1946, the last previous cycle year, some 100 patients had been treated.

At its October meeting the board was advised that the hospital continued to be crowded … "booked up until the 18th of November." However, the personnel situation was improved, with graduate nurses not quite so scarce and nonprofessional employees remaining longer. Dr. Gempel concurred that the nursing shortage had improved. He also reported that a group of doctors had purchased a new scientific camera for use in the operating room and in the hospital's educational program.

On November 19, 1949, Vice President Alben Barkley was married in St. Louis. The bride's father, Roy W. Rucker, was unable to attend because he was confined to Saint Luke's with a heart ailment. The nurses joined him in eating "a proxy wedding cake."

Also in November, the nursing school at Saint Luke's was rated in the top 25 percent of the nation's schools offering basic nursing education.

The schools at General Hospital and KU were in the same elite category. In the middle 50 percent were five other local schools—Research, General #2, Trinity, St. Mary's, and Independence Sanitarium.

Chaplain Bridges attended the board's November meeting and talked about the work of a chaplain. He was looking forward to bringing theological students and young clergymen to Saint Luke's, to work as interns or fellows under his guidance.

A special committee of Blue Cross trustees submitted a plan to correct deficiencies in payments to hospitals and expand Blue Cross benefits to the public. In December a new Blue Cross contract was approved with Group Hospital Service, Inc., implementing the new payment formula.

• • • • •

Although a Saint Luke's surgery residency had been established in 1940, the hospital's medical-education program was geared for general practice until after World War II. Among other things, it lacked the equipment and facilities needed for specialty training. However, change was in the offing. In 1949, Dr. Paul Gempel, Ferd Helwig, and the Executive Committee of the medical staff obtained AMA approval of an obstetrics/gynecology residency program at Saint Luke's for one year. Dr. Ehret O. Ramey was the first resident, entering the program in 1950.

The hospital assigned patient-care duties to fifty-four student nurses— a definite help in caring for patients.

On February 27, 1950, a retired Bishop Spencer conducted a service of confirmation in the hospital chapel for a twenty-year-old paralytic—a young man who had just begun his ninth year as a patient at Saint Luke's. It was the first time that Bishop Spencer had confirmed a patient of the hospital in the chapel.

Chaplain Bridges proposed that two theological residencies be established at Saint Luke's, with the hospital supplying room, board and laundry, and the auxiliary paying a stipend of $100 per month. Religious denomination would not be a factor, but rather "the applicant will be expected to give evidence that he is able to minister without restraint or prejudice to patients of any, or no, church affiliation." The proposed program was approved.

• • • • •

Bishop Spencer was succeeded as Bishop of the Diocese of West Missouri and President of Saint Luke's Hospital by the Right Reverend Edward Randolph Welles, Dean of St. Paul's Cathedral, Buffalo, New York. The new bishop presided at the board's April meeting.

• • • • •

An expansion of Hill-Burton became law, doubling the available federal funding for hospital construction. The new legislation allowed the federal contribution to range from one-third to two-thirds of the cost of a hospital project and also authorized the Surgeon General to furnish financial aid for research, experiments and demonstrations relating to use and development of hospital services and facilities. Encouraged, Saint Luke's resubmitted its architects' blueprints for the North Wing, an addition to the Children's Hospital, and alterations to the main hospital building.

The Saint Luke's construction project was approved by the State Advisory Council and presented to the Kansas City office of the United States Public Health Service the week of April 24.

Ms. I.E. Gutschke, R.N., the state director of Hospital Survey, Planning and Construction Services, wrote from Jefferson City that the chronic-disease category of construction funding was now being addressed "and your project has cleared this office and been placed on the eligible list." The federal share of estimated construction costs, if approved, would amount to $902,063.

The press reported on June 20, 1950, that Saint Luke's had received "the go-ahead signal" on the expansion program, aided by a federal grant. The project would make Saint Luke's a 500-bed medical center, the largest privately operated hospital in Missouri. A *Kansas City Star* editorial declared:

> "Newly reported building plans mean many more beds and better treatment facilities for hospitals in Greater Kansas City. When the extra space is available, the outlook is for easement of presently overcrowded conditions and a shortening of long waiting lists for admission to the hospitals here."

The editorial lauded the federal funding that contributed to hospital expansion otherwise beyond the reach of community resources. It cited this form of assistance as an important factor in the hospital growth demanded by increased population and medical requirements.

A construction-loan commitment for $750,000 was arranged with City

Bond & Mortgage Co. Despite the loan commitment, the hospital hoped to raise its share of the project funding through philanthropy. Baptist Hospital trustees, who also were conducting a campaign to raise funds for their new hospital, requested that Saint Luke's delay its effort. But on August 9, 1950, the Executive Committee meeting of the Saint Luke's board determined to proceed:

> "After a general discussion by all Members of the Committee, it was the consensus of opinion that the Baptist Hospital Trustees be advised that, since Saint Luke's had all plans ready to proceed, and that we find it necessary to start construction on, or before, October 1, 1950, that it is imperative that our campaign go forward starting in December and completing it after January 1, 1951."

A campaign to raise $1 million was undertaken and Ketchum, Inc., of Pittsburgh, Pennsylvania, was employed as manager.

When construction bids were opened on October 4, the low bidder was Swenson Construction Co., for the amount of $1,899,370. The Committee noted that this exceeded the estimate submitted to the federal government but assumed that the latter's grant would be increased to equal 50 percent of the project cost. However, the Missouri Division of Health declined to increase the funds above the amount previously approved. Swenson agreed to extend the time for awarding the contract to permit the hospital to sort this out. Meanwhile, the fund-raising campaign proceeded successfully.

The board was advised in its December meeting that the government grant had been increased in the necessary amount, and the Swenson contract was approved for execution subject to approval by the U.S. Public Health Service and the Division of Health of the State of Missouri. John Smiley was awarded a bonus in recognition of his services in negotiating the grant and assisting with the fund drive.

• • • • •

One of the directors expressed the opinion in December that "nurses are demanding too high a rate of pay." Herbert O. Peet concurred, saying "a person could not afford to be ill at home any more, as nursing care would amount to $36 a day … it would be cheaper to go to a hospital for care." He suggested that this would be "a good point to bring out when soliciting funds for the new wing."

In 1951, a separate ob/gyn department was established, and its residency progressed to a two- and then a three-year program. Ob/gyn residents began to provide care at the Florence Crittenton Home and also developed combined obstetrical and gynecological clinics at the Richard Cabot Clinic and the Jackson County Hospital as well as at Saint Luke's.

Saint Luke's obstetrical department was outstanding. Its physicians were instrumental in the development of the American College of Obstetrics and Gynecology.

The nursing school increased its enrollment to staff the North Wing and the expanded Children's Hospital and to alleviate the continuing shortage of nurses. Student nurses visited their alma maters, recruiting for the school; fifty-two high schools were visited over a two-week span. To entice recruits, a course entitled "Charm and Personality" was added to the curriculum.

The hospital remained "extensively engaged" in the training of residents and interns; the medical staff was "most cooperative" in giving lectures "to the boys." The teaching program was affiliated with Children's Mercy, Wadsworth Veteran's Hospital, and Richard Cabot Clinic.

Saint Luke's physicians also were involved in undergraduate medical education; one-third of the Saint Luke's medical staff were members of the faculty at KU, and seven of them were professors there. Saint Luke's doctors were not department heads, but the doctors who taught KU medical students in the University's clinics were largely from Saint Luke's. However, KU introduced a condition that all of its staff members be full-time academicians, a change that mirrored medical-school requirements elsewhere in the country but effectively ended the close relationship between the university and Saint Luke's.

Lucian Lane and Francis Bartlett were appointed to gather information about nurses' salaries and offer recommendations to the board. Mr. Lane, in an interim report in February, expressed concern over Saint Luke's low nursing salaries in comparison with other hospitals in the area. And in March there was an extensive report, warning that Saint Luke's was acquiring a reputation for the lowest paid staff in any of the major hospitals in Kansas City. The nurses' registry advised that it was unable to supply staff nurses to Saint Luke's at the hospital's existing salary scale. It was expected that the problem would worsen; several nurses were leaving to enter the armed forces, which paid considerably more. And the new

Veterans' Administration Hospital in Kansas City also offered salaries substantially higher than those at the private hospitals.

The president-elect of the American Medical Association declared that salaries paid in government hospitals threatened the solvency of private hospitals. He asserted that the government was building too many unnecessary institutions:

> "Tax-supported 'raids' on private and community hospitals for nurses, technicians, doctors and patients create a serious personnel problem."

He was particularly critical of the Veterans' Administration.

Because of a federal "wage freeze" it was necessary to obtain permission for nurses' salary increases, but they were implemented on March 1, followed by room-rate changes April 1 to pay for them. In May, Mr. Lane reported that "most of the nurses approved of the salary increases."

The fund-raising campaign enjoyed continued success ... David Beals advised in April that in view of gifts received and cash in hand it would not be necessary to obtain an interim loan for construction costs. Later, a check for $50,000 received unannounced in routine mail from the Kresge Foundation in Detroit put the campaign over the top.

The great flood in the summer of 1951 caused delay in construction when workmen were taken off the job to aid in the flood clean-up.

A *Kansas City Times* story on September 28 reported a $5,000 bequest for the maintenance of a private room for "gentle elderly women who could not otherwise afford such a room." Dr. Peter T. Bohan was to designate the beneficiaries, and after his death the board was to make the selection.

The October meeting of the Executive Committee was largely devoted to discussion of the hospital's overall financial situation and the past year's deficit. As a remedy, rates were increased again. About 40 percent of Saint Luke's patients had Blue Cross coverage, and another 15-20 percent had some other kind of hospitalization insurance.

Officials of the Florence Crittenton Home broke ground on October 28 for their new building on the Saint Luke's campus. The home would be equipped to treat twenty-four pregnant girls and later would be expanded to permit treatment of thirty-six more girls with serious emotional problems.

• • • • •

Mark Dodge was admitted to membership on the medical staff in November, 1951; he joined Dr. Arnold Arms in his flourishing internal-medicine practice. Dodge was a Navy flight surgeon during World War II. Mayo-trained, he was a superb endocrinologist and compassionate physician. Dr. Dodge also provided leadership and support for the hospital and his colleagues on the medical staff for many years.

Chaplain Bridges' ministry at the hospital was about to end. The new bishop had requested him to look for another position, stating that the hospital required a "more general type of chaplaincy than Chaplain Bridges wished to provide." The board sanctioned the bishop's action.

Improved admitting and reservation procedures for Saint Luke's were adopted in January. The new procedures shortened and made more convenient the admission process and also facilitated completion of hospital records. Once the new wing was finished, all room assignments would continue to be made through the admitting office. Executive staff members would be given preference for admission of elective cases, although patient welfare was to take precedence over staff status.

By March, construction costs for the wing had exceeded budget by $103,000, due to changes requested by the Missouri Division of Health and by the federal government. Part of this increase would be defrayed by the hospital's contingency reserve and part by a matching government grant. The balance would require a modest additional fund-raising effort.

· · · · ·

At the April meeting, David Beals urged that research and teaching efforts at the hospital be further emphasized, following the examples of Cornell University, the Harvard Medical School, and others. Dr. Helwig supported Beals, saying that the proper type of residents would be a credit to the hospital, and the proposal would enable Saint Luke's to obtain "an adequate number of men and better connections with schools in active teaching of medical students." It would be good for the students, the patients, and the medical staff. However, such a program would entail the considerable expense of providing nonpaying patients (teaching beds) for educational purposes, and it was not adopted at the time.

To avoid a costly addition to the present interns' quarters, the hospital purchased residential property located at 4406 Wornall Road to house the ten or twelve more interns needed to staff the North Wing.

Bishop Welles advised that dedication of the North Wing would take place on May 12, although construction work would not be completed by then. The addition to the Children's Hospital would not be ready either. However, it was the practice of the bishop to take a long vacation every summer at his summer home in Manset, Maine, and nothing stood in the way of that vacation. (His vacations lasted so long that at one point a resolution was introduced at a Diocesan Convention to the effect that if the bishop were out of the diocese for more than a certain prescribed period of time, the See would be declared vacant.) According to Ferne Malcolm Welles, the hospital historian who would later become the bishop's wife: "The construction was not completed, but that was the way it was. The bishop was about to leave on an extended vacation, and the dedication came off in May ... "

At the dedication, the bishop officiated in a service attended by about 300 persons. Afterward the $2,500,000 wing was visited by the guests, although it would not be open for business for several more weeks. Upon completion it was discovered that the rooms in the wing contained no built-in closets.

In May, there was a meeting at St. Joseph Hospital between hospital representatives and representatives of the Operating Engineers Union, concerning a new collective-bargaining agreement. A union request for a forty-hour work week was initially rejected but later approved, and a wage increase also was approved.

The Nursing Department needed office space, and the board's meeting room was converted to that use. Thereafter the board met in the new medical library.

There was concern over the high speed of Wornall Road traffic, past the hospital's west side. Signs were posted imposing a speed limit of twenty-five miles per hour.

In June, payment was approved of the tonsillectomy bills of Richard and Sherman Jones from the Drumm Farm.

The third floor of the North Wing opened July 1, with fifteen patients transferred there. The fifth floor, with five rooms for surgery and three for minor operations, opened a week later. There were also post-surgical recovery rooms ... before, patients were carted back to their rooms to be cared for by private-duty nurses. The fourth, second, and first floors followed in succession. Total additional beds: 117, bringing the hospital's announced capacity to 500 beds.

SEVENTEEN
1952-1954

socialized medicine ... medical education and research ...
financial constraints ... continued nursing shortage ...
Leslie D. Reid

*A*W. Peet had been absent from board meetings for some time due to illness, and he died July 22, 1952. His will included a final act of generosity—a $25,000 bequest to Saint Luke's Hospital for the building fund. An ornate memorial resolution eulogized him as a most devoted churchman, a highly successful businessman, and a philanthropist. It particularly praised his service to Saint Luke's, recognizing that:

> "His contribution to the building of this institution and its work were decidedly greater than those from any other individual."

A member of the medical staff pronounced him to have been "all wool and a yard wide."

The convalescent building was officially named the "Albert W. Peet Memorial," and Mrs. H.O. Peet's portrait of her father-in-law was relocated there. However, the building continued to be referred to as "the Annex" ... old habits were hard to break.

• • • • •

There were a number of news stories in September on the subject of socialized medicine, a concept steadfastly opposed by the American Medical Association. A prominent British physician told the International

College of Surgeons on September 5, 1952, in Chicago that Britain's national health service had been a "blunder" that lowered efficiency in medical care and entailed much more "welfare" than the country could possibly pay for ... the service was "splitting on the rocks of economics." He cautioned: "Put not your faith in politicians, of whatever party ... Medicine is your trust, not theirs. It is not safe in their hands."

Mac F. Cahal of Kansas City, executive secretary of the American Academy of General Practice, criticized nationalized medicine in England, saying that socialism would not mix with capitalism. He argued that the American way provided "perfectly adequate answers" through voluntary insurance and charity medical care of the indigent. On the same day, Harold E. Stassen, president of the University of Pennsylvania, spoke out against socialized medicine, saying that one of the essential requirements for the freedom of a people was that members of its major professions must be independent citizens and not subservient to the men in control of government through any scheme of socialized medicine.

Dwight D. Eisenhower, the Republican nominee for president at that time, also expressed opposition to socialized medicine:

> "I am opposed to a federally operated and controlled system of medical care which is what the administration's compulsory scheme is, in fact."

He stated that Americans receive better health care than anywhere else in the world:

> "We must not, in providing for the few, wreck the system under which so many can obtain adequate care."

Much of this rhetoric was generated by Harry Truman's appointment of a controversial "commission on the health needs of the nation"; also 1952 was an election year. Beginning in 1945, Truman had repeatedly advocated legislation similar to the Wagner-Murray-Dingell bill that would provide compulsory national health insurance.

Eisenhower's election to the presidency in November ended the advance of "socialized medicine" for a time.

• • • • •

David T. Beals was elected as first and executive vice president in September, succeeding the late A.W. Peet as lay head of the hospital.

It would not do for Operating Engineer's Union members alone to enjoy a forty-hour work week, so the same schedule was instituted for all other hospital employees.

· · · · ·

Saint Luke's was at the crossroads in medical education. It had been engaged in educational programs since the 1920s, but the commitment was relatively modest. To make it truly a teaching hospital, a major research and teaching program again was proposed.

Supporters of the expanded program argued that Saint Luke's was a "public" hospital ... the public gave the money to build it and the public used it as patients. The obligation of the board, it was therefore reasoned, was to the public. The choice: either organize adequate facilities for medical education and scientific research, and provide programs for preventive medicine, home care, and rehabilitation, or "be relegated to a first class nursing home."

It was said that an elite Saint Luke's bore a particular obligation to train doctors and engage in research. An excellent staff was already in place—trained and willing, and possessing prestige and community confidence as well as excellent "key men." The hospital would need a director of education, coordinator of research, supervisor of research, close board and staff cooperation, funded free beds, a laboratory and technician, and cooperation with colleges.

With the teaching ward disappearing in the nation's hospitals (one reason was the increase in prepaid health care), other ways had to be found to provide good training for medical personnel. Schooling would not be limited to nurses, interns, and residents but would be "for the entire personnel from top to bottom."

A scientific research program could be inaugurated using existing laboratory facilities and then expanded with financial support from philanthropic foundations such as the American Cancer Society and the Infantile Paralysis Foundation, as well as large manufacturers of X ray equipment and dairy products, and life insurance companies. Such a program would "sharpen the pride" of the medical staff and elevate "the whole tone of the institution."

Financial support for members of the hospital administration also was recommended, to enable them to attend conferences and educational seminars.

In conjunction with the proposed expanded program, an in-house appraisal of medical education and research was conducted at Saint Luke's. The report commended the nursing school highly as up-to-date ... a course entitled "Nursing in Atomic Warfare" had appeared in the nursing school's bulletin in 1952. However, the program for resident doctors and interns was said to lack desirable but very expensive state-of-the-art equipment ... a need described as complex and ever increasing. But the hospital had "the big essential things necessary to carry out an ever-expanding educational program for resident doctors, interns, and nurses." First and most important: a "correct attitude" on the part of hospital administration. Second: a medical library of sufficient size, and an up-to-date records department. Third: a hospital large enough to provide an adequate number and variety of acutely and chronically ill patients. There was a need for better staff performance "and tone" in matters of intern challenge and stimulus, teaching responsibility, research discussions, and talent development.

Ferd Helwig reiterated his support of an amplified program because if implemented it would aid in caring for the sick and also would aid "the intern problem." Another enhancement would be a charity clinic service, "which would benefit the nursing service as well as the training of interns and residents."

Dr. Helwig expressed concern over the lack of interns ... "staff men could never find one to make rounds." However, the solution did not seem to lie in more foreigners ... Helwig was outspoken that "for years we have had foreign men who were not capable of understanding the English language, nor of making themselves understood, which presented serious problems in taking patient histories—a situation which is bad for the patient, bad for the intern, and bad for the staff."

Dr. Helwig noted that training of the house staff could be improved: "Now these young men are literally hungry for more and better instruction from our doctors, and I believe our doctors are equally desirous of giving such help."

There was accord throughout the hospital that a major commitment to medical education and research was needed, including Saint Luke's residents and interns.

Support for medical education at Saint Luke's was not entirely altruistic. There were advantages for the medical staff and for the hospital. House staff demonstrated their worth during World War II, when the

Saint Luke's doctors were called into the service, and the demand for their services continued to grow. Interns and residents provided busy private practitioners with more thorough workups of patients and performed other functions, including coverage at night and on weekends. Most staff doctors wanted interns and residents around to take histories and handle physical exams and emergency calls, so they wouldn't have to. In return for the students' services, the medical staff taught.

Someone would be needed to manage this ambitious program. At about this time, Dr. David Gibson arrived at Saint Luke's Hospital. A protege of Ferd Helwig, Dr. Gibson had agreed to serve as associate pathologist. However, upon reporting for work he discovered that he was also expected to direct the medical-education program at the hospital. He would serve in that capacity for many years.

Hospitals throughout the nation were short on house staff—only about 60 percent of those needed were available. Fortunately, at Saint Luke's the shortage amounted to only about half that. The competition for available medical-school graduates was leading to increased compensation. Dr. Helwig commented that Saint Luke's intern salaries were not comparable to those in other hospitals, putting the hospital at a competitive disadvantage in recruiting, and he requested an increase. The board approved a salary of $150 per month for interns as well as a $25 increase for residents, beginning November 1.

Although it was a teaching hospital, Saint Luke's did not have a formal affiliation with any medical school. Such affiliation offered some advantages—in the preceding decade, medical schools had received large grants for research and training, while growing larger and more complex. However, there was a price that Saint Luke's found prohibitive: private hospitals usually had to grant the medical schools approval powers over staff appointments. So medical education and research at Saint Luke's remained autonomous—the individual effort of a private, community hospital.

• • • • •

Bed allocation according to service (specialty) was a novel concept in Kansas City. A study was commissioned to determine if designated areas of the hospital might be dedicated for use by the various specialties, such as internal medicine, surgery, and obstetrics. There was consensus among the Saint Luke's doctors that such allocation would improve patient care.

Plans were initiated, and a tentative date of January 1 was fixed for the allocation of beds by services, subject to approval by the medical staff and the board's committee on reservations and admissions.

The directors announced plans for spending several hours a week at the hospital. The chief of staff applauded ... in his opinion the medical staff would feel better if the board displayed more interest in the institution. There was a request that weekly visits by board members be at specified times so that department heads could plan for them.

In October, a quarterly supplemental payment from Blue Cross brought the latter's payment to 100 percent of billings, the first time in history that payment in full had been received from Blue Cross.

The polio ward, activated earlier in the year to meet the demands of another acute outbreak, was closed and the few polio cases transferred to other beds in the hospital.

The chronic nursing shortage continued. A recent meeting of the AMA had determined that the most important current problem facing hospitals was the scarcity of nursing personnel. In years past the nursing school had often supplied more than enough nurses to meet the hospital's needs, but the previous year, only eleven of the forty-five graduates had remained at Saint Luke's. There were a variety of nursing personnel employed: 194 nurses' aides, 133 nursing students, 24 orderlies, and 157 registered nurses. There might be a need to look for more help from practical nurses; they were subject to licensure in Kansas but not in Missouri.

Saint Luke's began to study ways to alleviate the cost of nursing education. In the course of the past fifty years, the time needed to adequately train a nurse had increased more than eightfold. Indeed, "the cost of all hospital education has increased to the point that we wonder if all such expense can justifiably be added to the room rate." Others were looking outside their institutions for financial support for educational expenses—to wit, philanthropy.

The maintenance of medical records was a recurring problem. It was suggested that an appropriate letter be written to the staff, advising them that the board was deeply concerned over the laxity accompanied by a reminder that "reappointment of staff doctors is annual." Trained personnel were added to the medical record room, to assist.

A *Kansas City Star* photo dated November 11 (Armistice Day) depicted three Saint Luke's student nurses being fingerprinted at the hospital "for special disaster duties." The accompanying story stated that 250 nurses, student nurses, practical nurses, nurses' aides, and orderlies had registered the previous day for civil defense duties in case of a disaster in the Kansas City area. This was the first step in the formation of a nurses' section in the Kansas City Civil Defense organization.

H.O. Peet spent a November afternoon at the hospital and determined that most of Saint Luke's problems had to do with personnel. He explained that in good hospital operation there are one-and-a-half employees per bed, and that keeping 750 persons employed at Saint Luke's was a "terrific problem" because of the unavailability of qualified people.

The recruitment of nurses posed a special problem ... the resistance to blacks. John Smiley explained:

> "We can get a lot of Negro girls and they are very capable, but the reaction we are getting from patients and other employees is causing a disturbance."

The committee on medical education and research met in November with several students from the KU Medical School, requesting that those who were interested in Saint Luke's "come over to look over the hospital, meet our staff, and look over our facilities." Eighteen students and twenty doctors toured the hospital, without results. (The Chief of Medicine at KU, a hero of all the medical students, applied pressure on the class leaders, insisting that they would be better served by doing their internships and residencies at university hospitals.)

To attract students it would be necessary to improve research efforts at Saint Luke's. The committee had three recommendations: 1) doctors should submit to the research committee projects in which they were interested, together with possible sponsors; 2) the research committee should work with the Crittenton Home on projects common to both institutions; and 3) there should be employed a technician to administer the research program.

In December, the board approved air conditioning for other parts of the hospital's first floor. Also, the John W. and Effie Speas Fund "which is sent to us in the amount of $2,000 each year for this sort of thing," would be used for treatment of a child with a malignant brain tumor. Bishop Welles reported that he had been working since the previous May to obtain a new chaplain for the hospital without any success but would continue his efforts.

When John Smiley's office was remodeled, he buried a "time capsule" in the wall. Its contents included his old gold watch and a bottle of Coca Cola. Smiley's secretary advised that they "secretly hid it where no one could find it until the wall was torn down." They made a good job of it— the entire building was later demolished without uncovering the capsule.

In January, 1953, Dr. E.H. Skinner died. He was a lecturer at KU in radiology and had participated in work at the Richard Cabot Clinic and in health care projects at Saint Luke's. For several months he had been treated intermittently for a blood disorder caused by exposure over many years to X rays, his medical specialty, and his death resulted from complications of that disorder.

Fee-splitting was a matter of concern. This practice, by which a specialist gave a part of his fee to the physician who referred a patient, was regarded as unprofessional. The American College of Surgeons directed a letter to the country's hospital presidents advising:

> "The Board of Regents of the American College of Surgeons has been forced to conclude that the nefarious practice of fee-splitting is on the increase in the United States."

Hospital boards, if uncertain as to whether their hospital was "entirely clear," were urged to confer with their chief of staff and their administrator. No problem was uncovered at Saint Luke's.

• • • • •

A proposal was submitted for rotation of board officers and directors, and the bishop appointed a committee to study and present recommendations respecting the proposal. The committee report offered suggestions as follows: 1) each year one-third of the authorized number of the total board should be elected for a three-year term; 2) a nominating committee should be appointed annually to offer nominations, to evaluate performance by members whose terms were expiring and resubmit names of those who had shown substantial interest but not more than three-quarters of the old directors; and 3) vacancies should be filled by the Executive Committee for unexpired terms. There was no recommendation for limiting the terms of officers.

The Saint Luke's directors also served as members of the hospital corporation, tantamount to shareholders in a for-profit corporation. Every year in January, there would be convened a regular meeting of the board to elect members, followed by a meeting of the members to elect directors, followed by another meeting of the directors at which officers were elected for the ensuing year. The cast of characters was the same for all three meetings ... characterized as a "Chinese fire drill" by some of the bewildered directors. In March, 1953, the board was expanded and it was necessary to convene not only a meeting of directors to elect an additional twenty members but also a special meeting of members to elect those same twenty as directors, after which there was reconvened the regular meeting of the board to get on with their normal business. When all was completed, the board had grown to fifty-four, its high-water mark.

· · · · ·

The board was advised in April that only one intern applicant had accepted a position at the hospital and that the deterrent was a lack of teaching beds. A committee was appointed to study the use of endowment funds to provide such beds.

The Reverend Thomas A. Simpson of Minot, North Dakota, was appointed chaplain of the hospital. Father Simpson, a jolly Yorkshireman, always had a twinkle in his eye. He occasionally invited young doctors to his home for dinner, where Mrs. Simpson served cherry pie made with unpitted cherries—diners removed the pits as discreetly as possible.

Twelve nurses were lost in May to the Veterans' Hospital, where the pay was $14 per eight-hour day as opposed to the $10 paid at Saint Luke's. John Smiley suggested a joint meeting with other hospitals regarding rates of pay for nurses "because if one hospital raises their rates, then the others must do the same." Helen Valentine (back again on an interim basis following the departure of Alicia Sayre in 1952) had submitted a memo to Smiley noting that several of the hospital's nurses had been hired from the Professional Registry at $12 per day out of necessity and in fact could find employment as private-duty nurses at $14 per day. Yet staff duty was much more strenuous than private duty. Two nurses had inquired about salary increases, and Miss Valentine was confident there would be others. A successor for Miss Valentine herself had still not been found, and it was anticipated that the hospital would have to pay considerably more for her successor than it was paying her.

A service at Grace & Holy Trinity Cathedral on May 25 celebrated the fiftieth anniversary of the School of Nursing.

Forty-three applications were received for the nursing school's next class. Eight of the candidates asked for financial aid, but only three scholarships were available ... the other six scholarships were in use. Tuition for three years' schooling was $450.

Scholarship recipients agreed to remain a year at Saint Luke's after graduation, in return for the financial support. Many of the nurses in training eventually would find jobs in industry, and it was suggested that perhaps business corporations would help to finance scholarships; Ford Motor Co. had recently given $7,000 to Saint Luke's for this purpose. There was a need for fourteen more scholarships, and it was proposed that board members help "sell" these.

At the June, 1953, board meeting there was further discussion of nurses' salaries. Smiley spoke of general unrest among the staff nurses, who were working alongside higher-paid private-duty nurses. Miss Valentine listed the new positions taken by the several nurses who had resigned since January 1—in addition to those who had gone to the VA Hospital, two had defected to industry, two had assumed private-duty work, and five had gone to doctors' offices. Also six were pregnant. She stated that a delivery room shortage was the most critical consequence of these losses. The board responded with a 7 percent salary increase for nurses.

In September the board charged various teaching cases to endowment funds, including the Linda S. Hall Fund and the Fund for Indigent Men, which was still being maintained by the churches of the Diocese.

A profit-and-loss statement for 1953 thus far reflected a serious financial problem: increased revenue had not enhanced the bottom line, and there had been significant losses to date ... particularly in the summer months, when salary expense was greater because of the need to provide vacation relief. It would be necessary to increase lab charges, reduce operating expenses in salaries and supplies, and generate greater occupancy. In discussing a proposal for increased room rates, hospital costs were debated. To illustrate that every area of the country was plagued with high costs, the board was shown a film prepared in the state of Indiana entitled: *High Costs of Hospitals.* According to the film, "the general opinion is that the trend isn't going to come down immediately."

The Finance Committee noted that the "rather disastrous" financial results reflected on the September statement would have been even worse if depreciation for the new building had been taken into account. However September occupancy was at 90 percent, and new room rates had become effective on September 20, so if occupancy held up, there should be "a little profit" for October.

A new Operating Engineers' contract would be negotiated soon, and representatives of the various hospitals involved were preparing to present "a united front insofar as possible."

· · · · ·

A community Hospital Master Plan Study published in October concluded that, with the additional beds at the new Baptist hospital and other area expansion, there would be excessive beds in the metropolitan area of Jackson, Johnson and Wyandotte counties. This was based upon a survey of the area using Hill-Burton criteria. Mr. Beals commented:

> "It would certainly seem that the enthusiasm to extend hospital construction is not justified. The government funds will be very difficult to get. That is not particularly good for us ... Transition is certainly evidenced in this survey. We do not need any more hospital beds and the situation of hospital occupancy is weak in places."

The prospect of overbedding led Beals to advocate a Hospital Planning Council in Kansas City. This advisory group would coordinate many aspects of health care among the hospitals, including purchasing, obtaining nurses, development of ideas on nursing and professional help, and in general funnel information through its offices. He advised that the Kansas City Area Hospital Association recommended the proposal and had requested Community Studies to examine its potential. That study was now completed and in the hands of the various hospital board presidents.

There were complaints by nurses staffing the nursery, not over salaries—which were now "commensurate"—but because narrow entrances and exits necessitated that all of the babies be hand-carried, a dangerous practice. A practical solution was found—smaller carts were introduced to transport the infants.

October showed a substantial net financial gain, in contrast to the results of previous months. The hospital also received donations of $10,000 from General Motors and $1,000 from Stewart Sand and Material Co.

· · · · ·

Mr. Leslie D. Reid of Chicago was a unanimous choice to succeed John Smiley as superintendent and chief administrative officer of the hospital. Smiley, now in his sixties, had "frankly stated" that he did not feel equal to the task of administration given his age and health. Reid commenced work on December 10 at a salary of $18,000 per year. Smiley remained in the hospital's employ as director of funds and endowments. The choice of a new director of nurses was deferred until Reid had assumed his responsibilities.

In January, 1954, there were the usual complicated annual meetings, with a regular business meeting and election of members, followed by a meeting of members to elect directors, followed by another, brief, meeting of directors to elect officers. New bylaws fixed the board at a maximum of fifty-four—not counting the president, Bishop Welles—and divided the board into three three-year classes chosen by lot. Directors were elected for one-, two-, and three-year terms. The whole proceeding took only forty-three minutes.

An open house was held in January in the interns' library, for all prospective interns. Only three of the invitees attended, all of whom, however, committed themselves to Saint Luke's for their internships. One of the problems was the interns' quarters—according to director George Reuland, they "presented a sorry situation and not one to attract new interns."

Leslie Reid, the new superintendent, disclosed that although various hospital articles and reports rated Saint Luke's at 500 beds, he had made a count and found the correct number to be 468, excluding bassinets.

A policy authorizing reduced rates for board members was discontinued by board action in the January, 1954, meeting.

In February, the hospital canceled its liability insurance except for coverage of hospital-owned automobiles. Saint Luke's was shielded by Missouri's charitable-immunity doctrine. However, there was an exception—the Supreme Court of Missouri recently had reinstated a damage suit against the Nettleton Home on the ground that a charitable organization was not immune to a damage suit when an accident occurred on property operated for-profit. Consequently, the committee recommended liability insurance for the three dwellings on Wornall Road, two dwellings on Broadway, and the Nurses' Home, all of which generated some income. This coverage was authorized by the board.

Scholarships for nursing students for the spring term had been provided "thanks to the splendid response from board members," but the question would come up again for the September school term. The employment of M. Jeanne Stickels as director of nursing education had brought stability to the helm of the School of Nursing.

At the March meeting, when remarks by Leslie Reid referred to hospital "profits," Bishop Welles asked "if it would be possible for the hospital to dispense with the word 'profit' and instead use the word 'gain' in relationship to the use of the hospital's actual profits." Semantics were important—the suggestion was accepted.

When a large unpaid campaign pledge balance was reported, a director asked if much of the arrearage consisted of medical-staff pledges. If so, "some specific and drastic action should be taken since not only the board but the public at large had so generously given to provide the doctors with a hospital from which they could earn a living." Subsequent review indicated that indeed unpaid pledges "are largely from our doctors." This was an aberration—the support and loyalty of the Saint Luke's Hospital medical staff over the years had been remarkable. Some of the construction projects had been largely supported by staff assessments on the basis of patient volume. In 1960, as another campaign was being organized, 96 percent of the staff responded generously.

Construction of a radioisotope laboratory had been under review for some time, and in April it was reported that "the Radioisotope Laboratory had been passed by the staff and that soon it would become a reality." This was the beginning of nuclear medicine at Saint Luke's ... an early application was treatment of diseases of the thyroid.

Papers were filed for the incorporation of the Hospital Planning Council championed by David Beals, and the new enterprise awaited the arrival of "an important man in the hospital field to assist us" as an employee of the council. Ford Motor Company and General Motors had indicated a willingness to lend financial support to the council.

Nursing school applications for the fall class indicated "a decided improvement in interest in the nursing profession." Five scholarships were donated, a $5,000 loan fund was established, and "by the fall term a definite plan of aid for girls interested in becoming nurses should be in motion." The nursing school was now fully accredited by the National League of Nursing; only 300 of the country's 1,100 nursing schools had achieved this distinction.

The Executive Committee in June recommended that the Insurance Committee include only one insurance broker as a member and that the hospital's insurance business "not go through him" ... his function being to advise the committee and the board, not to sell insurance. This was a sensitive issue, and the board procrastinated, deciding to continue "as is" until fall and then "talk about the question of appointment of personnel of the insurance committee." Ultimately the recommendation was implemented.

EIGHTEEN
1954-1955

foreign house staff ... Dr. Charles B. Wheeler Jr. ...
Hospital Planning Council ... more polio ... Salk vaccine

The Saint Luke's Hospital *Chronicle* for July 10, 1954, advised that a loan fund for laboratory students was established at the hospital. Among the donors were Roy Roberts and Ferd Helwig. The article produced an additional $1,200.

The *Chronicle* also reported that Saint Luke's pediatrician Edwin Schorer sailed July 2 for a two-month cruise of the Mediterranean, with visits to the Holy Land, Turkey, and Greece. In a radio sermon, Dr. Norman Vincent Peale spoke of encountering Dr. Schorer in Syria:

> "In one of the narrow streets of Damascus I saw a wonderful American man, a rotund, chubby pediatrician or 'baby doctor' from Kansas City. He and I had traveled on the same ship part way, and a more lovable man I never met. Children gravitated to him wherever he went."

A highly regarded physician, Dr. Schorer had been appointed Director of the City Health Department in 1933, where he refused to bend to political pressure in the performance of his duties. While a professor at the KU School of Medicine, he held afternoon tea in his laboratory for favorite students.

Dr. Schorer resided in The Walnuts, an expensive and prestigious address, employed a chauffeur, and was a friend of artist Thomas Hart Benton. (A small Benton painting of Dr. Schorer treating a young patient hangs in the second-floor pediatric section of Saint Luke's.)

Meanwhile, Chaplain Simpson, a man of more modest tastes, spent his summer vacation that year in Minot, N.D. His means also were modest; he commented that the retired rector of a nearby Episcopal church "is receiving more money in retirement than I am as a full-time hospital chaplain."

• • • • •

A *Chronicle* article for August 10, 1954, began:

> "With the arrival of eight new interns and residents, Saint Luke's house staff now numbers twenty-six—the largest in the hospital's history."

Despite Ferd Helwig's reservations about foreigners, they came from all over the world—Mexico, Iran, Philippines, India, Australia, Ecuador, and Brazil, as well as the United States. One American, Dr. Charles B. Wheeler Jr. (a resident in pathology), later served with distinction as mayor of Kansas City. A September article in *The Kansas City Star* noted that, of Saint Luke's thirteen interns, all but three were from medical schools outside the U.S.:

> "Getting interns has been an increasing problem for private hospitals. Young physicians naturally seek postgraduate training in public hospitals with a wide range of cases."

Another newspaper article reported five research projects underway at Saint Luke's and described this as a growing trend in major private hospitals:

> "They are adding research and teaching programs to their programs of patient care, in a fashion characteristic of medical school hospitals. The goal is better case results along with stimulation for the intern and resident physicians and the regular staff ... Private hospitals also are seeking ways to admit more free patients, in the interest of their teaching schedules. However, most pay patients welcome their own inclusion in a modern hospital's teaching rounds."

The Wall Street Journal published an article entitled "Sick Hospitals" ... financial stress was not peculiar to Saint Luke's. Blue Cross continued to pay 100 percent of billings, however.

Nurse staffing was again a problem; 60 percent of the Saint Luke's nurses were married and preferred not to work nights or weekends. To match raises in other hospitals, another round of salary increases for nurses was approved by the board.

Bishop Welles acknowledged receipt of a letter of appreciation to the hospital from Stine & McClure Undertaking Company!

• • • • •

By October, formation of the Hospital Planning Council was complete, with R.L.D.S. Bishop G.L. DeLapp of Independence Sanitarium elected president and two Saint Luke's representatives on the board of directors. The primary purpose of the new organization was areawide planning. The council had the support of presidents of hospital governing boards who recognized the need for orderly expansion of hospital facilities and the elimination of costly and unnecessary duplication. This was the first attempt at coordinating local health care. Its board consisted of the most influential people in the community, and it became a model for other voluntary health-planning organizations across the country.

There was need of planning. A recent study confirmed that there were adequate hospital beds in Kansas City but noted that, with group hospitalization and insurance subsidizing hospital care, the sick person who had his bed paid for would not be reluctant to use it even though his illness might not require hospitalization. "Thus the whole problem of hospitalization becomes more complex daily," said Mr. Beals.

• • • • •

Payroll was the hospital's biggest expense item, with salaries consuming from 70 percent to 75 percent of revenues. However, comparison of individual rates indicated that the for-profit sector offered higher salaries than the hospital paid. The problem lay in the number of employees, not the level of compensation. This would be painfully confirmed later when an increase in the federal minimum wage to $1 per hour necessitated a pay hike for a large number of Saint Luke's employees.

Superintendent Reid reported that Saint Luke's did a larger volume of business with Blue Cross than any other hospital. The average stay of Saint Luke's Blue Cross patients was 9.4 days for a six-month period. The rate of turnover was very important to profit and also in reducing pressure from the public and the staff for larger hospital facilities. A *Reader's Digest* article maintained that a significant part of the cost of a prepayment plan was "the cost of faulty use by fellow subscribers." Patient turnover and elimination of abuse would go a long way toward solving the bed shortage in any community.

Leslie Reid also commented on the sharp reduction in postgraduate medical education abroad; instead of doctors seeking experience in other countries, they now recognized the United States as the world leader in medicine. Alien doctors constituted 22 percent of the total house staff in approved hospitals, resulting in problems of language, orientation to American customs, and lack of assurance that their medical education had been in any way equal to that provided by American schools. Service in the armed forces was required of American men of military age, and many foreign physicians found places "because of the draft problem of the young doctor which still continues."

Reid advocated installing an intensive care unit at Saint Luke's … "we hope to work toward an acute surgical unit, concentrating our nursing care to meet that need." His interest had been spurred by an emergency visit to the crowded hospital that resulted in his being relegated to a bed in the hall. An ICU proponent told him that an intensive care unit would have beds and nurses set aside for such medical emergencies.

Dr. Helwig spoke in December about the function of the tissue committee in determining the justification for surgery based upon preoperative diagnoses. He also advised approvingly that the house staff as of July 1, 1955, would be made up almost entirely of graduates of American universities. This would bring about better service but also required an improved teaching program that would be attractive to American interns.

New staff bylaws formalized departmentalization at Saint Luke's—medicine, obstetrics and gynecology, orthopaedics, pediatrics, and surgery.

Saint Luke's was one of the first Kansas City hospitals to limit surgery to board-certified physicians, gradually phasing out general practitioners from this area of practice. High-quality surgery resulted, performed in operating rooms where a nurse coordinated activities and an anesthesiologist monitored the unconscious patient … enabling the surgeon to concentrate on the job at hand.

There was one problem, however. The surgeries at the time were not well ventilated, and Dr. Ralph Ringo Coffey commented that he "sometimes thought that the anesthesiologists were half-asleep over a half-asleep patient."

A January, 1955, *Kansas City Star* article featured the nursery that cared for Saint Luke's nurses' children. It operated from 7 a.m. to 7 p.m. daily in the North Wing of the hospital. The director of nursing stated that at least twelve nurses were attracted to the hospital because of this service, begun in 1953.

In February, the affiliation agreement with Missouri Valley College was discontinued. Such arrangements were not well regarded by the nurse's division of the State Department of Education. And only three Missouri Valley College students had come to Saint Luke's for clinical nursing instruction anyway.

Because of housing problems, it was suggested that there should be only one class admitted to the nursing school, in the fall of the year. Meanwhile, Saint Luke's was attracting larger classes of student nurses, due partly to referrals by counselors who preferred fully accredited schools such as Saint Luke's and partly to recommendations by graduates of the school.

• • • • •

In the hospital's early years, prominent Jackson County physicians officed in downtown Kansas City, traveling to offices, hospitals, and patients' homes by horse and buggy and later by trolley car and motor vehicle. After the new Saint Luke's Hospital opened its doors in 1923, a number of physicians relocated their office practices on the nearby Country Club Plaza—some as early as 1924. Now, in March, 1955, Saint Luke's physicians disclosed to the board an interest in the development of a medical office building across Wornall Road from the hospital.

Dr. Maxwell Berry, medical staff president, explained that there were several reasons for their interest: 1) most of the doctors had made up their minds "to sink or swim" with Saint Luke's as long as they continued practice; 2) owning and managing their own building would be cheaper than renting; and 3) there would be a decided advantage to the hospital in having doctors' offices in close proximity to the hospital.

Leslie Reid supported the project, citing advantages to be: 1) convenience to the physician; 2) assistance to the teaching program because of availability of the doctors to the interns; and 3) monetary gain for the hospital because of increased outpatient use of X ray, laboratory, and other facilities and equipment. Some hospitals paid for such buildings in entirety, said Reid. Herbert Peet had reservations, but general approval of the project was expressed by the board.

• • • • •

Dr. Helwig reported in March that Saint Luke's improved medical-education program had attracted a full complement of interns and that General was the only other Kansas City hospital enjoying such success. All were Americans.

Leslie Reid recited the following facts regarding hospitals across the country: more than 100 million people now were covered by membership in voluntary hospital prepayment plans; more than 47 million belonged to Blue Cross; and more than 90 percent of the babies born in the United States now were being born in hospitals.

• • • • •

Infantile paralysis was a scourge in the early and mid fifties. Although overall mortality rates were affected little by infantile paralysis, the disease was the leading crippler of children, and its incidence had been growing despite assurances by the March of Dimes that research was winning the battle against polio.

Dr. Paul Meyer of the Dickson-Diveley Clinic functioned as the Hospital's chief diagnostician for polio cases. Year after year, the polio cases were brought into Saint Luke's. Some left a week later and some stayed for months. A few died. One woman's first memories were of using Saint Luke's therapy pool. Macy's had an iron lung on display in the lobby of its downtown Kansas City store … it pumped away endlessly on a mannequin that lay inside. The shortage of iron lungs at Saint Luke's was relieved by Army and Air Force pilots transporting these life-saving devices to the hospital.

Heroism on the part of Saint Luke's personnel and volunteers was commonplace; they were seemingly unafraid of the dread disease. Occasionally nurses contracted a less virulent virus akin to polio, resulting in temporarily limp arms and legs but causing no permanent damage.

A feature story in *The Kansas City Star* recalled polio epidemics in Kansas City in those years. It began:

> "The neighborhood where I grew up in the '50s had all the necessities of childhood—lots of kids, a movie theater, a park, puddles for riding a bicy-

cle through, and a swimming pool that opened each Memorial Day. But in the heat of July and August the pool would close. The puddles were forbidden, the matinees half empty, and in the afternoon sun the dusty baseball diamonds at Ashland Square were deserted. If we were lucky we walked to school in the fall. Those less fortunate concerned themselves with recovering from polio. To most of us polio was a rumor, an inconvenience, an excuse our mothers used to get us to take afternoon naps. It struck a boy we vaguely knew in school. It would strike us too if we didn't go to sleep. The disease was lurking in those puddles that formed along the curbs after a summer storm. It was waiting for us in the crowd at the pool."

Dr. Jonas Salk of the University of Pittsburgh developed a polio vaccine, and the annual March of Dimes campaign raised millions of dollars to conduct field tests in 1953 and 1954. Millions of American families voluntarily participated in the trials; 7,500 Jackson and Johnson County youngsters were among those receiving the experimental shots.

On April 12, 1955, the public learned that Dr. Salk's wondrous vaccine was safe and effective ... an inoculation characterized as "the 'shot' heard 'round the world." Development of the vaccine was a great triumph in the never-ending battle against infectious disease.

Now that a miracle had occurred and success was achieved, the inoculation program got underway in the Kansas City public schools. Parental-consent forms were distributed in advance of the inaugural date of April 18, 1955. But the national demand was overwhelming, and no Salk vaccine was available in Kansas City at the scheduled time. Meanwhile, near-record warm weather reminded parents of the approach of another polio season. The vaccine arrived later in the week, and the shots commenced on Monday morning, April 25. Four thousand students received shots the first day, and by Friday about 26,000 youngsters had been inoculated.

The second shot was delayed because of problems with some of the vaccine produced at Cutter Laboratory, and Kansas City's allotment did not arrive until mid-July, during school vacation. Public school officials pleaded with parents to bring their children in for a second shot then, but many skeptical parents refused to allow their children to be immunized ... only 16,000 turned up, leaving thousands vulnerable despite the availability of the vaccine.

While the number of polio cases dropped off dramatically for the next several years, the potential still existed for a new epidemic. The Salk vaccine continued to be given in 1956, 1957, and 1958, but too many children remained unvaccinated, and sporadic cases continued to be reported. In the summer of 1959, the number of cases reported in Kansas City was double that of the previous year—214, the highest in the nation. Twelve died; 140 were paralyzed. Many of the victims were hospitalized at Saint Luke's. The epidemic frightened the skeptics into risking the Salk vaccine, and later when the Sabine oral vaccine was introduced, polio was further reduced. There were no more epidemics, but some children remained unprotected, and the long battle had not quite ended for that reason.

NINETEEN
1955-1956

corporate medicine ... Dr. David M. Gibson ...
all-Americans ... central blood bank ... Dr. R. Don Blim ...
Blue Cross/Blue Shield payments ... artificial kidney ...
Dr. Christopher Y. Thomas

Forty-two percent of Saint Luke's 1954 income had been generated from Blue Cross patients. For the month of March, 1955,
their hospital utilization was so high that Blue Cross temporarily with-
held $4,400 from payment due Saint Luke's. Part of the problem was that
Blue Cross policies reimbursed for hospital charges but not for less-
expensive outpatient visits to doctors' offices.

Only thirty-nine student nurses were graduated in May, a reduction
reflecting earlier recruiting difficulties.

Community Studies, surveying the status of the nursing profession in
Kansas City, released a report that concluded:

> "In comparison with school teachers and social service workers, the Nurse
> stands in the middle. On the basis of the questions asked of the Doctors,
> the conclusion was drawn that the older Physicians had a higher regard for
> the Nurse than do the younger Doctors."

The sixth-floor orthopaedic unit was down in census because its principal occupants were patients of the Missouri Crippled Children's agency
"and funds for this agency have run out ... no more patients will be
accepted until after July 1, 1955."

An expanded house staff, again made up entirely of American men, would arrive about July 1, and there was need to consider some provision for recreational and cultural activities. Board members were solicited for their spare tickets to baseball games, Starlight Theatre, or Philharmonic Concerts.

During the spring, discussion continued of the proposed medical office building and what encouragement Saint Luke's should offer the project. H.O. Peet, chairman of the responsible board committee, was not supportive. In June, when the question arose as to whether or not the board should take a position on the issue, Peet advised that he "did not feel that he had the time to go into the matter at this time." The board then appointed David Beals to chair that committee.

• • • • •

In June, there was resumption of an "old feud between organized medicine and hospitals over corporate medicine." The Iowa Attorney General ruled that, because hospitals billed for laboratory services, they were practicing medicine ... the implication being that all hospital lab services must be billed through a physician. Litigation resulted.

The president of a Boston hospital decried the dispute, saying that the doctors and hospitals needed to join hands and present a united front:

> "The modern hospital is no longer a workshop for individual doctors. It is a field for team play. And the team play is directed not toward the trustees or the administrator or the doctors or the aggregate entity called the 'hospital,' but toward the patient."

The speaker argued that it was quite proper for the hospital to employ doctors as its agents in carrying out its charter powers and that this did not constitute the practice of medicine by the hospital.

The board discussed this matter with its confidant, Ferd Helwig. All agreed that in opposing certain hospital services to patients "a minority group of the medical profession ... were trying to drive a hard bargain." Helwig declared that these doctors were "taking a position to which he was unalterably opposed," and he further felt that their stance "was not in the best interests of the public who support these voluntary institutions and use their services, nor was it in the best interest of the hospital."

It was later reported that an "unhealthy situation" similar to that in Iowa had developed in Missouri ... in St. Louis, where Blue Shield maintained that hospitals were engaging in the corporate practice of medicine by providing lab, X ray, and anesthesia facilities. In Kansas City, a hospital-supported committee had sponsored legal research which determined that under Missouri precedents this activity did not constitute practicing medicine. The Missouri Attorney General indicated informally that he would uphold the hospitals in the dispute. An opinion request was consequently withdrawn, and in St. Louis the doctors had "backed down." There was no problem in Kansas City, where Blue Shield had been organized under the hospital-friendly auspices of the Jackson County Medical Society.

• • • • •

An article in *The Star* announced that eighteen intern M.D.s, all recent graduates of the University of Kansas, and nineteen resident physicians now comprised the house staff at Saint Luke's "in its expanding training-teaching program," with July 1 being the "shift date for house staff." Dr. David M. Gibson, education and research director, was quoted at length. He noted that it was a major problem to secure an adequate house staff to insure proper patient care and that Saint Luke's was one of the few hospitals in the area to acquire its full quota of interns through the National Intern Matching Program, known as the "Match." (This was the process in which medical school seniors indicated their preferences among teaching hospitals for graduate medical education, and teaching hospitals selected graduating seniors for their programs; the choices were then compared, in the hope of finding a match.)

With its new complement the house staff was significantly better, not only in the view of Saint Luke's senior physicians but also from the patients' perspective as reflected by compliments on the improved care. It appeared that Saint Luke's had a very good chance to continue to fill all house staff positions with American interns.

Because of academic casualties, the nursing school was more selective in accepting students in 1955. Only fifty-six out of 104 applicants were chosen, but fifty-five of these were still in school.

The nursing school would have its 1,000th graduate in the 1955 class. Scholarships were still being encouraged … the Nurses' Scholarship Fund had grown from $1,200 to $4,200.

By November, it appeared that Blue Cross would break the enrollment records set the previous year. Not coincidentally, occupancy at Saint

Luke's was running at about 90 percent. Some nights only one or two beds were empty, allowing no selectivity for persons who "might like certain accommodations."

The federal minimum wage was increased to $1, a raise that affected hospitals throughout the country; 40 percent paid their employees less. This had a significant financial impact upon Saint Luke's, where 394 employees earned less than the new minimum.

An ordinance passed by the City of Kansas City imposed a $100 annual license fee on hospitals. Hospitals felt that as nonprofit institutions they should be immune, and resisted payment. Letters were written by hospital officials to the mayor and council, to no avail.

Dr. Max Berry lauded the "all-American" house staff as "one of the best helps that Saint Luke's staff has had." The outlook for filling positions the following year was excellent; members of the medical staff attended a meeting at KU and discussed with seniors their plans for future "schooling." Medical staff members also planned to visit six or eight other medical schools and interview students.

Dr. Helwig presented the board with a summary of the teaching program. Since the policy of admitting interesting teaching patients was instituted, 144 of such cases had entered the hospital, and fifty-seven others were treated on an outpatient basis. Two hundred eighty-eight members of the house staff had seen the 144 patients. In all instances, medical or surgical care was directly supervised by a member of the medical staff.

Saint Luke's did not purport to offer psychiatric services, though a board member urged that mental health care be provided as a means of increasing occupancy. Leslie Reid pointed out that psychiatric treatment was expensive, necessitating extremely high rates, but it would benefit the School of Nursing, whose students now had to go elsewhere for their thirteen weeks' psychiatric training. Reid noted that half of the country's hospital beds were devoted to the care of mental patients:

> "Like many medical problems, this is a growing problem because of the aging of the population. Progress is being made in the care of such people, but treatment will not be as spectacular as the Salk Vaccine, which has greatly encouraged the population in the dreaded Polio Disease."

Meanwhile, Reid acknowledged that psychiatric patients were in fact admitted to the hospital:

"We do not have the facilities, nor equipment, to handle these patients, but
are constantly getting them regardless of wanting to limit ourselves."

The Saint Luke's Nurses' Choir made several public appearances during the holiday season. And the December *Chronicle* reported the death of the legendary Dr. Peter Thomas Bohan at the age of eighty-two.

A survey by Community Studies had determined that, despite an abundance of hospital beds in Kansas City, one segment of the populace was underserved: Kansas City "had an extremely limited number of places where Negro patients and doctors might go." However, now Kansas City's private hospitals were being desegregated, and within a few years, black patients would be treated in all of them. This was accomplished without fanfare, and it is difficult to determine when the first black patient was admitted to Saint Luke's. It is clear that conversations among Dr. Max Berry, Medical Staff President in 1954 and 1955, David Beals and Leslie Reid addressed the issue and that by 1956, there were black patients at Saint Luke's Hospital.

A $235,000 grant to Saint Luke's Hospital by the Ford Foundation was used to extend services and improve facilities, as well as for research.

In the closely watched "corporate medicine" case, the Iowa court issued an opinion that the employment by Iowa hospitals of technicians and pathologists constituted illegal practice of medicine. This was a serious blow to Iowa hospitals, which intended to appeal the decision to the Iowa Supreme Court. If carried to its logical conclusions, Iowa hospitals would be unable to operate an ER, employ technicians, or even provide interns or nurses. This had grave implications for a high-tech, tertiary-care, teaching hospital such as Saint Luke's.

• • • • •

A local American Legion post had urged the Red Cross to establish a central blood bank in Kansas City in 1949. The Jackson County Medical Society reviewed the concept of a single source for all blood needed in area hospitals. It appeared to physicians that such a facility would cost more per transfusion than the present system, but Community Studies was retained to conduct an impartial review of the matter.

If established, the blood bank would be operated by area hospitals, with its only function being the recruitment of donors and the drawing of blood. Pressure was exerted by many groups—"particularly labor"—interested in placing credits with the bank for future withdrawal. But whole blood is perishable. And there were other complexities.

Pathologists were apprehensive about the proposed blood bank, anticipating higher costs for patients. Also, in the event of a shortage, the bank might buy blood of an inferior quality ... hospitals always used blood from known professional donors or from the patient's friends or relatives, who would not mislead the pathologist as to the donor's medical condition.

Despite such reservations, the Community Studies survey supported the enterprise, and by February, 1956, formal steps had been taken to incorporate a community blood bank that would meet the requirements of a four-county area for blood and plasma. A thirty-nine member advisory board was created, composed of thirteen members each from the medical profession, the hospital association, and the public at large. This body in turn selected from among its number a twelve-man board of directors, four from each of the three groups. There was a contractual relationship between area hospitals and the blood bank.

• • • • •

A significant quantity of blood was needed for transfusions at Saint Luke's, where acute illness and high occupancy were the norm. The high level of occupancy was due in part to increased length of stay. The baby boom also was contributing to the congestion; the department of obstetrics was enlarged to accommodate the newborns. Over the previous decade, close to thirty-six million babies had been born in the United States, with an average of 225 births per month at Saint Luke's.

Community Studies arranged for a grant of $132,000 to fund the new Hospital Planning Council for a year, and additional grants were committed for another two years. The council had made little progress due to lack of funds but now would go forward, with an executive director appointed.

For its next intern class Saint Luke's sought eighteen men from the Match program but received only ten, with the possibility of four more. Other Kansas City area hospitals fared even worse. This shortfall was representative of an acute problem for hospitals throughout the country.

Bishop Welles expressed the hope that Saint Luke's could establish a home for older people located conveniently near the hospital. He also announced the anticipated departure in August of the avuncular

Chaplain Simpson, now old enough to qualify for a church pension and desirous of either outright retirement or some less-demanding job.

At the May, 1956, meeting of the board, Leslie Reid submitted that in view of the many services performed by hospitals there was no need to apologize for rates. Of the charge of $22 to $23 per patient day, $16 went for salary expense, and the remainder supported ancillary procedures such as emergency care, X ray, and laboratory services in addition to room and board.

Use of the old Kansas City Cradle building was discontinued following completion of a one-story addition to the Children's Hospital connecting to the Annex, and the Cradle became the site of the nursery school for nurses' children.

In June Mrs. A.W. Peet and the indestructible Ursulla Burr received pins recognizing thirty-five years of service to the auxiliary.

Across the country there was an increase in the number of hospitals and patients, and a decrease in the number of schools of nursing and number of nurses in training. Only one-half of the graduate nurses worked in hospitals. The hospital nursing shortage could only grow worse.

During the summer, the usual seasonal reduction in occupancy did not occur. This was attributed to air conditioning and indicated that consideration should be given to air conditioning the remainder of the main hospital building.

Meanwhile many patients were cooled by electric fans placed behind tubs of ice. Dr. Arnold Arms felt at times "that it was nothing more than a steam room at Saint Luke's." On one occasion, employees in the central supply room threatened a walkout because of the heat in their work area. The air conditioning would also be welcomed by the hospital's laundry workers, who sought relief by chewing on ice manufactured by the hospital's large ice machine.

Leslie Reid compared Saint Luke's rates with the much higher rates in California, suggesting that "when people complain about hospital rates you can indicate that there are others in the country that are greatly in excess of that which we charge." He advised that beds were being added throughout the country, and "as we add these facilities we certainly will be using them, and this means that insurance will have to keep up with the demands of the public."

· · · · ·

The medical care at Saint Luke's was worth the money. Dr. R. Don Blim, later president of the national Academy of Pediatrics, joined the staff in 1956. Although he considered the pediatric facilities to be "woefully inadequate," he chose Saint Luke's because he wanted to be associated with the hospital's premier medical staff. In his view:

"It is not the bricks and mortar that make the hospital an excellent hospital."

Young Dr. Blim immediately was encouraged to work in the Cabot Clinic, which he found to be "a delightful experience:"

"I used to go over every Wednesday morning and see children—always felt very guilty in leaving and felt as though we should be spending more time there than we did. We would frequently see twelve-year-olds bring in their younger siblings because mom was still in bed."

• • • • •

Central air conditioning for the remainder of the hospital was approved in September in order to "maintain the excellent reputation of Saint Luke's."

Teaching cases continued to be admitted to hospital beds under the intern and resident training program, and several outpatient cases were cared for under the program as well. Various charitable funds were charged for the expense.

Jeweler Ernest Jaccard's will provided a trust fund of $50,000 to be used for the care of indigent old men. Also, the board approved an amendment to the contract for care of crippled children, permitting transfer of some young patients to convalescent centers and making more hospital beds available for acute patient care.

• • • • •

Blue Cross increased its rates repeatedly, citing higher hospital charges and greater utilization by members. The Kansas City area length of stay was eight-tenths of a day above the national average, and utilization also exceeded the norm. Further adjustments in the rate structure as well as changes in hospitals' contracts were in the offing. There would be a time lag in implementing these adjustments, and Blue Cross maintained that hospitals would have to share in the interim deficit. A reserve, or contingency fund, was being created out of Blue Cross income, and hospitals were being paid less than 100 percent of billings.

Bishop Delapp of Independence Sanitarium, now president of Blue Cross, was invited to the September board meeting. There, Blue Cross was urged to recognize that creation of adequate reserves by withholding payments to hospitals would not benefit subscribers if hospitals had to curtail or discontinue service as a result. Both Blue Cross and participating hospitals needed to be financially strong, but not at the expense of each other.

Moreover, as donors witnessed the increase in Blue Cross and other contract business, hospital income from philanthropic sources might well be reduced ... "the shift to contractual service within the hospital population may lessen the philanthropic support which hospitals have enjoyed for inpatient service."

Initially established through philanthropy to care for the sick and the needy, Saint Luke's patient-care income had never met the cost of maintaining the hospital. Outside sources had always kept the hospital active and effective.

It was now recognized that there had been many mutually beneficial results from nearly two decades of Blue Cross operation:

> "Doctors have enjoyed the experience of seeing cost of medical care become a diminishing problem in extending their services. The hospitals have enjoyed in a similar fashion a broadening in the scope of hospital care. Fewer empty beds and fewer charity cases and improved services for all patients have been a direct and natural result of the service. And last, but perhaps most important, the general public has benefited."

However, despite the insurance-generated revenues, hospitals had never escaped their struggle with the dollar.

The problem created by withholding payment was particularly acute at Saint Luke's, where Blue Cross patients now represented 46 percent of the patient population. Blue Cross was constantly in arrears, a situation quite disturbing to the directors of the hospital. "They are in a sense building up this fund at the expense of unpaid hospital credits."

Saint Luke's urged that Blue Cross use its reserves to pay all hospitals 100 percent each month while rates were in the process of being adjusted. The situation was characterized as "one instance where conservatism is working to no one's benefit."

Bishop DeLapp responded in generalities, without directly answering the proposal that the contingency fund be used to permit full payment to hospitals. Leslie Reid then declared:

"The hospital was built for all persons to use, and when Blue Cross does not pay its full charges, then, some question must be raised as to whether the hospital is giving charity to members of Blue Cross who could well afford to pay their bill in full ... It would certainly seem that the contingency reserve set up by Blue Cross should be used in the present situation to meet the plan's obligation to the hospital."

The argument in favor of full payment of hospital bills prevailed. At the board's November meeting, it was reported that Blue Cross had accepted as a basic premise that it should resume full payment of billings for 1954 and 1955, and it was anticipated that 100 percent would be paid for 1956 (although completion of payment was in fact delayed until 1957).

• • • • •

Dr. Helwig commented on the recent use by Dr. Christopher Y. Thomas of a revolutionary new artificial kidney to treat a Saint Luke's patient. Within a few hours the patient had "returned to reasonably normal conditions," whereas without the equipment the patient "would certainly have died."

Dialysis for acute renal failure developed during the Korean War, and the artificial kidney came to the attention of Dr. Thomas while he was taking his surgical residency at the Cleveland Clinic. Dr. Thomas there became acquainted with Dr. Willem J. Kolff, the machine's inventor, and learned how to use the equipment in a renal-dialysis procedure. When Dr. Thomas discovered that the Travenol Co. was going to manufacture a dialysis machine for Dr. Kolff, he persuaded Travenol to make a second machine for Saint Luke's.

The equipment was funded by a gift from Kenneth and Helen Spencer. The second artificial kidney to be manufactured, it bore serial number 0002; it was the first such machine to be used in a hospital setting anywhere.

While in Cleveland, Dr. Thomas also encountered the first models of Dr. Kolff's heart-lung machine, which he later introduced at Saint Luke's.

As much as anyone, Chris Thomas was the personification of Saint Luke's. He was born at the then-new facility in 1923, and, during a distinguished medical career spent entirely at Saint Luke's, he contributed much to the development of the hospital as a tertiary-care center.

TWENTY
1957-1958

Robert A. Molgren ... tornado ... heart-lung machine

• • • • •

*N*ursing students continued to visit their high school alma maters in early February each year to promote the Saint Luke's School of Nursing. Well over half the students who enrolled in the school were lured by these recruiting efforts.

• • • • •

Leslie D. Reid died of stomach cancer on March 7, 1957, at age 48. He was succeeded in May by Robert A. Molgren, the administrator of the KU Medical Center.

Noise in the hospital moderated due to a 40-percent reduction in the number of doctors' pages, a change in which the doctors cooperated by promptly answering their summons. Another improvement in the noise level resulted from under-the-pillow speakers for the fourteen-inch television-and-radio combination sets available for rental to hospital patients—a service sponsored by the auxiliary.

The air-conditioning system now operated in all parts of the hospital except for the sixth floor and two floors of the North Wing. There was a modest increase of fifty cents per day for beds in areas that had been recently air-conditioned.

On May 20, a tornado struck the neighboring Jackson County community of Ruskin Heights, resulting in forty-four deaths and more than 200 injured. Many of the casualties were treated at Saint Luke's. The metropolitan area in general was not well prepared to handle this emergency.

Unsupervised ambulance drivers brought people to the closest acute-care hospital, Menorah, which soon was overwhelmed—while doctors and nurses waited in vain at Saint Luke's to receive victims. Police blocked the Menorah driveway and redirected ambulances. Area hospitals learned a valuable lesson about the need for disaster drills and improved mass-casualty plans from the experience.

In June, medical education received a boost when the hospital received $85,000 from L. Russell Kelce to establish a research, education, and equipment fund.

· · · · ·

The H.O. Peet Foundation contributed $1,500 to the heart and lung fund, for the purchase of the new "heart-lung machine … under consideration by some of our staff men." Saint Luke's would be the only Kansas City hospital with this equipment, first observed at the Cleveland Clinic by Dr. Thomas and described by Dr. Helwig as "a machine which permits by-passing the heart and lungs, greatly facilitating surgery on the heart."

Dr. Helwig stated that "if we can get enough experience on it, we may be the first group in Kansas City to use it on an actual patient." He described other equipment designed for this purpose as "outlandishly expensive" and subject to rapid obsolescence. The new machine was "not research equipment primarily for a large educational institution but actually practical clinical equipment for doing a procedure on patients who need it."

Dr. Helwig told the board in September: "The men who are working with the heart-lung machine are quite enthusiastic, are progressing very nicely, and feel that they will soon be able to use it in the care of patients." And in October, Drs. Thomas and Clarke L. Henry presented and narrated a film showing the progress of the heart-lung project. In addition to the film they used slides and a diagram to explain the operation of the heart-lung machine.

· · · · ·

House staff were being housed at 4408 and 4410 Wornall Road, quarters described as "not too acceptable at the moment," but improvements were planned. A Ford Foundation grant of $198,000 permitted a number of improvements in hospital facilities. Meanwhile, Blue Cross brought its 1957 payments to Saint Luke's to 100 percent by reducing its reserve from 5 percent to 3 percent.

Maurice Johnson of the Saint Luke's board, serving as president of the Kansas City Area Hospital Association, reported: "Both Research and St. Joseph hospitals are in a race to get before the public with a drive to raise money for extra facilities. Research has to build a completely new building, and St. Joseph has to add to their facilities." They solved the problem with a joint drive for funds.

There was a labor dispute with the Operating Engineers' Union, the only union recognized at Saint Luke's. Negotiations with several area hospitals for a new collective-bargaining agreement had broken down, and a strike was called. However, when the union learned that Saint Luke's was preparing to operate hospital machinery with management engineers, it reduced its demands, and a settlement was reached.

Saint Luke's had one of the largest boards on record, with some committees functioning well and some not at all. The area of hospital operations in which the directors should participate was hard to define. A survey noted: "They do not belong in the day-to-day operation of the hospital or the Medical Staff."

Saint Luke's bylaws stated that not more than 75 percent of the hospital's directors should be renominated unless the board found "good cause" to do otherwise. The nominating committee took this provision seriously. The previous two years had seen some of the members attending the annual meeting in January anticipating re-election, only to discover to their surprise that they were being dropped from the board. In some cases this occurred after they had paid their dues for the ensuing year.

December, 1957, saw a continued increase in patient-care activity. As a result, the hospital experienced difficulty trying to serve all of the patients who wanted to use it. Reduced length of stay improved matters, however.

• • • • •

In January, 1958, 420 people attended a dinner honoring Dr. Ferdinand C. Helwig for his thirty years' pathology service at Saint Luke's. Reminiscing, Dr. Helwig attributed his choice of a career in pathology to Dr. A.E. Hertzler, for whom he had been a surgical intern. Dr. Hertzler had told Helwig that he lacked the temperament and the hands to be a surgeon and advised him to stop trying to become one, characterizing his efforts as "a waste of time." He said that Helwig was "unique" in his shortcomings, and that he (Hertzler) "must have been blind" when he thought that he saw the potential for a surgeon in him. Hertzler advised Helwig to "stick to the microscope" and become a pathologist.

Helwig co-authored (with Walton Hall Smith) a book entitled, *Liquor, the Servant of Man*. A satire, it argued that alcohol was the greatest single blessing ever bestowed on the human race. The book was popular in some quarters, especially with those who believed that liquor had been socially acceptable throughout history and in moderation possessed virtues not to be scorned by physicians. But Helwig was accused by others of being a renegade to the "dry" state of Kansas.

• • • • •

The KCAHA maintained a close relationship with Blue Cross, which helped to fund the Association, and it was in the interest of member hospitals to nurture this relationship. Blue Cross was continuing to pay 100 percent reimbursement, an achievement not without some hardship for the insurance company in the face of steady increases in hospital rates.

There was a trend in writing health insurance to institute deductibles of $50, $100, or $200 and to tailor policies to fit the needs of particular groups. Instead of one premium charge for all, Blue Cross set differing rates for various groups commensurate with experience, which helped make possible the improved level of reimbursement.

It was reported in March that Saint Luke's had "matched" twelve interns out of a requested eighteen, the best percentage in the city. "There is some question as to whether or not it will be necessary to seek the services of foreign interns."

The president of the medical staff commended his colleagues for making Saint Luke's more attractive to interns. Medical lectures ("Grand Rounds") were reorganized for Thursday mornings, and the medical staff scheduled interns' work so that they could attend. Rounds were held in the medical library.

A shortage of "charity cases the interns are actually able to work on" was a detriment. Funds were available "to a degree" to admit, as such teaching patients, people who lacked insurance or private funds for hospital care. The problem was also being addressed by utilizing patients from the

Richard Cabot Clinic and rotating interns through Children's Mercy and General hospitals. And under consideration: possibly allowing house staff to care for ER patients who did not have a personal physician.

The hospital's finances were sound. In remarks to the board, David Beals "cautioned members not to brag about our present financial condition, where we have in advance the means to pay for projects, as it would not set well with other organizations who do not find themselves in that condition."

Saint Luke's medical-surgical beds experienced an occupancy rate of 98 percent in 1957. Pediatrics conformed to the area-wide 60-percent range for that specialty. Total occupancy of general hospital beds in Kansas City: 86 percent. Existing plans, calling for 700 more beds in area hospitals, would reduce occupancy in Kansas City to 74 percent.

One problem that the hospitals faced was extended care of the elderly. At Saint Luke's, a few long-term geriatric cases required an average of thirty-six acute patient days' hospitalization. There was a great need for facilities for the chronically ill and the aged, which would lower the demand for acute-care hospital beds. The rapidly increasing numbers of aged persons made this imperative. Hill-Burton funds might become available to remedy obsolescence in metropolitan hospitals.

A community wide nursing shortage occurred in 1958; Saint Luke's had twenty-two positions open, due in part to a lower salary scale than prevailed at other hospitals. Nursing personnel comprised nearly 50 percent of the hospital-employee complement and 55 percent of payroll cost. Molgren proposed a salary increase, financed by a $1 per bed per day rate increase. "These salary ranges have been agreed upon by hospitals in this area and some have implemented these ranges as of the first of May," he said. The medical staff president supported the increased charges, commenting that he seldom heard any complaint about costs, and there often was favorable comment about the service rendered.

An Asian flu epidemic was exceedingly severe, leading to a significant number of patients suffering from staphylococcus infection. Staph infections were a worldwide scourge, caused by organisms resistant to penicillin. The physicians' Committee on Contagious Diseases formulated a plan to combat such infections at Saint Luke's.

The sixth floor (orthopaedics) was razed beginning in June, to be replaced by a medical floor.

By June, there had been an increase of nearly 200 admissions over the previous year, but 1,260 fewer days of patient occupancy—the result of reduced length of stay.

Fourteen interns and twenty-four residents began house-staff service in July, and all were graduates of American schools. Fifty-eight freshmen student nurses were enrolled, and almost seventy percent of the recent graduating class remained at Saint Luke's. In addition, Saint Luke's was one of twenty-four hospitals offering clinical experience to men enrolled in the Hospital Administration program at the University of Minnesota.

Clinical use of the heart-lung machine was introduced at the hospital in August. Volume would steadily increase because there were only two such machines in Kansas City (the other was at KU). This was an expensive procedure, and, although life-giving, the hospital lacked the funds to subsidize it; the cost was an individual family responsibility.

Conforming to a recommendation by the Insurance Committee, the board purchased general coverage against liability for negligence in case the Missouri Supreme Court should abolish the state's charitable-immunity doctrine.

The board was advised in October, 1958, that, surprisingly, the average stay of the patient with prepaid hospital insurance was now less than those without insurance. Molgren speculated that insured patients underwent early diagnostic and therapeutic treatment which detected and corrected medical problems before extended stays in the hospital were required.

A KCAHA committee studying hospital costs identified three reasons for cost increases: 1) inflation; 2) public demand for the best available in hospital care, which was becoming increasingly complex (the report suggested restraint in purchases of equipment until it was tried and tested); and 3) abuses resulting more from general prosperity than from prepaid insurance, characterized as a minor factor in rising hospital costs. The report urged voluntary cost containment by hospitals in order to avoid forced controls.

The KCAHA's separate, autonomous Hospital Planning Council included a voting majority composed of community leaders who had no relationship with hospitals. At the November Saint Luke's Board meeting, Nathan Stark, a Hallmark executive, presented a report in behalf of the council. He noted that in communities that had overbuilt on beds, money was spent on hospitalization which could have been better used for other community programs; that hospitals would be imperiled by reduced occupancy; that length of stay and admissions would rise; that hospital costs would increase; that Blue Cross charges and other insurance rates would have to go up; and that personnel shortages would worsen. Hence the need for planning, in order to avoid overbedding.

Nathan Stark later became vice chancellor for Health Affairs at the University of Pittsburgh and thereafter was appointed Health and Human Services Undersecretary during the Carter administration.

Admission of black patients to Kansas City's private hospitals eliminated the need for the General Hospital #2, which had served the black population; it was remodeled and became the Western Missouri Mental Health Center.

TWENTY-ONE
1959-1961

teaching beds and charity care ...

union activity ... Medical Plaza Corporation ...

open-heart surgery ... cardiovascular laboratory ...

Dr. Ralph R. Hall ... fund-raising

*I*n January, 1959, Dr. Mark Dodge urged that the hospital establish a charity ward of at least twenty beds to provide continuing resident training, to assure survival of the surgical residency in particular, and to attract interns to Saint Luke's. Dr. Dodge suggested starting with nine beds at an annual cost of $75,000.

Dodge was a staunch advocate of the teaching program: "If you have young minds to criticize you, you don't make as many mistakes."

Forsha Russell, chairman of the board's Endowment and Gifts Committee, reported on the availability of the hospital's charity and endowment funds for the teaching program. One fund, for indigent crippled children only, was seldom used, owing to the Infantile Paralysis Foundation and accessible state funds. None of the funds had any restriction as to the patient's religion, politics, or race ... the only stipulation was that the beneficiary be without money for medical care. To Russell's knowledge, Saint Luke's had not turned down a single deserving case in the past five years:

> "By deserving, I mean that they must qualify as to financial need and be the type of case that can be dismissed, as far as is foreseeable, within a reasonable length of time; and in that I have reference largely to elderly patients who should properly be in an old persons home or a convalescence center."

He also acknowledged that the services of an adequate and qualified house staff were "so important to the operation of our hospital," and that the availability of teaching patients (charity patients provided by the endowment funds) had been one reason why this program had succeeded. Russell added that no deserving case recommended by clergy, staff, or board had been rejected whether or not a "teaching case." He expressed reservations regarding the expense of the proposed charity ward. Additional unrestricted endowment funds totaling $1,500,000 to $1,750,000 would be needed to support it.

• • • • •

Pending legislation was a source of concern to the hospital:

House Bill No. 415 would repeal the charitable-immunity doctrine in Missouri. Some fifty persons representing Missouri charities had appeared at the Jefferson City hearing in opposition, citing the resulting cost to their institutions.

Senate Bill No. 50 seemed to resurrect the "corporate medicine" problem. It was introduced by the Missouri State Medical Association and opposed by the Missouri Hospital Association. According to the hospitals, the legislation could forbid employment by hospitals of all paramedical personnel, including occupational therapists, physical therapists, X ray technicians, laboratory technicians, and nurse anesthetists. Also, a state board of healing arts could introduce regulations that would make it illegal for hospitals to use pathologists, radiologists, anesthetists, and physiotherapists unless there was an agreement leasing the department involved. And it could become illegal for hospitals to operate group practices or hire physicians to head various services. Hospital trustees were initially urged to oppose the bill. However, it was concluded later that the legislation dealt with a problem of the medical profession and would not be interpreted or applied to outlaw hospital activities in paramedical areas. The bill was signed into law.

• • • • •

Twenty-four members of the medical staff formed "The Medical Plaza Corporation" to erect the medical office building first discussed in 1955. The enterprise was viewed as a demonstration of loyalty to Saint Luke's:

"These doctors entered into this venture primarily as an investment to establish for themselves an equity in this building. All are closely associated with Saint Luke's Hospital and look upon it as the institution in which they do most of their work ... Several fields of medicine are represented and each field is represented by more than one man in the corporation. The fact that Saint Luke's is the only privately owned hospital in the city that has a fully accredited intern and residency program was also a consideration, as they feel that it is a step forward to make themselves more accessible to the interns and residents for teaching. It is not the intention of this group to compete in any way with the services offered by this hospital, nor will they insist upon beds at this hospital any more than at the present time."

• • • • •

Efforts to unionize Saint Luke's dietary, housekeeping, and laundry employees in March failed. However, organizational activity continued and by May also included nursing orderlies and aides. A meeting called by the AFL-CIO Retail, Wholesale, and Department Store Union was attended by some 100 employees. The activity was believed to be limited to Saint Luke's, partly because of its "longest experience" with the Operating Engineers Union. A meeting of the board's Executive Committee was scheduled to review the organizational activities and also the anticipated negotiations with the Operating Engineers in June. "Mr. Molgren felt that a positive and aggressive attitude on the part of management might be the best course to follow."

The hospital's refusal to recognize the Retail, Wholesale, and Department Store Union was followed by a series of union-sponsored meetings with steadily declining attendance by Saint Luke's employees. Management's stern response was reported by Robert Molgren:

> "We have attempted to determine who were agitators or disrupting influences in the departments and to terminate employment of those who gave just cause."

A "strike vote" meeting was conducted by the union in July, attended by thirty-seven people. The majority in attendance voted to strike, should this "become necessary." The meeting was followed by a letter from the hospital to employees of involved departments listing benefits and pledging continued improvements. A salary adjustment for all hospital employees was authorized. The union responded by again rejecting the hospital's position and demanding that "something" be done in the near future.

Area hospitals were attempting to establish a uniform response to union activities. Saint Luke's remained the primary union target, although organizational efforts were underway at Menorah, Trinity, and St. Joseph. Meanwhile, negotiations continued with the Operating Engineers; settlement of that contract was reported in October.

The KCAHA established a steering committee to coordinate the strategy of the eighteen hospitals most likely to be affected by intensified organizational efforts. Fourteen hospitals agreed that they would not negotiate if contacted by a union and would defer to the steering committee for advice in public relations matters. Similar commitments were expected from the other four hospitals.

The Saint Luke's board resolved to make every effort to discourage further union organizational activity, stating that "personnel in the affected departments should be notified that any future evidence of such activity on the part of any individual shall be cause for dismissal." Another request for recognition by the Retail, Wholesale, and Department Store Union was rejected, and management held many meetings with employees to develop and build relationships. One employee "whose actions and comments have had an unhealthy influence and have disrupted the functions of the department" was terminated. A letter was prepared for mailing to employees of affected departments should this become necessary.

• • • • •

A May 24, 1959, article in the Sunday *Star* described an operation on a seven-year-old resident of Emporia, Kansas, a ward of the state of Kansas, who had undergone corrective surgery to repair a hole in a partition between the chambers of his heart:

> "At Saint Luke's Hospital, where a team of surgeons and technicians have the only artificial heart-lung machine actually being used in operations in a private hospital here, it was decided to take the little boy's case."

Members of Phi Sigma Epsilon fraternity at Emporia State Teachers College had agreed to donate the blood required for the operation; a dozen persons gathered at the Community Blood Bank the day of the operation. A team of four trained surgeons (they first began using the machine in operations the previous August at Saint Luke's after spending two years in a laboratory perfecting their technique) stood over the patient as two other surgeons manned the pumps of the artificial heart-lung machine. Two trained nurses completed the team. The small patient's expensive bills were paid for by the Louetta M. Cowden Fund.

• • • • •

A number of generous gifts were received from Mrs. Louetta M. Cowden. A fund established by her contributions was "a very significant part of our teaching program." Mrs. Cowden's philanthropy had much to do with the survival of the hospital's medical-education program in the early years.

As previously requested, a section of the hospital was set aside for teaching cases. Members of the medical staff were encouraged to keep these beds occupied "within financial limits" with cases to meet the needs of the surgical residency program.

A record freshman class of eighty-eight enrolled in the School of Nursing, and more than 70 percent of the previous graduating class stayed on to work at Saint Luke's. A new group of interns were thoroughly indoctrinated, the resident staff was "well-filled," and the house staff generally was "functioning effectively."

In response to depleted nursing scholarship funds, the auxiliary contributed $1,000 for two scholarships and $500 for student loans, as well as $160 worth of Starlight Theatre tickets for student nurses.

In January, 1960, Saint Luke's was granted $5,000 by the Missouri Heart Association for a research project by Dr. Helwig to investigate whether viruses could inflame heart muscle by causing allergic reactions.

Twenty-five applications for internship were received for the next year, an increase over the prior year's seventeen. It was hoped that there would be a full house-staff complement as a result.

Following a February visit by the Joint Commission on Accreditation of Hospitals, Robert Molgren advised David Beals:

> "Our inspector from the Joint Commission has been here and gone. I feel sure that after the sessions with him on last Wednesday and Thursday there were a number of the medical staff quite willing to tell him where to go."

Chaplain Simpson retired, effective the end of the month of April. William N. Beachy, M.D., a rare combination of Episcopal priest and medical doctor, was appointed to succeed him.

In May, Robert Molgren discussed five challenges to hospitals of the future cited at a recent hospital convention: the need for hospitals to work jointly to avoid wasteful duplication while planning service improvements; the need for Blue Cross to broaden its coverage, organize itself nationally, and control the abuses of its services which unjustly burdened hospitals; the need to find better ways to care for the elderly and the indigent; the need to clarify relations and improve cooperation among doctors, trustees, and administrators; and the need to thwart unionization by providing better pay and morale among employees.

• • • • •

A report from the medical staff recommended the development of a cardiac catheterization laboratory as well as arrangements for interpretation of electrocardiograms. Molgren supported the cath-lab project … it was essential to the continued evolution of the hospital as a referral point for specialized services. A cardiologist would be needed to direct the program. The same person could also interpret electrocardiograms on a fee-for-service basis.

The cath-lab project was approved, and Molgren announced the employment of Dr. J. Tenbrook King, "an exceedingly competent cardiologist." July 1, 1960, Dr. King arrived to assist in the development and implementation of the CV lab. There was no office available for "Tim" King, but someone recalled a unisex public toilet off the lobby with extra space immediately inside the door. Into this area were shoehorned a desk, filing cabinet, chair, and telephone. This "office" served adequately for a time, except for the occasional interruption when a woman needed to use the facilities—whereupon Dr. King retreated to the hall.

The same month another $50,000 Cowden donation was placed in the fund for education and research.

• • • • •

John F. Kennedy was elected to succeed Dwight D. Eisenhower in the American presidency. He had campaigned in support of health care for all of the elderly, using Social Security as the financing mechanism. A December KCAHA communication anticipated some changes on the health care front:

"It is obvious that the new administration will push aggressively for a massive medical and welfare program out of the next Congress, with particular emphasis on health care of the aged, financed through Social Security."

This smacked of socialized medicine, and both the American Hospital Association and the American Medical Association were opposed.

A decline in the number of obstetrical patients was troublesome. Five new obstetricians were invited to join the medical staff.

Pediatric additions also were discussed, but none took place; pediatricians already on the staff felt that their own specialty was well represented. Indeed "the possibility of Mercy Hospital relocating in this area might reduce our occupancy still further, and in that event it might be more expedient for Saint Luke's Hospital to close its Pediatric Department."

For the first two months of 1961, occupancy in medical, surgical, and orthopaedics exceeded 100 percent.

The Match produced ten new interns out of a complement of eighteen, of whom nine were from KU. This compared very favorably to the other Kansas City hospitals.

A new hospital entrance was built to the west off Wornall Road, eliminating the series of steep steps on the Mill Creek side known to panting pedestrians as "cardiac hill." There was also a new ambulance drive. No longer, after a winter snowfall, would ambulance drivers be confronted by a slippery incline that forced them to carry patients up the hill on stretchers.

The new emergency entrance featured a porte-cochere for ambulances, extending over the adjacent driveway ... the roof had to be raised when ambulance drivers discovered that it was not high enough to accommodate their vehicles.

Ralph R. Hall, M.D., joined the staff July 1, 1961, as the new director of medical education and research. He spoke of house-staff-recruitment problems, one of the difficulties being that medical schools did not believe that private hospitals offered adequate graduate education. However, their attitude was changing with respect to some hospitals, particularly those where a research program accompanied medical education. Such a program also benefited the hospital and its patients ... it stimulated the house staff to learn more, brought the latest techniques to the hospital, and attracted financial aid.

The surgical department participated in the planning for proposed new operating-room facilities at Saint Luke's, having complained that in the construction of the hospital's existing facilities "to their surprise and frustration their suggestions and recommendations were almost completely ignored." Their involvement was significant this time.

At local and national hospital meetings, considerable thought was given to the likelihood of more third-party payers reimbursing on the basis of the provider's cost. Many governmental agencies, and in certain areas Blue Cross, already used this method. The Missouri Crippled Children's Service was the only agency having such a cost-based contract with Saint Luke's.

• • • • •

The Hospital Planning Council determined that Kansas City needed better beds and better hospitals rather than more beds. A united hospital fund campaign was organized, and the KCAHA asked hospitals to submit lists of their requirements to correct problems of obsolescence. Large corporate contributors such as Ford, General Motors, and Chrysler preferred the planned community-wide effort to individual hospital drives. A professional fund-raising organization was selected.

The Saint Luke's board approved the campaign and authorized the hospital treasurer to advance $25,000 in operating funds, with the understanding that this money would be returned as soon as gifts were in hand to permit this.

Several osteopathic hospitals would be included in the United drive, because many industrial firms would not support the drive otherwise. Asked to comment on the virtues of osteopathy:

> "Dr. Helwig said his remarks might not be generally accepted by many medical men, but he felt that over the last 40 years there had been a continual upgrading of the academic requirements for osteopaths, until today it is somewhat comparable to what is demanded in medical schools, and they are practicing an acceptable caliber of medicine and do have a large practice. Many states require that they take the same Board of Examination as medical doctors. In the state of Missouri, a great number of smaller hospitals permit them to use their facilities—otherwise the small hospitals would not be able to operate; and in some localities, only osteopaths are available to care for patients."

Final approval of Saint Luke's participation in the United Hospital Fund drive was contingent on participation by 80 percent of the major hospitals in the area—Research, Trinity Lutheran, Menorah, St. Joseph, and St. Mary's in particular. H.O. Peet opposed becoming a part of the drive because he did not believe Saint Luke's was "getting a fair deal" in the proposed apportionment of the funds to be raised. Nevertheless the motion to approve carried by majority vote.

After several months' effort, the United Hospital Fund campaign floundered. Fifteen business leaders were invited to a meeting to determine the public's attitude regarding continuation or abandonment of the campaign, and their response to the invitations was poor. Campaign finances were almost exhausted, and it was decided not to ask the hospitals for more money.

Medical-surgical occupancy in October was at 103 percent, and the medical staff was pressing for more beds. But the UHF campaign offered no relief; it was abandoned … a failure. The hospital decided to proceed with an independent fund drive to raise $1,500,000 to $2,000,000 … approximately the amount which Saint Luke's would have received from the UHF Campaign. Robert W. Wagstaff was chosen to chair the campaign.

Saint Luke's private campaign was criticized by KCAHA's Hospital Planning Council, which believed that 104 more beds for Saint Luke's— already the largest private Kansas City hospital—would result in lower occupancy at other area hospitals, increasing patient costs and possibly causing some to close their doors. Several hospitals now planned separate drives, and for hospitals to compete for funds could only result in chaos. Community planning would suffer a setback; with no increase in demand, one hospital's gain was another hospital's loss. And as occupancy dropped in some hospitals, the aggregate hospital bill went up along with Blue Cross and other insurance rates.

Saint Luke's countered that its action was in response to public demand, in the only way open to it since the suspension of the UHF drive. Robert Wagstaff, ever the combatant when Saint Luke's interests appeared to be threatened, went on the offensive—charging that the hospital's effort to raise funds was hampered by the criticism. He attributed the latter to two or three persons doing everything in their power "to smear Saint Luke's Hospital by innuendo in an attempt to hurt the campaign and cloud the issue."

TWENTY-TWO
1962-1964

congestion ... Louetta Cowden ...
Saint Luke's Hospital Foundation ... Code Blue ...
nursing school accreditation ... integration ...
charity clinics ... Kitty Wagstaff

*D*uring 1961, patient occupancy frequently exceeded "capacity," a feat made possible by utilizing corridors, alcoves, and sun porches. Waiting lists and cancellations were routine occurrences. This was one of the real underlying, pressing reasons for the campaign ... "the need for funds is extremely urgent," said Bishop Welles.

Meanwhile efforts to revive the moribund UHF Campaign were pushed by a special committee. The Hospital Planning Council met with Saint Luke's representatives on February 9, 1962, in a last-ditch effort to head off Saint Luke's expansion program. Council representatives recognized the need to revitalize the UHF campaign but argued that the campaign's success or failure should not affect council planning. They acknowledged the pressures upon Saint Luke's generated by patient demand but contended that the solution lay in redirecting the patients to other hospitals able to provide adequate care, despite lacking certain advantages:

"It is worth considering the reasons why Saint Luke's Hospital is reaching an optimum utilization while other hospitals are not. Some of these are undoubtedly the following ...

"Saint Luke's has a favorable location, in the central city and in one of the good areas of the core. It is on a main traffic artery with good transportation.

"Saint Luke's has over the long years of its fine services been a 'status symbol' hospital, considered as the one used by the top economic and social segment of the population.

"Saint Luke's bigness of itself has attracted an excellent medical staff in the specialist category.

"Saint Luke's has problems of obsolescence, both physical and functional, but these are nowhere nearly so evident to the public eye as is the case with a number of other hospitals in the area. To the public it remains a fine building in a good location, whereas other hospitals have borne the brunt of population shifts, deteriorating neighborhoods, and other factors over which they have had little control, such as entirely new hospitals entering the picture and draining off patients.

"We do not believe that Saint Luke's has reason to feel complacent over these points ... or to assume that all of these factors are totally a direct result of their own good management, while problems of other hospitals are an equally direct result of poor management. By and large, we firmly believe that most of the major institutions in the Kansas City metropolitan area are well managed and that their boards and administrators are working earnestly to make that management ever better."

Saint Luke's representatives were not persuaded. They were aware of the tensions and problems resulting from suspension of the UHF campaign and regretted its failure. However, Saint Luke's had subordinated its own needs to support the campaign and now had to proceed with an independent effort.

In March, Robert Wagstaff announced that the Saint Luke's campaign goal of $1,500,000 was more than 95 percent achieved; he was optimistic about reaching $2,000,000 the following month.

• • • • •

A June *Kansas City Times* article disclosed grants from the Missouri Heart Association to Saint Luke's for heart studies. One of these funded research by a member of the house staff.

Despite the generosity of Louetta Cowden and others, the cost of medical education and research at Saint Luke's was borne largely out of patient-care dollars. (Paying patients were charged more to cover this expense, a practice known as "cost-shifting.) If these programs were to flourish, other funding support had to be found. Consequently, the Saint Luke's Hospital Foundation for Medical Education and Research was created in September. The general purpose:

"To assist financially furtherance of post-graduate medical education of the house staff; fellowships for training residents or others whose training may be considered important to the board of directors of the foundation; and the administration of research grants which might be available to the visiting or house staff of Saint Luke's or to other physicians interested in research that would be designated by the board of the foundation."

Dr. Helwig became the first president.

The Louetta Cowden Foundation contributed $10,000 to the new foundation. This grant was followed by other Cowden Foundation grants over the next thirty years, totaling $1,355,000.

• • • • •

The Community Blood Bank performed well until the summer of 1962, when an attorney from the FTC appeared on the scene to investigate whether the hospitals were conspiring together or otherwise committing unfair trade practices in the handling of the blood supply. This was the first instance in which the Federal Trade Commission had concerned itself with nonprofit corporations and was the result of complaints by the blood bank's commercial competitors.

Patient admissions continued to be "exceedingly high" … more than 1,000 patient days above those of a year ago, with related increases in ancillary services.

During August and September, occupancy constantly exceeded the normal bed complement. Thirty or forty overflow patients were cared for daily in alcoves and sun porches, admitted directly to the recovery room, or held in the ER. This shortage in accommodations would only be exacerbated by interruptions in service resulting from the building program. Meanwhile, the hospital lacked sufficient nurses, technicians, and house staff.

The first four floors of the Medical Plaza Building were completed. The board approved a proposal by the doctors in the building to widen Wornall Road, the street that divided the hospital from the medical offices. The hospital and doctors underwrote the cost in proportion to their ownership along the street.

In December 1962, ground was broken for a multi-story parking garage to replace the small parking lot south of the hospital. This inaugurated the new building program to be supported by the recent fund drive. Architects were completing working drawings and final specifications on the remainder of the project, to wit, an eight-story East Wing and a new building entrance that would face Wornall Road and connect with the second floor of the existing structure. The new East Wing would extend from the existing east front of the hospital toward J.C. Nichols Parkway. (Mill Creek Parkway had been renamed in honor of the pioneer developer.) Besides patient rooms, it would contain expanded surgical, radiological, laboratory, and ER facilities.

• • • • •

A novel emergency procedure, external cardiac massage, saved several lives. The procedure, cardiopulmonary resuscitation or CPR, utilized an innovative cart equipped with an AC defibrillator discarded by the surgery department and Dr. Max Berry's electrocardiograph as well as other equipment, special drugs, and supplies. The cart itself, an ordinary metal one, was purchased at Sears, Roebuck by Dr. Berry—medical manufacturers had yet to produce such equipment. Dr. Ralph Hall was responsible for training the house staff of twenty-four residents and six interns in the new procedure, named by its Saint Luke's practitioners "Code Blue."

The first patient—in the first such resuscitation performed west of the Mississippi River—was an elderly lady from near Osceola, Missouri. A few months after her recovery, the woman called Dr. Berry and asked him to come to Osceola and confirm to her friends and neighbors that she had been raised from the dead. The experience converted her into an evangelist who went about telling people what it was like in heaven; it was her belief that she was recalled from the hereafter for that express purpose. However, she instructed Dr. Berry: "If I ever die again, I don't want you to try to resuscitate me because it is so nice there."

Dr. Berry and Dr. Tim King, aided by the Saint Luke's house staff, later published the first paper on cardiopulmonary resuscitation—*CPR in a Community Hospital.*

• • • • •

The Executive Committee voted to establish a new intensive-care unit in accordance with a medical-staff recommendation, to be implemented as determined feasible by administration. The new twelve-bed ICU was opened in February.

• • • • •

David Beals died—a great loss—and the March board meeting adopted an appropriate commemorative resolution. In April, H.O. Peet was named first and executive vice president, the position occupied by his father for so many years, and Robert W. Wagstaff was elected second vice president.

The FTC investigation of alleged restraint of trade by blood-bank activities in the Kansas City area continued. In May, it was reported that hearings then in progress involved—among many others—Saint Luke's, together with Dr. Helwig as hospital pathologist and Robert Molgren both as Executive Director of the hospital and as an officer of the Community Blood Bank. The prosecution's presentation continued for weeks, and the proceedings were fully reported in the newspapers.

Also in May, legislation permitting hospitals and physicians to refuse to perform abortions in Missouri was approved by the Missouri House.

Dr. Hall identified specialty training offered at Saint Luke's through residencies as: internal medicine, general surgery, pathology, obstetrics-gynecology, orthopedics, radiology, and urology. The following year there would be thirty-nine members of the house staff.

Dr. Hall stated the case for medical education at Saint Luke's:

> "First, it is felt by many that there is an obligation to teach young physicians in the atmosphere of private practice and so to foster the private practice of medicine. Second, there would be an ample opportunity for training interns and residents in Kansas City in order to assure an adequate supply of well-trained physicians for this area. Third, but certainly as important or more important, the presence of a good house staff improves general patient care. It does so for several reasons. They are in the hospital at all times. Outstanding and rather dramatic examples of what can be done are techniques such as external cardiac massage. Some of the patients who would have expired only two years ago are now going home because of our newly acquired knowledge and the availability of the house staff. The number of people who have gone home from Saint Luke's Hospital after having cardiac arrest is almost equal to that of any large medical center in the country. We have in mind particularly the Johns Hopkins Hospital, where this concept originated. In addition the teaching program is likely to attract more highly qualified staff physicians."

Dr. Hall warned that the AMA's Council on Medical Education was drastically reducing the number of internships and residency programs; only the "sound" programs would survive. Other Kansas City hospitals already had seen their programs discontinued for failure to keep up with existing standards. There was no special dispensation for private hospitals. The same rules applied to them as to university hospitals. In order to continue to meet standards, Saint Luke's would have to make changes from time to time.

The arrival of hot weather brought no relief from the overcrowded conditions consistently reported for several months; because of air conditioning there had not been any seasonal slump in elective patient activity.

• • • • •

There were accreditation problems with the National League of Nursing and the Missouri State Board of Nursing, due in part to Saint Luke's inability to hire qualified faculty for the School of Nursing. It was necessary to increase the number of qualified faculty, and salary ranges for faculty recognizing academic preparation would have to be adopted in an effort to attract them. Meanwhile, the Saint Luke's school was operating under temporary approval.

Miss M. Jeanne Stickels, director of nursing education, presented a written report on "Problems in Nursing Education." She stated that a hospital such as Saint Luke's, with the number and variety of its patients and the excellence of its medical staff, had a responsibility to educate nurses for the community as well as for the hospital. And although many people said that hospitals with nursing schools had access to cheap labor, the converse was actually true … "it is costly to have a school of nursing."

Nursing education had changed for many reasons. With the advances in medical techniques, more and more work was imposed on the physician, who in turn delegated more to the nurse. Not too many years before, nurses did not do blood pressures, intravenous puncture, or intramuscular injections. Now, instead of the old apprentice-type training or rote learning, schools had to equip students to apply basic principles and exercise prudent judgment. The nurse was legally responsible for her actions now—no longer just an agent of the hospital or a servant of the physician.

The accreditation process itself also contributed to the changes. Although accreditation by the National League of Nursing was voluntary, accreditation by the State Board of Nursing was mandatory if graduates were to be licensed as registered nurses.

It would be necessary to adequately prepare students for their state boards. Experience must be balanced with sufficient classroom work. And at Saint Luke's, maintaining a planned rotation of clinical service presented great difficulties in view of the hospital's belief that this required nursing experience at all hours and on weekends and holidays.

A Student Nurse Handbook, published by Saint Luke's in August, 1963, provides insight into the deportment expected of nursing students of that era.

Freshmen were allowed six "overnights" per month; juniors and seniors were allowed to be away overnight "as their judgment permits." However, advance parental arrangements were required:

> "A signed statement by the parent giving the student permission to use her own judgment as to where she spends her overnights must be on file in the Nursing Office before a student will be granted an overnight leave."

Parental control was to be exercised over matrimony as well; marriage by students was permitted upon submission of a letter from parents indicating knowledge of matrimonial plans.

The receptionist conducted a bed check after 12:30 nightly and was expected to "use a flashlight to identify occupants in darkened rooms." Other miscellaneous regulations:

> "Students will conduct themselves in a lady-like manner at all times."
> "There will be no calling out of windows to persons outside the residence."
> "There will be no use of 'crude' language."
> "Alcoholic beverages will not be permitted in the residence. Merely the presence of a bottle, empty or otherwise, in a student's room will be grounds for suspension or dismissal."
> "Students should be aware that conduct in parked cars is particularly vulnerable to criticism. Unbecoming conduct will not be tolerated."
> "Smoking on the streets is unwomanly and is not acceptable."
> "The student is expected to use sound judgment in her exposure to the sun ... Absence from class or clinical experience as a result of sunburn will be considered unexcused."
> "For the safety of the student, baby-sitting is not allowed."

• • • • •

A September article in the Chamber of Commerce magazine *Kansas Citian* described how the assistant vice president of the Chamber was restored to life through Saint Luke's Code Blue procedure. "Steele is alive today because of a method of external heart massage relatively unknown three years ago."

Robert Molgren reported on the progress of open-heart surgery at Saint Luke's and of the cardiovascular laboratory, now conducting five or six procedures a week. A new pump oxygenator had been purchased, using funds from Russell Kelce.

In October, area hospitals agreed to assume the legal expense for defense of the KCAHA in the continuing FTC blood bank proceeding, apportioning it on the basis of patient days. There were now three separate categories of defendants: the KCAHA, the pathologists, and the Community Blood Bank. The Saint Luke's board approved this apportionment. "Although hospitals are not legally responsible or liable for any damages as a result of an adverse decision of the hearing, nevertheless, it is costing them a substantial amount to defend themselves."

The hospital's acute shortage of beds and of nursing personnel continued. Overworked Saint Luke's employees were exhausted. To avoid damage to the hospital's image for quality, it was necessary in November to reduce the bed complement—to stop placing patients in alcoves, emergency rooms, recovery rooms, and ICU units—and also to initiate a five-days-per-week operating-room schedule. Meanwhile, the nursing shortage continued.

The foundation agreed to expend $10,000 (in addition to its existing $18,000 annual commitment) for the teaching program and obtained an IRS ruling to insure donors that their contributions to the foundation were tax deductible.

A disheartening survey by a representative of the State Board of Nursing found changes introduced in order to satisfy earlier criticism of the School of Nursing to be inadequate. Curriculum adjustments had already had a "telling effect" upon the hours and quality of nursing on floor assignments, and now even further adjustments were being required.

> "There appears to be a deliberate effort on the part of certain groups and agencies to bring about the demise of the diploma or hospital school of nursing."

The greatest deterrent to efforts to fill the position of Director of Nursing Education was that qualified candidates were "rather openly discouraged from becoming associated with anything other than the degree or baccalaureate program."

Saint Luke's had company in its "plight," but "the number of schools sharing our philosophy of nursing is fast diminishing." Upon her return from World War I, Miss Eleanor Keely had predicted: "The day of the diploma nurse is over." Now, forty-five years later, her dire forecast was apparently coming true.

· · · · ·

At the September board meeting, Bishop Welles had pleaded eloquently for adding black physicians to the medical staff. He noted that Saint Luke's was founded by Christian men and that the Executive Council of the diocese had adopted a resolution requesting the admission to the staff of qualified black physicians. The council resolution complimented the hospital for accepting black patients and for its role in training black physicians in surgery but characterized these as "minimal steps." It sought acceptance for internship of qualified black graduates of approved schools of medicine and admission of black nurse candidates to the school of nursing. "There was no discussion by the board of this matter," according to meeting minutes. However, the bishop asked the chief of staff to present the council resolution to the medical staff.

When by December no black doctors had been presented for appointment, Bishop Welles "suggested to the board that if CORE or the NAACP should ever place pickets in front of Saint Luke's Hospital because they felt Negroes were being denied what to them seemed fair, that feeling his Christian duty as strongly as he does, he would probably join them."

Herb Peet replied that he did not anticipate any such picketing, that the hospital employed black people and that its restaurant was "completely integrated." Peet said that requests for application forms by Negro doctors had been filled and that if some doctors were better qualified than others of whatever color, their chances for staff appointment were good, "but to appoint them just because they are Negroes would be discriminating against the white doctors who are qualified and have been waiting for staff appointments."

According to Peet, the nursing school had few black applicants. It had not enrolled black girls, but it had also turned away qualified white girls because of limited facilities. "Perhaps in time, we will be in a position to accept qualified colored girls for nurses' training, and this would be a great service to medicine in view of the critical nursing shortage." There had been some adverse publicity on racial issues, which Peet felt was unfair; he responded that "the accomplishments of the hospital and its board of directors during the past year with regard to civil rights was commendable."

Bishop Welles answered that he was proud of Saint Luke's and of Mr. Peet. "He wished to add, however, that there are some really fine Negro doctors in this city, that the colored people would like to have the best medical care possible, that some believe that Saint Luke's Hospital offers the best medical care, and that they would like to have Negro doctors to admit them."

The employment record at Saint Luke's with respect to numbers of blacks gradually improved and would continue to do so. Over the years, blacks had filled service jobs—cooks, housemen, laundresses, janitors. Now more professional roles would be theirs. Noting the progress, a black Saint Luke's laundress later would remark:

> "The barriers to jobs throughout the hospital broke down a little bit at a time. It is more fair for the children than it was for me."

Bishop Welles continued his integration efforts, inviting Dr. Starks Williams to speak to the board in January, 1964. Dr. Williams was past president of Queen of the World Hospital and was also a member of the medical staffs of St. Mary's, St. Joseph's, and Menorah Hospitals. Williams said that he was not a public speaker, not a crusader or a "civil righter," but a "mixed-blood" American who found it necessary to fight for his rights in a way which he felt was contrary to the American dream. "The Negro, as a mixed-blood American, has been fighting for his rights to develop his talents, to express his ideas, wants, and needs, since 1620," he said. The institutions of Kansas City could not render a service for the public good and the public welfare if that service was not available to everyone. If a Negro had something to give, he should be able to give it. Continued Dr. Williams:

> "If he qualifies and can do the work, he is not asking for special privileges but the right to practice his profession; and his patients want a place to be cared for, a place for babies to be delivered, and not be asked whether they are black or white ... "

Dr. Williams noted that ten years before, when he came to Kansas City, all of the city's hospitals were completely segregated. There was one institution for Negro private cases, and there was one public hospital for Negro patients. The staff of Queen of the World, the former St. Vincent's Maternity Hospital, was integrated as an experiment, to see if Negroes and whites could work together, and it proved to be "an enormous success." More recently (as of January, 1964), staff appointments had integrated the medical staffs at Research, Menorah, St. Mary's, St. Joseph's, Mercy, and the new consolidated General Hospital. When Wagstaff cited the critical overcrowding at Saint Luke's produced by its existing medical staff, Williams replied:

> "He had discussed this situation with a colleague, who had suggested that he tell the members of this board that the future is more important than the present and to set the stage for the next generation so that they will not have to fight the battle that the present generation has fought so that Negroes who are newly trained nurses, technicians, and doctors may come to this city with the knowledge that Kansas City would have an open heart."

There the matter rested. However, members of the medical staff executive committee subsequently engaged in a special recruitment effort, identifying several black physicians who joined the staff.

• • • • •

Meanwhile, at Saint Luke's there was a waiting list of qualified applicants and insufficient beds for the patients of existing staff members. Letters of recommendation were part of the admission process and were not limited to professional qualifications. One doctor was described as "rather difficult … to get to know well, but … he has always been pleasant when I have seen him on the golf course."

In January, 1964, Dr. Frank Dickson died at age eighty-one.

The low bidder for the building program was J.E. Dunn Construction Company. After extensive negotiations to reduce the cost of the project, Dunn was awarded a contract for $5,750,000. The entire program, including various interim charges, parking garage, and professional fees, totaled nearly $7,000,000. Construction of the new East Wing got underway.

The other area private hospital with internship and surgical residency programs lost its accreditation. The various councils and accrediting groups clearly preferred that medical education be conducted in university-affiliated hospitals.

Saint Luke's remained independent of university affiliation. There seemed little to be gained and much control to lose from such affiliation. If it became necessary to follow that course in the future, no problem in finding a university partner was anticipated.

The Nearly New Shop, a secondhand thrift store, was opened for business by the auxiliary in February, 1964, at 4414 Wornall Road, across the street from the hospital. Zoning problems had frustrated the auxiliary but finally were overcome.

A February article in *The Kansas City Star* reported on the "quiet revolution" that had opened the doors of all Kansas City hospitals to black persons over the previous ten years. A KCAHA spokesperson said: "Today there is not a general hospital in the Kansas City metropolitan area which does not admit Negro patients, staff Negro doctors, or hire Negro technicians." Hospitals were no longer keeping records of black patients … "They are just patients." The absence of black doctors from hospital staffs was not so much the result of exclusion as of a lack of black doctors. Only 3 percent of the 1,500 medical and osteopathic physicians in Kansas City were blacks.

However, Saint Luke's still maintained a segregated nursing school. The KCAHA representative was critical:

> " … applicants must be female caucasians … which I resent not only for its discrimination against races, but for its discrimination against men. A whole new field of nursing opportunities for men is now open."

A device called a cardioverter restored a man's normal heartbeat at Saint Luke's. His arrhythmia occurred after surgery to repair a hole in his heart. The cardioverter, developed a year earlier, had been applied in 200 cases in Boston and New York with a 90-percent success record. Now Saint Luke's patients were benefiting from the invention. There were also continuing successes by Saint Luke's Code Blue team.

• • • • •

The March board meeting featured another presentation on medical education, this one by Dr. Christopher Thomas. He began by explaining that the interest of KU and MU in a graduate medical-education program at Saint Luke's resulted from concern that if their graduates went out of town for postgraduate work, they might also set up their practices out of town and be lost to the community.

Thomas applauded an educational concept called an "externship." The extern was an undergraduate medical student with elective time but no vacation opportunity, who came to Saint Luke's to gain experience under careful supervision of qualified staff men in lab research, surgery, medicine, CV lab, or ER. It was mutually beneficial: externs earned money, and medical-staff men were assisted in care of their patients. There would be twelve externs at Saint Luke's that summer and twelve to fourteen in the hospital on weekends during the year.

Dr. Don Blim later recalled his own earlier externship experience while a KU medical student:

> "We would come over to Saint Luke's Hospital in the late afternoons, take histories and physicals on the new admissions, and, hopefully, get a chance to make rounds with some of the attending physicians. We all did this, and it provided significant income for starving medical students who were on the G.I. Bill."

Thomas also explained a "clinical clerkship": education for some twenty undergraduates per month in disciplines where the university lacked qualified instructors.

In addition, there were twenty-seven medicine residents.

To provide the necessary volume and variety of clinical experience for its house staff, Saint Luke's had arrangements with other institutions:

> At Jackson County Hospital, one intern per month cared for thirty-five patients hospitalized in a "Saint Luke's ward." Residents also staffed the County Hospital's surgery clinic one morning per week, its medical clinic once per week, and one gynecology clinic per week. In addition, there was the County Hospital's outpatient clinic. The county had treated 700 indigent patients per year in this clinic, and now with Saint Luke's help it was able to treat 7,000 patients.
>
> At Children's Mercy Hospital, one surgical resident and two interns from Saint Luke's staffed the outpatient clinic and helped take night calls. Crittenton patients received increased ob/gyn care from house staff under medical staff supervision, with 135 babies delivered the previous year. And at Richard Cabot Clinic, house staff manned two medicine clinics per week, one surgery clinic per week, one diabetes clinic per week, and one ob/gyn clinic per week.
>
> When tax-supported General Hospital did not fill its quota of interns, Saint Luke's made some of its house staff available to keep one ward open … a tremendous clinical experience.
>
> If hospitalization was required, house-staff physicians made the arrangements, and patients were admitted to Saint Luke's through the teaching program.

All of this was charity care. Jackson County paid travel expenses and 60 percent of the cost of hospitalization. The other costs, including house-staff salaries, were covered by Saint Luke's teaching and charity funds.

Dr. Thomas echoed earlier comments by others concerning the

improved patient care resulting from the presence of house staff at Saint Luke's. Without their residents' constant attendance, for example, the Code Blue operation would not be effective in saving lives.

The staff also provided a constant interchange of ideas with senior physicians regarding patient care. Dr. Hertzler ("Pa" to the house staff) addressed his residents as "Boy" unless they were in hot water, in which case the appellation "Doctor" warned: "beware." Dr. Bohan kept his residents up half the night doing lab work; all of his patients had to undergo a weekly urinalysis. Both left a legacy of well-trained physicians.

The highlight of the April board meeting was another presentation on medical education and the role expected of the foundation in its support, this time by Dr. Mark Dodge. He described the benefits derived by the hospital, reiterating the example of coronary emergency care. Without the house staff's presence to restart a stricken heart, a patient's chances of living "would be practically nil" within three or four minutes. Another example: a patient admitted at 2 a.m. with a bleeding ulcer would be seen at once by house staff and started on his way to diagnosis and treatment, whether or not his personal physician could treat him promptly.

As a teaching hospital, Saint Luke's had an obligation to provide state-of-the-art equipment. It still had the only artificial kidney in Kansas City. This equipment—combined with the hospital's fluid and electrolyte service—had saved fifty to one hundred lives in a decade.

Dr. Dodge did not shrink from cost-shifting—increased charges to financially responsible patients for the hospital's excellent services were necessary to pay for medical education and research. He argued that Saint Luke's should not be afraid to charge patients a premium for the advantages in their care that accrued from these programs. Without a business-like approach to research and development, Saint Luke's would be as outmoded as most of the other community hospitals in Kansas City. Accordingly, Dodge suggested an increase of $4 per day in the room rate to help pay for the teaching program. However, the need for expanded foundation contributions was increasingly evident. If the foundation were properly supported, each year would see decreasing education costs borne by the patient; the foundation's procurement of endowments and development of research grants was just beginning.

• • • • •

The State Board of Nursing issued a list of recommended requirements and regulations that were untenable for private-hospital nursing schools. When Robert Molgren questioned the new requirements, the Missouri Hospital Association appointed a committee to meet with the state board. The board was made aware of the concerns of the nursing schools, doctors, and hospitals about the proposed changes. Similar concerns existed with respect to the policies of the NLN, and Molgren urged the exercise of greater Saint Luke's influence at the national level.

In June, the FTC hearing examiners issued a "discouraging" decision in the protracted blood-bank proceeding, finding restraint of trade on the part of participating organizations. An appeal to the full Commission would be filed, to be followed by an action in federal court if necessary.

· · · · ·

The June 19, 1964, board meeting saw an historic policy change. The Executive Committee had recommended racial integration of the School of Nursing, believing that this progress in race relations could be accomplished "without too much friction." Director Edward S. Washburn offered a motion to approve the recommendation. The motion was seconded, and during discussion it was pointed out that this was a change of the policy which heretofore had permitted only "Caucasian females" in the School of Nursing. Mr. Peet called for a vote. There being dissenting voices heard, he asked for a show of hands. The motion carried by majority vote.

A year later (May 21, 1965) the board minutes contained a significant entry:

> "It was reported that the School of Nursing has accepted two Negro girls for enrollment next fall."

The nursing school was again the principle topic at the August, 1964, board meeting. The National League of Nursing had revoked the school's accreditation, finding fault with its emphasis on clinical experience—particularly its assignment of students to floor duty on weekends and for evening and night shifts. Current trends in nursing education, as reflected by the league's criteria, stressed administrative duties and paperwork at the expense of patient-care experience. This was disturbing to the physicians, especially senior staff members, and to Robert Molgren, who felt that if the program were revised to comply with NLN requirements, it would produce a nurse inferior to the present graduate.

The revocation prompted disappointment but not deep concern. NLN compliance was voluntary, and it would be possible to operate the School of Nursing without league accreditation. Non-accreditation by the NLN had no effect on eligibility to take state board exams or on license reciprocity in other states.

An August article in *The Kansas City Times* discussed the difficulties local hospitals were experiencing in hiring nurses. One example cited: an RN airline stewardess working between flights at Saint Luke's. Reasons listed for the shortage were: forsaking nursing for marriage, low salaries, personnel "piracy" by states that lacked schools of nursing, increased technology resulting in higher entrance standards for nursing schools, high mobility of nurses who were deserting the hospitals that trained them for the armed forces or other more-attractive places, and loss of glamour by the profession.

Congress enacted a bill to support nursing schools financially, with funds to be available by July 1, 1965. Meanwhile, the RN shortage at Saint Luke's persisted.

Fifty Saint Luke's nursing-school graduates took the state board exams … of these there were eleven failures, with psychiatry the stumbling block for the majority. There was limited opportunity for affiliation in psychiatry with other institutions, and the school was dissatisfied with that particular educational experience. However, class enrollment was at an all-time high. The absence of NLN accreditation was no deterrent. There had even been a number of transfers from accredited institutions.

• • • • •

Hospitals utilized a market-based approach to their patient billings, with rates influenced by competing hospitals' charges. Now Blue Cross was introducing a cost-based approach. Conversion to such a system depended on an ability to determine with uniformity various hospital costs, a modification difficult to achieve. However, this approach would make it much easier to explain hospital charges to patients, to third-party payers, to governmental agencies, and to the general public.

Unions had some success in organizing nonprofessional personnel in two Kansas City osteopathic hospitals. And overtures were made to employees of two other hospitals. A meeting was scheduled for officers and administrators of area hospitals.

Mrs. Robert W. Wagstaff announced that the auxiliary would sponsor a "Holly Ball" in December, to be a biennial event. This was the revival of a tradition after a hiatus of many years. The ball cleared some $16,000. Kitty Wagstaff would head this premier social event for the next thirty years, as chairperson and later as honorary chairperson.

TWENTY-THREE
1965-1967

teaching beds and cost-shifting ... Medicare ...
Robert W. Wagstaff ... KU affiliation ...
Charles C. Lindstrom ... dialysis

*H*ousekeeping was a frequent source of complaints in hospitals. At the January, 1965, board meeting, Lucian Lane proposed creating a housekeeping committee, saying he recently had received criticism of housekeeping at Saint Luke's. Robert Molgren was asked to investigate and report. Bishop Welles said he received surprisingly few complaints and many compliments despite all of the construction work at the Hospital.

In February, Molgren responded to Lucian Lane's earlier comments. A major portion of the reported housekeeping difficulties at Saint Luke's arose from distorted or incomplete facts, and Molgren related various controls and inspection procedures followed at the hospital.

H.O. Peet announced in March the receipt of $7,500 from the William Volker Fund, to defray the cost of a cobalt unit ... an important weapon in the fight against cancer.

Plans for the Annex included converting the former day nursery to an animal laboratory, and this was approved subject to review of costs.

Robert Molgren reported on recent Congressional actions that would have significant future consequences for Saint Luke's, including Taft-Hartley labor-law amendments, unemployment insurance, minimum-wage increase and, most of all, the enactment of Medicare.

Dr. William Mixson, medical staff president, and his colleagues endorsed the establishment of twenty-five teaching beds as necessary to the medical-education program, particularly to a full four-year surgery residency. These beds were provided in stages; sixteen beds activated July 1 and the remainder one year later. The foundation furnished financial support.

Expanded foundation support was needed. Saint Luke's was committed to medical education and its benefits ... an outstanding medical staff and better patient care. But it was difficult to defray the program's ever-increasing expense. Simply raising rates would have a far-reaching effect on Blue Cross and other third-party payers and on the cost of hospitalization to the general public. It also would lead to eventual scrutiny by the federal government under the impending Medicare program.

The usual summer nursing shortage was alleviated by the use of part-time RNs, some help from student nurses, and double shifts. Of the School of Nursing's graduating class of seventy-five—the largest ever—thirty-two remained at Saint Luke's; of these, twenty-four accepted the unpopular evening and night shifts, where the most critical deficiencies existed.

• • • • •

On July 30, 1965, President Lyndon B. Johnson signed Medicare into law over the strenuous objection of the American Medical Association. Recognizing Harry Truman's earlier support for such legislation, LBJ traveled to nearby Independence, Missouri, to affix his signature to the law while the former president and Mrs. Truman looked on approvingly. They were presented with the first Medicare cards.

Part A of Medicare provided compulsory hospital insurance and Part B provided for payment of physicians' fees. It was predictable that a sharp increase in the use of medical services would result, in outpatient activity as well as inpatient volume.

Medicare emulated the Blue Cross practice of paying hospitals on the basis of cost and introduced a generous initial formula for calculating those costs. One consequence not fully anticipated at the time: the Medicare program and its promise of free-flowing dollars spawned a for-profit hospital sector that looms large a few decades later. Health care providers who treat patients in order to make money compete with those who make money in order to treat patients.

• • • • •

In September, Herbert O. Peet submitted his resignation as first and executive vice president, asking to be elected an honorary director. Robert W. Wagstaff, then the second vice president, was thereupon elected to succeed him as lay head of the hospital.

It became apparent that the prestige of the School of Nursing was suffering from lack of NLN accreditation; the joint-conference committee recommended the expenditure of every effort to regain NLN accreditation, even though restrictions on student nurses' duty hours would "aggravate our nursing shortage for the present and will increase the cost of operating the hospital." The committee also wanted to reactivate and upgrade programs for training LPNs, nurse aides, surgical technicians, and other paramedical personnel in light of the acute RN shortage.

Board treasurer C. Humbert Tinsman urged that increased expense for teaching beds be subsidized by philanthropy rather than by patient-care revenues. The foundation was providing some financial assistance and hoped to contribute much more in the future. Director Max L. Marshall, with an insurance-man's insight, supported Tinsman, saying that there would be repercussions with third-party payers should hospitals continue to raise the costs of their services.

A new chapel off the lobby was opened. Due to an engineering miscalculation, the level of Wornall Road outside the chapel's west wall had to be adjusted and the road was torn up for a considerable time.

During October and November, various floors of the new East Wing were opened for patient care.

By November, the foundation had $100,000 in its treasury and was becoming "increasingly active."

The noble experiment in medical-staff integration lauded by Dr. Starks Williams came to an end. Queen of the World Hospital was "deactivated." Its bed occupancy had slipped badly, and the few remaining patients were almost all black. In December, Wagstaff announced that St. Andrew's parish was sponsoring a clinic in the Queen of the World building and that Saint Luke's physicians would staff the clinic one day per week.

A special budget presentation directed attention to the imponderables to result from Medicare implementation in 1966:

> "Under the Medicare program hospital charges will be subject to some type of control, the details of which are not yet known. It is possible that not all of the costs included in our budget will be allowable under the program."

Accordingly the budget now being adopted for 1966 would have to be reworked sometime before July 1, 1966.

• • • • •

The federal government introduced its first health planning legislation in 1966. The expanding federal stake in financing health care delivery dictated this. Once Uncle Sam engaged in health planning, it would become difficult to obtain funding for voluntary community planning groups because of duplication, even though the new law made community efforts optional.

The first edict of the federal Department of Health, Education, and Welfare under Medicare dealt with hospital-based physician reimbursement. At Saint Luke's, this applied to the pathologists and radiologists. Two billings would be required, one for hospital services (payable out of the hospital insurance fund) and the other for the physician's services (to be paid from the physician insurance fund). If the patient had not elected Part B Medicare coverage for physician cost, he would be billed directly for the doctor's fee.

The hospital board approved a contract with the school district of Kansas City, Missouri, to establish an LPN training course at Saint Luke's, commencing in February with an initial student enrollment of twenty-five. The board also joined the Medical Plaza Corporation in obtaining a zoning change that would permit additional stories for the neighboring medical office building.

The medical staff established a Utilization Committee, the first such committee in the Kansas City area. Its purpose was to reduce patients' length of stay to the absolute minimum, consistent with good medical care. As a result of the committee's efforts, the length of stay of Blue Cross patients was about the same as uninsured patients at Saint Luke's, the only Kansas City hospital with this experience. The committee attracted the attention of hospitals around the country.

Attempting to alleviate the nursing shortage, the hospital instituted a refresher course for retired RNs desiring to return to practice and a training course for senior aides, and hired fourteen ward clerks to help RNs in the evening. The LPN training program was delayed pending approval by the State Board of Nursing. Meanwhile, staff doctors were made aware of the severity of the nursing problem. This resulted in nine office nurses accepting part-time employment at the hospital as well as the employment of the wife of one board member and the wives of two medical-staff members. Physician practice habits also were modified to eliminate time-consuming details plaguing nurses on evening and night shifts, and nursing services were restructured to relieve RNs of some of their duties. The shortage was aggravated by the addition of more beds and the accrediting bodies' restrictions on the number of duty hours to be performed by student nurses.

In April, a meeting was convened at General Hospital to inform other area hospitals of financial problems at General and what this might mean to the city's private hospitals. The meeting's sponsors hoped to generate support for increased city funding of General; otherwise there would be reduced inpatient, outpatient, and emergency care there and an increase in indigent cases at private hospitals. However, despite their efforts, General Hospital was forced to reduce bed utilization from 700 to 400 because of lack of funds; private hospitals took up the slack in indigent care in the community.

About 60 percent of hospitals applying for Medicare participation were rejected. One reason: participation in Medicare required compliance with the Civil Rights Act of 1964. The application inquired as to the degree of racial integration of hospital employees, medical staff, and patients.

In accordance with a recommendation from a U.S. Public Health Service team that surveyed Saint Luke's with regard to civil-rights compliance, the following resolution was adopted:

> "Resolved, That Saint Luke's Hospital shall continue to operate in such a manner as to provide medical care on a nondiscriminatory basis to all persons without regard to race, creed, or national origin. It also shall be the policy of this hospital to be nondiscriminatory in assignment and use of all facilities and in administration of all employment policies."

Robert Molgren then signed the hospital's application for approval as a provider of services to Medicare patients.

Saint Luke's was approved as a Medicare provider, and within a few months Medicare patients comprised 33 percent of Saint Luke's patient load. The hospital's patients of Medicare age increased 5 percent in the short time following the approval of the program.

• • • • •

A July 6, 1966, article in the *Kansas City Times* announced a new relationship between Saint Luke's and KU—a limited agreement to share facilities and teaching staffs as part of their graduate medical-education programs. The joint effort was confined to internal medicine and psychiatry. Saint Luke's did not offer a residency in psychiatry, and the affiliation allowed Saint Luke's residents and interns to take instruction in that specialty on an elective basis at the Medical Center. The associate dean at KU noted that the two institutions had shared educational programs for many years.

A KU publication minimized the new arrangement, characterizing it as but one of several such relationships. It declared: "Another affiliation between a community hospital and KUMC began July 1." It noted that KU had affiliated programs with Menorah, the VA Hospital in Kansas City, Children's Mercy, and General as well as the Wadsworth VA Hospital in Leavenworth, Kansas, and three hospitals in Wichita.

• • • • •

The resignations of Robert A. Molgren as Executive Director and Miss Jeanne Stickels as director of nursing and nursing education were presented to the board. In August, Charles C. Lindstrom of Minneapolis, Minnesota, was hired as the new administrative head of the hospital with the title of Executive Director. Chuck Lindstrom would perform in an exemplary manner at Saint Luke's for the next twenty-eight years.

Three ophthalmologists received staff appointments in anticipation of a residency program in ophthalmology.

An innovative minimal-care unit was opened "as a means to alleviate staffing problems by concentrating in one area those patients needing lesser patient care."

At the board's October meeting, medical staff president Dr. Andrew Mitchell—a urologist—described the use being made of the artificial kidney machine and the expansion of the dialysis program that additional funding could support. The foundation was investigating whether grant money for this purpose might be available through the U.S. Public Health Service. A subsequent gift of $20,000 from Richard C. Green helped establish a dialysis room within the hospital.

The Episcopal diocese wished to establish an extended-care facility in the Saint Luke's neighborhood, and the hospital offered to seek a site for this purpose. A "Joint Committee on the Diocesan Home for the Aging Chronically Ill" was formed ... its members included several clergy, Drs. Dodge, Mitchell, and Thomas, and influential board members.

• • • • •

The arrival of Dr. James Crockett at Saint Luke's signaled a higher level of cardiology expertise at the hospital. In November, Saint Luke's embarked on seven four-week courses in intensive coronary care under the direction of Dr. Crockett for nurses from all over the country. Enrollment for all sessions was full.

The FTC issued its final order in the Blood Bank case, directing Saint Luke's Hospital (among others) to cease and desist from engaging in anti-competitive activities. An appeal to the federal Eighth Circuit Court of Appeals was authorized.

The new administrator, Charles Lindstrom, attacked the nursing short-age, recommending increases in the salaries of nurses, the payment of overtime, and premium-pay increases for evening and night shifts as well as shift-differential increases for LPNs, aides, and orderlies. In support of his recommendations he cited increased militancy on the part of nurses and the nationwide salary increases in response. He also noted the criti-cal problems experienced at Saint Luke's in covering nursing shifts around the clock. The proposed increases were approved.

The 1967 hospital budget reflected the "dramatic" raises given to RNs, as well as a new minimum wage of $1.40 per hour. Blue Cross was noti-fied of a substantial escalation in Saint Luke's charges—approximately 10 to 15 percent.

The gracious service provided by small kitchens on each floor of the hospital was discontinued. No longer would food be brought to patients' floors in bulk in a heated cart, with orders then carefully filled with each patient's prescribed menu. And no longer would eggs or toast or meat be specially cooked to individual taste and presented on fine china decorat-ed with that floor's particular design or pattern.

The second biennial Holly Ball was held on December 9 in the Hotel Muehlebach's Imperial Ballroom. Proceeds covered the cost of one teach-ing bed for a year.

Occupancy for 1966 averaged 80 percent. In December, 1966, 42 per-cent of the adult patient days were Medicare-generated. The impact of

Medicare was largely felt in average length of stay ... it increased by one entire day in just six months.

Saint Luke's Children's Hospital benefited from fourteen auxiliary volunteers and a group of "candy stripers"—forty high school girls who spent 788 hours during the summer months working with 1,281 children in crafts and occupational therapy.

Paul Meyer of the Dickson-Diveley Clinic was the new medical-staff president. For years he donned a Santa Claus suit and added holiday cheer to the stark hospital halls. One icy Christmas Eve, twelve slip-and-fall cases crowded the orthopaedic clinic, where jolly old Saint Nick fitted them with casts.

Dr. Meyer informed the board that the effect of Medicare on utilization was a constant challenge for the medical staff, but that due largely to the efforts of the physicians' Utilization Committee, Saint Luke's length of stay was shorter than that of any other local hospital. Nevertheless, February occupancy was 89.3 percent compared to the previous February's 85.1 percent.

In April, 1967, Charles Lindstrom reported a continuing increase in patient days. This generated a need for more timely business information, both financial and statistical, and the hospital employed a director for the data processing center. The present system was being redesigned to meet future needs ... the computer age was dawning.

Saint Luke's was the only hospital in Missouri or Kansas to fill its intern-matching quota in 1967. Twenty new interns came from seven different medical schools ... ten from nearby KU and, surprisingly, four from distant Saskatchewan University in Canada.

The nursing crisis was somewhat alleviated by the hospital's recruitment of seventeen out of twenty-three graduates from its first class of practical nurses.

• • • • •

Dr. Louis Scarpellino, the hospital's chief of radiology for twenty-five years, died. He was replaced by Dr. Gerhard Schottman, who would serve the hospital well for the next quarter century.

At the May meeting, the board was advised that the Joint Conference Committee had placed "Doctor 8B-5" on probation. As a result of litigation elsewhere, the need for due process in disciplining doctors was gaining recognition; the medical staff's procedures had proven to be "quite clumsy" in this case and were to be reviewed by the physicians.

During April, 42.1 percent of the medical-surgical days were accumulated by Medicare patients. The percentage would be identical in May and again in July.

A brochure celebrating National Hospital Week noted:

"Saint Luke's Hospital conducts a three-year program for nursing students and now has a total enrollment of 170 girls—and boys!"

As the result of a Midwest Research Institute recommendation, menu planning by computer was initiated in June; this would produce substantial savings in the cost of food. And the board approved the auxiliary's proposed "Baby Photography" service. At subsequent board meetings there were reports of the considerable profits generated by the auxiliary from this project.

A bolt of lightning struck a hospital chimney early on September 13, 1967, showering the new ambulance drive with debris and breaking windows, but no one was injured. However, this led the board to purchase a $3.5 million business-interruption insurance policy.

The LPN class conducted in concert with the School District of Kansas City graduated its second class, nineteen, and half of them remained at Saint Luke's.

The National League of Nursing submitted a report on its observations during a recent visit. It was favorable, and there was optimism over the prospects for restored NLN accreditation. But formal notification would wait until the first of the year.

• • • • •

Newspaper reports reflected an absence of community awareness of the "good work" being done at Saint Luke's with artificial kidneys. Publicity was needed. In October an article in *The Star* remedied this. It reported that an estimated twenty-five persons per year were stricken with kidney failure in the Kansas City area, and there were hospital facilities for only a fraction of these. The crux of the problem was money—a lack of funds for technicians, machines, and hospital space. Under existing circumstances it was necessary to select the patients most likely to survive, described by the reporter as "a delicate, heart-breaking task that most physicians find generally distasteful but necessary." Programs to train patients to operate their own machines at home were not widely available, but General Hospital and Saint Luke's hoped to develop such systems. Both hospitals had been doing chronic kidney dialysis for several years. Saint Luke's had four machines and treated five patients per week.

Use of the machines was at best a "holding action," pending the perfection of kidney transplants. The obstacle to successful transplantation lay in the body's immune system, which put up a protective battle against the foreign organ. Almost all of the work done at Saint Luke's was supported by private money, mostly by Saint Luke's Foundation for Medical Education and Research.

• • • • •

The first prenatal instruction in the Kansas City area was offered to expectant West Side mothers by Saint Luke's Dr. David Broderick in 1915. Now, on October 10, 1967, formal prenatal classes were initiated at Saint Luke's to inform prospective parents about prenatal and postnatal care and acquaint them with the hospital. Films were shown explaining pregnancy, birth, and care of the newborn. There was also a defense of the high cost of health care.

The Insurance Committee, chaired by Herbert A. Sloan, thought that Saint Luke's should continue to carry general liability insurance; the Legal Committee, chaired by Dick Woods, believed it to be an unnecessary expense in light of Missouri's charitable-immunity doctrine. The Executive Committee sided with the Legal Committee, and the board followed suit. The board did, however, adopt a resolution providing for indemnification by the hospital of Mr. Lindstrom and his administrative associates.

In November, 1967, the board accepted the generous gift from the Dickson-Diveley Clinic of the clinic building and its underlying land. The two-story structure was immediately adjacent to the hospital. Its staff of four physicians and twenty-five employees moved to the Medical Plaza Building.

Earlier that year Drs. William F. Benson and Theodore L. Sandow, both Mayo-trained orthopaedic surgeons, had joined Dr. Frank Williams of Dickson-Diveley and Dr. William Medlicott to form the Midwest Orthopaedic Clinic.

Foundation assets now amounted to approximately $200,000. RN staffing was a comfortable 96 percent, and a continuing shortage of LPNs would be relieved as more students graduated from the Licensed Practical Nursing Program.

Diploma nursing schools such as Saint Luke's still had their champions in Washington, where two helpful bills were pending. The objectives were to boost training resources and staff by annual grants, provide tuition for pupils, and improve library resources with matching-fund grants. Directors were encouraged to write Missouri and Kansas congressmen and senators in support.

An ailing Ferd Helwig announced his retirement as director of pathology effective December 31, 1967. Dr. Helwig suffered from emphysema, the result of smoking, and the labored breathing of this revered physician was painful for his colleagues to witness. The board adopted a resolution at its December meeting naming the hospital's medical laboratories in his honor.

Saint Luke's Hospital was advised by the National League of Nursing on December 21, 1967, that its School of Nursing was accredited for three years. This would not only aid recruitment but allow the school to become eligible for certain government grants.

The foundation presented its first guest lecturer, Dr. John S. Stehlin of Baylor College of Medicine, who spoke on "Regional Chemotherapy for Cancer."

A post-year memorandum from Charles Lindstrom stated that Medicare patients comprised 43.2 percent of the medical-surgical patient days in 1967, a 5-percent Medicare increase for the year. For the same period the hospital received $2,465,875 from Medicare.

TWENTY-FOUR
1968-1969

experimental medicine ... hyperbaric bed ...
UMKC School of Medicine ... Board Presidency ...
Everett P. O'Neal ... kidney transplantation ...
Homer McWilliams ... MACHPA

*I*n January, 1968, the board directed that procedures for admission to the medical staff be reviewed in light of recent litigation elsewhere in the country, fomented by physicians denied hospital privileges. A protocol evolved devoting greater attention to due-process considerations.

The hospital continued to be congested. Nonemergency patients were on a waiting list—five to six weeks for surgery—and the need for expanded acute-care facilities was evident. Robert Wagstaff declared: "Saint Luke's Hospital will soon have to move ahead to satisfy the community and medical-staff needs."

A comprehensive study by the Midwest Research Institute in 1967 had forecast a need for 3,327 more beds in the area by 1980. Meanwhile, an addition of eleven beds on Main 5 had increased Saint Luke's bed complement from 462 to 473. Despite the addition the hospital's medical-surgical occupancy was 98 percent.

A consultant recommended the addition of 230 beds at Saint Luke's— eighty-five general acute, fifteen surgical ICU, eighty extended care, twenty minimal care, and thirty psychiatric. The addition of psychiatric services was urged in order to "offer a well-balanced program" to patients and house staff alike. Expansion of educational programs also was recommended.

Staffing in nursing remained good, although an influenza "episode" left the hospital understaffed for several days. Increased authority was given to head nurses; they now could dismiss subordinates who were not performing properly.

Dr. Mark Dodge, now medical-staff president, pressed for more teaching beds to attract young physicians and keep the teaching program strong. Also, the hospital needed a department of psychiatry to provide a well-rounded medical education for the house staff. And there was a lack of proper housing and clinical research facilities.

The fact that the physician complement at Saint Luke's continued to be heavily weighted on the side of white Christians led to suspicions that medical-staff admission procedures were biased. The matter was discussed at the March board meeting:

"During the last week an inspector from the Department of Health, Education and Welfare, Office of Civil Rights, visited with Mr. Lindstrom regarding a formal complaint against Saint Luke's Hospital regarding the admission of Negro and Jewish physicians to the medical staff. Although there are members of both groups on the medical staff, the number is thought to be so small as to be labeled 'tokenism.' Mr. Wagstaff stated that the Board and Medical Staff must use a thoughtful approach to these problems so as not to impede the development and future progress of the hospital."

The Midwest had fared poorly in matching interns for the coming year—many medical-school graduates were entering the military directly from college and completing their internship there. And the West Coast was attracting others. However, Saint Luke's would have thirteen of the twenty it sought, comparing favorably with other hospitals in Missouri and Kansas.

The administrative resident for the next year was a Roman Catholic nun, Sister Maria Brandner, from the University of Minnesota. Upon completion of her program, she received a master's degree in hospital administration.

Applications were submitted for federal grants of $24,000 through the Nursing Education Opportunity Grant Program and $60,000 through the Nursing Student Loan Program. The grants, financing nursing education, were received in due course.

• • • • •

At its February, 1968, meeting, the board was advised of a joint research project with Midwest Research Institute involving experimental dog surgery. The research was conducted by thoracic surgeons Clarke L. Henry and Patrick G. Graham in the Annex laboratory, with MRI underwriting all expenses and assuming responsibility for housing the animals. The program aided efforts to develop an artificial heart, by testing artificial aortas in the abdomens of dogs. It was conducted discreetly, to avoid protests by animal-rights activists.

Interest in the development of an artificial heart continued at the March board meeting:

> "Dr. (Robert) Allen gave a brief presentation of some of the new surgical techniques being practiced at Saint Luke's hospital in the area of thoracic surgery. He commented that it is most likely that artificial heart transplants offer the greatest potential for the future rather than the transplanting of hearts from human to human."

· · · · ·

On April 4, 1968, Martin Luther King was assassinated in Memphis, Tennessee. This ignited riots all over the country. Kansas City was not spared. The effect on Saint Luke's, and staff response, were noted:

> "The performance of our hospital employees during the recent episode of civil disorder was extremely gratifying. Employees in key positions were asked to remain at their stations until such time as relief people were present. This was done in each instance and when necessary, nursing personnel worked double shifts to cover patient needs. Student nurses helped prepare patients for bed when the complement of nurse aides fell below minimum needs. Due to the curfew and the fact that some of our employees lived in the area of strife, each night during the week 15-20 employees slept at the hospital. The nursing supervisory personnel performed exceptionally well and worked many extra hours to insure that the nursing needs of the institution were met. The performance of our staff was extremely pleasing, but not surprising."

During the week following the riots, Public Service Employees Local #1132 attempted to organize nonprofessional employees in Kansas City hospitals. The same union had struck the KU Medical Center the previous year, closing it down for several days. Area hospitals now banded together to resist the union threat, employing Harry Browne, dean of labor-relations attorneys in Kansas City, to advise them. At Saint Luke's, the activities of nurse aides and housekeeping employees were especially scrutinized with a view to eliminating union sympathizers. This could have consequences, as was noted at the May board meeting:

> "Usually when a reduction of staff occurs there is a slump in morale in the department for a short time, which is followed by a resurgence of good morale as those remaining realize they are capable of performing the duties. It is also evident in most instances that employees are generally happier when they are doing a full day's work."

• • • • •

A hyperbaric bed, looking much like a single-passenger space ship, arrived from England ... "the only one of its kind in the country." It was obtained through the efforts of Dr. Leslie Thompson with funds supplied by the Saint Luke's Foundation. In the course of treatment, the patient was sealed inside the bed's chamber, which was then filled with pure oxygen. Studies indicated that the equipment might be helpful in improving the survival rate of some heart-attack victims. There were also other applications of the bed.

Rose Marie Hilker, R.N., M.A., was named Director of Nursing and would serve in that capacity for the next seventeen years.

At the annual meeting of the American Nurses Association, several actions were taken with ominous financial overtones for Saint Luke's. A salary resolution set base salary for graduates of diploma schools such as Saint Luke's at $7,500. A second resolution abolished the ANA's "no strike" policy, in effect since the late 1940s. The association also recognized state nurses' associations as bargaining agents for nurses in negotiating salaries and fringe benefits.

Through a program financed by the U.S. Public Health Service, 5,943 indigent patients were screened for cancer at Saint Luke's from September 1, 1966, to December 31, 1967. Ninety-three of those examined actually had the disease.

Six patients were currently receiving dialysis treatment at home, and a grant was sought to support this cost-effective program.

Saint Luke's outpatient teaching program treated 3,600 adults at the Richard Cabot Clinic (that clinic also generated an additional 2,000 - 2,500 pediatric patients), 10,300 at Jackson County Hospital, and 4,600 at Saint Luke's own clinic.

The annual board-medical staff dinner was held June 26, 1968. Robert Wagstaff's remarks were reported in a subsequent *Kansas City Times* article. Among other things, he predicted: "By 1990 the hospital will have a bed capacity of 1,000 and will double its ambulatory and special-care units."

• • • • •

Apparently, physicians would be available to staff an expanded Saint Luke's Hospital. President Lyndon B. Johnson announced that the country needed 50,000 more doctors and would pay medical schools to train them. More than eighty new schools would be built, and it was proposed that a new medical school at the University of Missouri-Kansas City be among them.

In July, Robert Wagstaff suggested that Saint Luke's serve as "back-up" hospital for the proposed UMKC medical school. Dr. Ralph Hall explained that the proper clinical facilities in medicine and surgery must be available in the community to facilitate the establishment of such a medical school, and while General Hospital could be used for obstetrical cases, Children's Mercy for pediatric cases, and the Psychiatric Receiving Center for psychiatry, a hospital was needed that could supply 250 medical-surgical beds and could demonstrate a willingness to underwrite a residency program, support the concept of teaching beds in a private hospital, and provide student laboratory facilities. The alternatives to a Kansas City medical school were either enlargement of the University of Missouri's school in Columbia or financial support for other existing colleges in the state, to wit, Washington University and St. Louis University, both in St. Louis, and for two colleges of osteopathy.

The board approved the proposed affiliation in principle with a resolution expressing "the hospital's willingness to designate such necessary teaching beds, programs, services, facilities and financial support as required for the successful exploration, development, and operation of such medical-school relationships."

Meanwhile in July representatives of the Saint Luke's medical staff joined Charles Lindstrom in a visit to Hartford Hospital in Hartford, Connecticut, one of the first community hospitals to offer a formal medical-education program. That hospital was preparing to affiliate with Connecticut's first school of medicine, to be opened in the fall. Valuable information was gained from the site visit.

The Jackson County Medical Society in August designated Saint Luke's as the "back-up" hospital for the University of Missouri-Kansas City. A careful review by two medical-school deans, consulted by the Medical Society, facilitated Saint Luke's selection.

The Saint Luke's house organ, *Intercom,* applauded:

> "In terms of education, patient care, and research benefits, the relationship promises to be of immense value to Saint Luke's Hospital and the community. It opens up a new era in the hospital's medical-education program, paving the way for expansion of teaching facilities ... Saint Luke's research program, so greatly supported by the Saint Luke's Foundation for Medical Education and Research, will be enhanced."

The medical residents would all be graduate physicians; the role of Saint Luke's Hospital in undergraduate education, if any, had yet to be determined.

Negotiation of the affiliation agreement's terms extended into October and beyond. Meanwhile, with the promise of Saint Luke's back-up role, Kansas City was named as the location for the new medical school. And the MU affiliation generated excitement and interest among the members of the medical staff.

• • • • •

A board motion to add two more floors to the East Wing passed unanimously, as did a motion to construct a fifteen-bed surgical ICU as soon as possible. These additions were recommended by the hospital's consultants, James A. Hamilton & Associates, who also recommended that Saint Luke's size on the existing site be limited to 700 beds. Charles Lindstrom contacted the Hospital Planning Council to advise them of the proposed additions to the hospital, and the Council requested a study to assess the proposal's impact on the community.

Dr. Willem Kolff discussed with the medical staff the feasibility of organ transplants. He reviewed the issues relative to organ transplants and stated that Saint Luke's was qualified to perform organ transplants and particularly kidney transplants in the very near future. Having a dialysis unit was considered essential for these programs. In a community such as Kansas City there was probably the need for twenty-five kidney transplants per year. The cost of such a procedure was great, and the life expectancy of the patients following transplants was relatively short ... kidney transplants were in their infancy.

Dr. Dodge reported to the board that preliminary work to learn the techniques of kidney transplantation was being carried out in the dog laboratory of the hospital. He stated that the performance of heart transplants at Saint Luke's Hospital was also a possibility in the near future. The surgical techniques were relatively simple, but the legal and ethical questions were complex.

After discussion the board enthusiastically pledged their support of organ transplants at Saint Luke's.

December, 1968, saw another successful biennial Holly Ball. Kitty Wagstaff was assisted by Mrs. Kenneth M. Dubach, auxiliary president, as co-chair.

• • • • •

At the December board meeting, Bishop Welles declared his conviction that the president of the hospital should be a layman, with the bishop of the diocese serving as board chairman. The necessary revisions to the hospital's Articles of Incorporation and bylaws were prepared. Robert W. Wagstaff became the first lay president of Saint Luke's Hospital.

Meanwhile, questions were raised again about the ethnic composition of the Saint Luke's medical staff:

> "Mr. Wagstaff reported that the Missouri Commission on Human Rights has asked for information regarding nondiscriminatory policies and practices relative to physicians on the Medical Staff of Saint Luke's Hospital. Mr. Wagstaff stated that we will meet to discuss our position with them."

Wagstaff and Charles Lindstrom subsequently met with a representative of the Missouri Commission on Human Rights. The commission sought assurances that physicians would be added to Saint Luke's medical staff without regard to race, creed, or ethnic background. A list of qualifications was sought, to be applied equally and fairly. Answers were prepared to questions raised by the commission as well as a written statement regarding the hospital's policies and practices relative to nondiscrimination.

Everett P. O'Neal, a prominent black Episcopalian, was elected to the Saint Luke's board on January 17, 1969.

Negotiations culminated in purchase of the three-and-a-half-acre Sweet Lumber Company tract lying immediately to the north of the hospital across 43rd Street. Opportunities to acquire a tract of this size for land-locked Saint Luke's were rare.

The Eighth Circuit Court of Appeals issued a favorable opinion in the Blood Bank case, reversing the earlier adverse Order of the Federal Trade Commission and vindicating area hospitals, including Saint Luke's. After a six-year struggle, the case finally was laid to rest.

An ice and snow storm in February, 1969, prevented many hospital personnel from reporting for work. Nursing students were pressed into service to assist in the care of patients. The result was "an interesting and rewarding experience for the students."

Occupancy in February was 90 percent, with Medicare patients accounting for 43.4 percent. Several young physicians reportedly were shifting the bulk of their practices to other hospitals because of a five-week wait for routine patient admissions. This was a serious problem—these doctors represented the hospital's future. All emergency cases were cared for immediately, although patients might be held in the emergency room and recovery room if beds were not available elsewhere.

A formal pediatric nursing affiliation with Children's Mercy Hospital was established to enrich the experience of nursing students. Both the National League of Nursing and the Missouri State Board of Nursing had encouraged this relationship because of the small pediatric census at Saint Luke's. The board also approved affiliation with Avila College for a first-year nursing student's academic work, with Avila providing thirty-three credit hours of basic science and other general-education credits. These college credits could be applied later toward a nursing degree.

It was important to teach young physicians to provide outpatient care, in an attempt to keep patients out of the hospital. The work load in the outpatient resident clinics—Saint Luke's, Richard Cabot, and Jackson County Hospital—was increasing rapidly. Also, General Hospital wanted Saint Luke's help to supplement its extremely limited house staff. The total number of clinic visits at the hospital and at the offices of attending staff exceeded one million per year; grant money might be available to support outpatient programs.

In April the Saint Luke's Foundation approved the purchase of a second hyperbaric bed for the hospital.

• • • • •

Dr. Raymond Stockton, a urologist, presented to the board a brief history of the hemodialysis program at Saint Luke's and plans for its future. He noted that the program, which began in 1955, was first used to treat patients with acute renal failure and had proved to be very successful. It was later extended to patients with chronic kidney diseases. Then in 1966, more sophisticated artificial kidneys were added to the program, and through the outstanding efforts of Dr. Christopher Y. Thomas, a thousand dialyses subsequently were performed. The next step, largely an economy measure, was a program of home dialysis.

Now the hospital prepared to perform kidney transplants, and Dr. Thomas again provided splendid leadership. There were methods to prevent organ rejection, but success depended largely upon close tissue typing. The primary problem, however, was the supply of organs. In any event, it seemed certain to Dr. Stockton that "kidney transplants will be done at Saint Luke's in the very near future."

Dr. Stockton was clairvoyant; on April 29, a two-hour operation transplanted a healthy kidney into a 30-year-old mother at Saint Luke's, immediately following the donor's death at Bethany Hospital. Dr. Thomas performed the operation. The tissue matches were perfect. The Saint Luke's team had perfected their technique on laboratory animals and had visited transplant centers. Much of this was financed by the Saint Luke's Foundation. Dr. Thomas later advised that the recipient was no longer in isolation, was walking, and had a "great desire to return to her family and home."

A kidney transplant had been performed at Saint Luke's in 1963, but the patient lived for just twenty-three days. And another had been performed between twin brothers at KU in 1958, but the recipient died in a few months. Now surgical techniques and methods of thwarting rejection had improved, and the Saint Luke's operation was the beginning of a highly successful kidney-transplantation program.

• • • • •

The Episcopal Diocesan Council was advised of a hospital-board decision against proceeding with an extended-care facility for the present, even though this would result in the use elsewhere in the state of diocesan money designated for such a facility.

• • • • •

A May, 1969, article in *The Kansas City Star* reported a lawsuit testing the terms of the $8 million hospital trust fund established by the last will and testament of Homer McWilliams. Mr. McWilliams, a bachelor, had died at age ninety-eight after spending the last eighteen years of his life in Kansas City's Trinity Lutheran Hospital. In the case *(First National Bank vs. Danforth),* the bank sought construction of McWilliams' will, "so that all hospitals ... may have an equal opportunity to establish in court their eligibility to receive these funds."

The terms of the will restricted the McWilliams beneficiaries to non-profit "Protestant Christian" hospitals contributing to the maintenance, support, and care of patients "born of white parents in the United States of America." Despite the restrictions, almost every hospital in the area claimed eligibility.

In a decision dated January 13, 1975, the Missouri Supreme Court would decide that the income from the trust should go to Saint Luke's, Trinity, Baptist Medical Center, and Independence Regional Hospital, all of which qualified as Protestant Christian hospitals. In the course of its decision, the court noted that each of the qualifying hospitals admittedly did not limit its patients to those born of white parents in the United States but rather cared for sick and infirm patients of all races, colors, creeds, and nationalities. However, the court ruled that this did not disqualify them from benefiting from the trust funds.

Since then, Saint Luke's has received significant sums over a period of many years from the trustee bank (now Boatmen's First National Bank). This money is used for the hospital's high-risk maternal and infant-care program, serving residents of Jackson County. The obstetrical teaching patients who benefit from the McWilliams trust are indeed of every possible religious creed (or of no religious persuasion whatsoever) and of all races, colors, and nationalities. Thus, a trust established under an instrument with clearly discriminatory racial and religious overtones is in fact applied for the benefit of all and sundry, and black mothers and babies receive a disproportionately large amount of the resultant care.

• • • • •

The AMA recommended the admission of osteopaths to hospital staffs. Two osteopathic students sought to enroll in Saint Luke's intern program, but their applications were filed too late for the upcoming class.

The following year, osteopathic students were included in the Saint Luke's Match.

Dr. James E. Keeler, now president of the medical staff, advised the board in May, 1969, that the MU negotiations were nearing completion. The medical-education programs would be managed through UMKC, but persons appointed to Saint Luke's staff as a result of the program also would have to be approved by the Saint Luke's medical staff and board.

In September, in joint Operating Engineers' negotiations with Menorah, Research, and St. Joseph, the Saint Luke's representatives voted to reject a union proposal that the other three found acceptable. Saint Luke's later reluctantly agreed to it since independent action was impractical.

Four kidney transplants had been performed by September. And the home-dialysis program received a $45,000 grant from the Missouri Regional Medical Program, in response to a grant application submitted by the foundation.

A site-visitation team from MU visited Saint Luke's; their favorable report facilitated federal funding for the UMKC medical school.

Dr. E. Grey Dimond, UMKC Provost for Health Sciences, presented his concepts of medical education to a general meeting of the medical staff. The most controversial feature was a proposal to engage in an accelerated program combining B.A. and M.D. degrees. The Saint Luke's physicians were reported to be "very excited" about Dr. Dimond's ideas and looking forward to the affiliation with the university.

In its recruiting efforts, the nursing department began advertising in *The Call,* Kansas City's black-owned and published newspaper, as well as in suburban newspapers.

The Legal Committee reversed its previous position and recommended the purchase of general liability insurance to protect the hospital and its personnel. They were influenced by the likely elimination of the charitable-immunity doctrine in Missouri, either by judicial decision or by legislation. The insurance was approved. The quoted premium was not exorbitant but would in all likelihood be doubled or tripled should the protective doctrine in fact be abolished.

A Midwest Research Institute report concluded that Saint Luke's could expand to 950 beds on its present site, including an extended-care unit of 200 beds. A pending master plan for such expansion would cost $20 million to implement. The report supported the program from the standpoint of community need and hospital financial strength, and could be used to seek the necessary financing.

Two classes of LPNs graduated annually through the program with the Kansas City school district. ICU staffing was greatly improved, with personnel receiving training in coronary care through the Kansas Regional Medical Program.

The KCAHA presented salary guidelines to the various hospitals, recommending minimum wages and starting nursing salaries, and also deferring the date for implementing adjustments until later in the year rather than the customary March 1.

Teaching beds continued to be financially burdensome. Support for the patient care came from three sources: the foundation, endowment funds, and hospital operating income. However, the program was worth the cost. The availability of teaching beds had led to the development of an outstanding staff and attracted interns and residents. Patients accepted for the teaching program were selected primarily for educational value, with the choice being made by Dr. Hall and the referring attending staff. Bishop Welles stated that the program began with indigent Episcopal families referred by clergymen; solvent private patients were not considered for house-staff attention.

As feared, the charitable-immunity doctrine was struck down on November 10 by the Missouri Supreme Court. The hospital would experience significant liability-insurance premium increases.

A November *Kansas City Star* article announced a $3 million construction contract for a four-story addition to the eight-story East Wing, adding 144 patient beds and bringing the hospital's size to more than 600 beds. The hospital planned a second phase to commence the following year involving various departmental expansions and some extended-care facilities.

• • • • •

The National Health Planning and Resource Development Act established organizations called Health Systems Agencies or HSAs, as the basis for a new planning system. HSAs would control large blocks of monies, and there was competition among several local organizations for designation as the HSA for the Kansas City area. These included the KCAHA's Hospital Planning Council. The Stanford Research Agency recommended Mid-America Comprehensive Health Planning Agency (MACHPA), and

MACHPA subsequently was named the Kansas City-area planning agency.

By December, 1969, MACHPA was in business with an enormous board of sixty directors. At a luncheon of presidents of major Kansas City hospitals, it was agreed that institutions financing their own development should use the agency only as a reference and information source and not solicit its approval before pursuing their plans. However, approval should be sought if a proposed expansion involved federal funding or a community fund-raising effort. The presidents also agreed that planning should be employed to assure adequate services and facilities in the Kansas City area and avoid unnecessary duplication, although it was contended that "some duplication and rivalry between the hospitals is good."

• • • • •

The board approved the affiliation agreement with MU, formally establishing Saint Luke's as the back-up hospital for the new medical school planned for UMKC. It would be a year-to-year relationship, however. The Missouri legislature voted $1,026,100 for construction of the new facility, and the federal government contributed an additional $8,856,843.

TWENTY-FIVE
1970-1972

Spencer Center ... Wilbur Mills ...
price increases ... Dr. William A. Reed ...
Dr. Gerald Touhy ... Arthur Anton Vogel ...
challenge to tax exemption ... Hometel

O n January 21, 1970, occupancy was 96 percent, with 385 of the 388 medical-surgical beds occupied, most ICU beds filled, and forty-eight of fifty-one obstetrical beds and twenty-one of thirty pediatric beds occupied. For the year 1969, Saint Luke's teaching program had served 1,102 inpatients and 3,824 outpatients, with most of the expense being covered by patient-care revenues.

A Medicare auditor from the Missouri Department of Health reviewed the hospital's utilization plan in February and pronounced himself satisfied that it complied with federal regulations.

A reduction in nursing-school tuition was the apparent reason for a large increase in the school's enrollment ... eighty-nine in 1970 versus forty-two the previous year.

In February, another $45,000 grant from the Missouri Regional Medical Program was received in support of home dialysis training for patients.

At a building-campaign banquet on March 17, a goal of $3 million was announced to fund the first phase of a $7 million expansion program. The remaining $4 million would be financed by debt. The improvements would include 144 new beds, a fifteen-bed surgical-ICU unit, and a fifteen-bed coronary-care unit. Dr. E. Grey Dimond said that plans for the new UMKC medical school were on schedule, and declared: "The facilities you're discussing are the strength that will make this a great medical school." At the same time a gift by Mrs. Kenneth Spencer from the Kenneth A. and Helen F. Spencer Foundation was announced, for the purpose of constructing a building to house an auditorium and library. The structure would be called The Helen F. Spencer Center for Education.

The new center would be across the street from the hospital and require demolition of the Nearly New Shop. The auxiliary would have to relocate.

The board was advised at its March meeting that for the first time since 1967 the hospital's complement of twenty interns was filled.

Also in March, board member Lucian Lane asked about the racial make-up of the medical staff.

> "In response to a question by Mr. Lane, Dr. Hibbard stated that he knew of no physician who had been refused medical-staff appointment due to ethnic considerations. He also stated that he did not think the Medical Staff should go out and seek persons from other ethnic groups which are not now members of our staff."

Dr. Hibbard chaired a KCAHA committee reviewing emergency services in the Kansas City area. Although Saint Luke's was identified as a major resource, capable of handling any crisis, it was designated a "minor facility" due to its outlying geographic location.

In April, 1970, the Louetta M. Cowden Fund presented the foundation with a gift of $500,000. This was unrelated to the pending capital-fund drive but rather reflected a continuing interest in medical education and research.

In May, 1970, the School of Nursing at Saint Luke's graduated its first male nurse. He reported complete acceptance from female classmates and patients … "That was my biggest surprise … ."

• • • • •

An article in the May 15 *Kansas City Times* stated that Wilbur Mills, chairman of the House Ways and Means Committee, was proposing sweeping changes in the Medicare and Medicaid programs aimed at controlling "skyrocketing hospital costs." His proposals followed a "scathing report" on the two programs issued by the Senate Finance Committee in February. Since Medicare and Medicaid had gone into effect in 1966, the cost of the nation's hospital services had risen more than four times as fast as the cost-of-living index. The two programs would cost about $13 billion in 1970, some $5 billion more than was anticipated when they were enacted.

A review of Saint Luke's experience over the ten years preceding the adoption of Medicare reflects a gradual escalation in the hospital's charges—most frequently at an annual rate of one dollar per day per bed.

The primary cause of these pre-Medicare increases was wage and salary boosts. Hospital pay scales never were overly generous, and during this decade payroll raises were triggered by periodic changes in the minimum wage prescribed by federal law, with a ripple effect throughout employee ranks. The same was true to a lesser extent of employee benefits negotiated with the Operating Engineers' Union, such as holidays, funeral leave, and insurance. However, hospitals are very labor-intensive institutions, and even in the high-tech, major teaching hospital that is Saint Luke's, the cost of wage and salary adjustments outstrips the cost of advances in equipment, facilities, and programs, not to mention supplies and other expenses.

During Medicare's first six months, the percent of total occupancy by patients aged 65 or older in Saint Luke's grew by 5 percent, to 33 percent of the total. The following year, 1967, the Medicare percentage exploded—to 42 percent. In 1969, it was 43.4 percent in February, 44.3 percent in April, 45.3 percent in October, and 47.2 percent in December. The trend continued in 1970, when, not coincidentally, June set a new total occupancy record for Saint Luke's—98.7 percent

The rate of increase in hospital charges also escalated rapidly.

The Wilbur Mills tirade in May, 1970, did nothing to repress hospital charges generally, and Saint Luke's was no exception. The 1971 operating budget presented to the board in October, 1970, proposed rate increases that would produce an increase of $14.22 per patient day in total costs over the 1970 budgeted costs. This included a room-rate increase of $6 per day and an ICU increase of $10 per day as well as selected rate increases among other revenue-producing centers.

Advanced medical procedures helped to fuel the rate increases. At Saint Luke's these included an electroencephalogram for tracing brain waves and a gastrointestinal laboratory (formerly available only in the Medical Plaza building).

• • • • •

An article in *The Kansas City Times* discussed pressures to create more group practices. Occupants of the Medical Plaza Building were in the forefront of this movement: "The physicians in that building are already in a group practice, a 'referral' group practice" ... the doctors there usually directed patients to specialists in the building rather than elsewhere. Other group practices described in the article included the Mayo Clinic and the Kaiser Foundation Health Plan.

Although the board might rely on the medical staff to provide high-quality care at the hospital, the ultimate accountability for such care was not delegable and rested with the directors. However, it was comforting to know that the medical staff could avail itself of peer review, problem-oriented medical charts, and medical audits to insure excellence. The medical audits established standards and measured the physicians against those standards. It was a continuous system, based within the hospital.

American medicine was under fire as overly specialized and overbuilt, and lacking in concern for the inner-city poor. However, Saint Luke's needed its specialists as a tertiary-care institution and its facilities to accommodate the patient load. And the hospital provided access to health care without regard to socio-economic status—to a considerable extent through its emergency room. Outpatient services in the emergency area had increased rapidly in recent years, making it difficult for physicians to handle patient demands there. The ER functioned as an outpatient clinic where the public could come for medical attention, with the evening hours and weekends being especially convenient for members of one-car families. Unfortunately, it was a constant struggle to find employees willing to work at those times.

Saint Luke's personnel assisted in transferring patients from the old Children's Mercy Hospital to its new Midtown building on what came to be known as "Hospital Hill." Satisfaction was expressed with the new facilities for area children.

• • • • •

William A. Reed, a thoracic surgeon based at the KU Medical Center, joined the medical staff in December, 1970. Dr. Reed's open-heart surgery results were outstanding, and his appointment constituted a giant step forward for Saint Luke's heart program. The continuing success of cardiology and the excellence of Reed's cardiac-surgery program strained hospital resources but led to nationally recognized, high-quality cardiac surgery at Saint Luke's and ultimately to the hospital's superlative heart-transplantation program.

Hubert H. Bell and Lynn H. Kindred were approved for medical-staff appointments, further strengthening the hospital's cardiology program.

• • • • •

At the hospital's annual meeting in January, 1971, Maxwell Berry and Blaine Z. Hibbard became the first area physicians elected directors of a private nonprofit hospital when they joined the Saint Luke's board. Dr. Hibbard was president of the medical staff at the time; both were staunch Episcopalians.

Blaine Hibbard deserved much of the credit for the early utilization measures initiated by Saint Luke's physicians, and he was active at the national level in the American Society of Internal Medicine.

• • • • •

To provide complete surgical- and obstetrical-anesthesia coverage, Saint Luke's needed the services of a full-time anesthesiologist. Dr. Hibbard reported in February that "the addition of Dr. Gerald Touhy as Chief of Anesthesia has been of great assistance to the operation and function of our surgery department." Dr. Touhy established a nurses' training program ("certified registered nurse assistant") and a residency, both in anesthesiology.

• • • • •

The occupancy crunch continued, with "extreme shortage of beds and waiting lists for admission." No favoritism was shown; patients were accepted on a "first come, first served" basis.

In April the board was advised that students in the hospital's LPN Program ranked in the ninety-eighth percentile in an NLN achievement test. And twenty-five of the forty-three graduating seniors in the school were staying on at Saint Luke's. Meanwhile, the hospital received an additional $22,000 for the nursing scholarship and loan funds from the federal government, bringing the total from that source to $48,000.

At the May meeting it was reported that national health insurance programs were being considered in Washington. "The inevitability of such health insurance systems was noted." The idea of health care as a matter of right, not privilege, had gained general acceptance. Dr. Hibbard and Dr. Blim testified before the U.S. Chamber of Commerce in Washington, D.C., later in the year on the subject, and Dr. Blim also testified before Wilbur Mills and his House Ways and Means Committee on the elements of national health insurance that should be present to protect children.

The Kidney Center at Saint Luke's was one of twelve such facilities in the country, made possible largely through a U.S. Public Health Service grant. Of the ninety-seven dialysis patients treated at Saint Luke's from 1966 through April, 1971, fifty-three were from Missouri and forty-two from Kansas; and surprisingly, one each from New York and Pennsylvania. The main purpose of the centers was to train people for home dialysis while they awaited transplants, a more permanent solution to renal disease. In June, 1971, a thirty-seven-year-old man who had been receiving treatment on the artificial kidney since March became the fifteenth kidney-transplant recipient at Saint Luke's.

•••••

Arthur Anton Vogel, a Harvard Ph.D. and internationally acclaimed theologian, became Bishop Coadjutor of the Diocese on May 25, 1971, insuring that he would succeed to the office of Diocesan Bishop and the hospital board chairmanship following the retirement of Bishop Welles, scheduled for December 31, 1972.

In August, 1971, President Richard M. Nixon imposed a general wage-price freeze that was modified in December to single out hospital charges for special treatment ... limiting them to a 6-percent increase.

The Nixon administration's national health strategy—like that of President Lyndon B. Johnson before him—called for an increase in the supply of physicians. Medical schools would benefit.

Despite the fact that the new UMKC medical-school building would not be completed until 1974, Dr. E. Grey Dimond welcomed ninety-four students to the school's first classes in the fall of 1971.

Although the affiliation agreement with the University was approved, financial negotiations were conducted annually, and medical education at Saint Luke's remained autonomous and independent to a considerable extent. Educational programs fell into three categories: integrated (with certification and recognition vested entirely in the university); coordinated (with parallel programs and an active exchange of students); and independent (each institution conducting its own program). The university established standards for the integrated and coordinated programs. The hospital's director of medical education was subject to mutual approval by the university and the hospital; Dr. Ralph Hall was the initial director.

Saint Luke's absorbed many of its other trainees. Of the eight radiology technicians graduating from Saint Luke's in August, four remained at the hospital as registered X ray technicians. Five of the six medical-technology students graduating in June also stayed.

· · · · ·

At an October 13, 1971, meeting, the Mid-American Comprehensive Health Planning Agency board adopted a resolution imposing a moratorium on additional acute-care beds in Kansas City. A letter to Charles Lindstrom from MACHPA, also dated October 13, explained that there was general overbedding and overutilization in Kansas City (Saint Luke's "occupancy crunch" was an exception). MACHPA accurately forecast that utilization of acute beds would decline as a result of increased emphasis on outpatient services, financial incentives promoting alternatives, and stringent utilization-review programs. It also correctly predicted that an HMO under development in the area would ultimately reduce bed demand. In November, Lindstrom reported that the moratorium did not preclude replacement of existing beds or the development of satellite services by existing institutions; but meanwhile Blue Cross would not pay increased hospital charges for new beds lacking MACHPA approval.

A committee of the medical staff, appointed to study "division of beds between medical and surgical patients," investigated the possibility of further division—dedicating beds throughout the hospital according to types of service. The result was a proposal for allocation of 171 beds to internal medicine, 145 for surgical patients, 67 to the ob/gyn department, 30 to pediatric patients, and 60 to the orthopaedic surgeons. Dr. Reed expressed concern that his cardiac-surgery program be allowed room to grow, and it was recommended that any such allocation be postponed until after the new East units were opened.

At the January, 1972, annual meeting of members, Saint Luke's accepted the provisions of the Missouri Not For Profit Corporation Law, modern legislation that allowed greater flexibility in the hospital's governance. Also the number of directors was reduced to the present fifty-one from the previous high of fifty-four. At the annual board meeting, the bylaws were amended to create the office of vice chairman of the board—to be occupied by Coadjutor Bishop Vogel.

During 1972, when the four additional floors of the East Wing begun in 1970 were completed—increasing the number of patient-care beds by 147 to a total of 634—the medical staff was able to implement the division of services into medical, surgical, orthopaedic, obstetrical, and pediatric floors—an important step in providing specialized nursing care for patients.

The Dickson-Diveley group temporarily moved their outpatient crippled children, participants in the Missouri Crippled Children's Program, from the hospital to the Dickson-Diveley offices because of parking problems—problems exacerbated by the opening of new beds in the East Wing.

Contracts were signed for additional construction—Northeast and East of East buildings, to be built on a cost-plus-fee basis with a guaranteed maximum of $4,641,608. Occupancy of the existing expanded facility was 900 patient days below budget, but was expected to build slowly as the institution grew into the recently completed additional floors. The new construction program would add surgical suites, improving the low census. There also would be new medical ICU units and a new postoperative recovery room, as well as facilities for pathology and diagnostic radiology.

Cost-containment efforts focused on reduced length of hospital stays, economies of scale in purchases, and scrutiny for unnecessary tests; these initiatives enabled Saint Luke's to conform with the Nixon price freeze without adversely affecting the hospital budget.

The Urban League of Kansas City awarded a certificate to Saint Luke's for making strides toward equality of opportunity—board member Everett O'Neal was instrumental in achieving this recognition.

Dr. Raymond Stockton, now medical-staff president, offered a lengthy report on the relationship with the UMKC medical school, noting that third- and fourth-year undergraduate students now rotated through Saint Luke's medical-education program for elective subjects in medicine. Dr. Ralph Hall was assistant dean of undergraduate education, and Dr. Max Berry was named associate provost for graduate medical education. Approximately forty Saint Luke's doctors were associated with the new school.

A joint committee was formed by Saint Luke's and the doctors' Medical Plaza Corporation to eliminate duplication of services performed at both locations.

In April, the board approved a $9 million loan, concentrating in a single transaction the financing required for previous and pending construction work. Also in April, the Helen F. Spencer Center for Education was dedicated, with an open house to introduce the public to the magnificent new center. The building included a spacious boardroom where the directors would henceforth conduct the hospital's business.

At a May meeting of the Saint Luke's Hospital Foundation, a fund-raising goal of $20 million was announced to endow medical education and research efforts at Saint Luke's. However, despite recognition of the need, no campaign was initiated to implement this goal. It would be another two decades before an effort of such magnitude was mounted to relieve patient-care revenues of this burden.

At the same meeting Dr. William A. Reed stated that, of the last 400 open-heart surgical patients at Saint Luke's, 97 percent had been restored to good health.

> "He said that there are 25 hospitals in the country performing as many coronary-bypass operations as Saint Luke's, but that the hospital 'is second to none in results.'"

● ● ● ● ●

Bishop Welles announced that he would retire to Maine earlier than previously announced and gave his "farewell address" at the May board meeting. He recited all of the changes since April 23, 1950, when he attended his first directors' meeting in the old boardroom. He named the seventeen laymen who, with him, comprised that earlier board, noted that hospital assets then approximated $3,500,000, and quoted from board minutes stating that "the work of healing the sick in mind, body, and soul is one of the things that no one reading the New Testament could doubt was the center of our Lord's life and ministry." He praised the way the board continued to successfully cope with "the more intricate, complicated, and sophisticated operational problems and requirements of Saint Luke's." But he devoted the major part of his remarks to urging the board to continue to entrust responsibility for the hospital's future to laymen rather than to health care professionals. His concluding sentence:

"In summation I believe that the Presidency and policy-making decision power should remain in the hands of unpaid, voluntary laymen of the Episcopal Diocese of West Missouri if Saint Luke's is to continue its quality and existence."

His address was followed by an ovation.

• • • • •

Expectations were great respecting the level of occupancy in the hospital: Grant Cowherd, Chairman of the Budget Committee, described the hospital's 83-percent occupancy over the first four months of 1972 as "disappointing but not fatal." In May, with the average occupancy at 85.6 percent in medical-surgical, a program was implemented to reduce operational expenses by 7 percent ... the hospital had budgeted for even higher occupancy, and occupancy directly affected profit in those less-complicated times.

Because of the early retirement and departure from the city of Bishop Welles, Bishop Vogel presided at the June, 1972, board meeting. At the conclusion of the meeting, the new chairman praised Saint Luke's as a "hospital that cares."

There was much discussion of pending labor negotiations with the Operating Engineers Union representing the hospital's maintenance and engineering employees. Saint Luke's was preparing to "take a strike" if necessary, by training nonunion boiler operators and drawing up contingency plans. There also was concern over the possibility of other union organizational activity, which led to the adoption of a policy statement forthrightly declaring:

"Any organization which imposes the threat of labor disputes and the possibility of walkouts, shutdowns, or strikes ... has no place in hospitals, where the care of patients depends upon the stability and continuity of a work force."

It was reported in June that a leasing arrangement with Hometels Corporation of America was under negotiation for the construction of a hotel on the former Sweet Lumber Company property lying across 43rd street to the north of the hospital.

• • • • •

Congress extended Medicare benefits to victims of end-stage renal disease under age sixty-five, a development that greatly increased the volume of dialysis treatments and the national cost of health care. But now providers were relieved of the heavy burden of "playing God," in deciding which patients should receive the life-saving treatment.

Saint Luke's dialysis and kidney transplantation program experienced an operating deficit, largely attributable to the high cost of transplantation. A June article in *The Kansas City Star* noted variances in prices charged by the city's three kidney-dialysis units, ranging from a high at Research Hospital for a single treatment of $200 to a low at Saint Luke's of $120: KU charged $160. The article began:

> "Chronic kidney disease patients in Kansas City apparently need a shopper's guide to help them determine where they can most economically have their lives saved."

Saint Luke's Dr. Chris Thomas commented:

> "There are always two sides in every business endeavor. Either you're on the side of constant cost reduction or you're on the side of continually passing the costs to the consumer. We have got to start getting some economy into this field."

• • • • •

At the September board meeting, President Robert Wagstaff commented on a recent *Star* article noting the expansion of Kansas City-area hospitals and attributing higher costs to patients as the result. Earlier in the year, Congress had given HEW the power to deny full Medicare reimbursement to hospitals for capital investments that lacked planning-agency approval; Wagstaff, a rugged individualist, pointed out that hospitals were increasingly coming under the control of various planning agencies, a development that might interfere with Saint Luke's ability to "determine our own destiny."

Responding to Wagstaff, Dr. Stockton encouraged cooperation with the local Mid-America Comprehensive Health Planning Agency. Its head, Kenneth Bopp, recently had informed the medical staff of the goals and objectives of that agency and provided a better understanding of it. Dr. Stockton briefly reviewed the reason for MACHPA's creation, its area of geographic jurisdiction, and its financial support by the federal government and by local matching contributions. He pointed out that

MACHPA was recognized as an authority on health matters with which consumers and health providers alike must work in the future. For example, General Motors and Ford executives conferred with the agency about proposed projects, and MACHPA was instrumental in influencing major changes in one of them. Planning agencies were increasing in number and in authority over hospital decisions, and Saint Luke's should acknowledge their existence and work with them in a cooperative spirit.

Wagstaff replied that although the hospital's board might confront and resist planning agencies on certain critical issues and policy decisions, Saint Luke's must and would change with the times and situations. He agreed that there were costly and needless waste and duplication in the health care field that had to be brought under control, but the controls should not "impinge on our basic freedoms of institutional operation."

The Executive Committee approved a revision of the affiliation contract with UMKC, insuring that Saint Luke's expense reimbursement was commensurate with the hospital's commitment to the medical-education program.

The nursing school enjoyed its greatest enrollment ever, with eighty-four freshmen, eighty juniors, and sixty seniors.

In October a delegation of Chinese physicians visited Kansas City, thanks to the efforts of Dr. E. Grey Dimond and the regard in which he was held by the Chinese. They had lunch at Saint Luke's, the only private hospital on their American agenda. Security was total. It was a warm and informative occasion, with many expressions of mutual respect and descriptions by the Chinese of their medical practices in rural communities.

• • • • •

An October hearing before the State Tax Commission resulted from a Jackson County challenge of the tax-exempt status of Saint Luke's, Research, and Baptist hospitals. The principle at stake was major, but the immediate monetary consequences were seductively minor. Saint Luke's equipment and fixtures were assessed a token $100 by the Jackson County Board of Equalization; the same was true of Baptist Hospital's real estate and of Research Hospital's residence quarters for nurses and physicians. The issue was charity care, and Robert Wagstaff, the first witness, testified that in his twenty years on the hospital board he never had known of a deviation from the board's unwritten policy against excluding patients on financial grounds. Charles Lindstrom's subsequent testimony confirmed this.

The county's challenge contended that because financially responsible patients were required to pay for medical treatment, the three hospitals were not charitable institutions. There also was evidence that the hospitals had realized net operating profits before depreciation (which went into their reserves for growth and development) and that the value of charitable services in relation to total patient billings for Research and Baptist was small (figures from Saint Luke's were not available.) Also, it rankled the county to be charged for indigent patients transferred by it to Saint Luke's for further treatment.

The KCAHA and the Missouri Hospital Association, while not parties to the proceeding, were permitted to express their concern that a bad legal precedent might be established with statewide or even nationwide repercussions, if the taxes were imposed.

The tax commission took the case under advisement.

Later in the month a New York lawyer, speaking at a meeting of the National Association for Hospital Development, said that taxing hospital property would reverse fifty years of congressional policy as well as challenge recent Supreme Court decisions. A church-related hospital should be particularly protected because of decisions maintaining the separation of church and state ... "the power to tax is the power to destroy."

• • • • •

A new three-year contract—much more satisfactory to the hospital than in the past—was signed with the Operating Engineers' Union representing Saint Luke's maintenance workers and engineers.

The Hometel contract was signed, and in November the City Plan Commission recommended approval of an eight-story, 215-room hotel. It would meet a need for nearby accommodations—30 percent of Saint Luke's patients came from outside the five-county area, and it was difficult for rural families in particular to visit patients. However, approximately two years passed before the hotel was in business and the hospital realized any income or lodging benefits from the project. In the meantime, the auxiliary's Nearly New Shop, which had moved to the Sweet site when the Spencer Center was built, would have to move again.

There were staffing problems in the ER, and two solutions were under consideration: 1) hire a full-time ER physician; 2) utilize additional residents and interns to staff the area, improving coverage at all hours.

There was vindication on the tax front. It was reported at the December, 1972, meeting that the State Tax Commission had ruled that Saint Luke's and the other two hospitals were not liable to pay property taxes. However, the county filed an appeal, a routine recourse not taken very seriously at the time by the hospital community.

A description of the extent of Saint Luke's educational efforts in 1972 noted that some 400 students studied at the hospital annually (including more than sixty residents and interns) in medicine, surgery, obstetrics and gynecology, orthopaedics, pathology, radiology, and nursing. The surgery program became affiliated with the UMKC medical school that year, and Saint Luke's department of surgery has been a teaching forum for UMKC medical students ever since. The hospital also served as an affiliated clinical facility for university programs in pharmacy, physical therapy, medical technology and hospital administration. A formal educational program in X ray technology was offered, and a year-long LPN program was conducted in affiliation with the Kansas City, Missouri, Board of Education. There were affiliations with the Wadsworth VA Hospital, Jackson County Hospital, Children's Mercy Hospital, Richard Cabot Clinic (where more than half the patients were seen by Saint Luke's house staff and attending staff), the Florence Crittenton Home, Avila College, Western Missouri Mental Health Center, and the University of Missouri (for physical therapy).

TWENTY-SIX
1973

price controls ... informed consent ...
Don's World of Beef ... CV program growth

*P*resident Nixon's wage-and-salary guidelines complicated fiscal planning for the hospital. For most of the nation's economy, price controls ended in January, 1973, but regulations remained in place for the health care sector, where conditions—in the opinion of the Nixon administration—threatened renewed inflation. At Saint Luke's, a contract was agreed upon with the hospital's pathologists, but their compensation exceeded the guidelines and was being revised. The hospital prepared a 1973 budget report for the federal government ... although it did not need approval prior to implementation, it was required to report the budget figures because some items were subject to "exception reporting" even though cost justified under the guidelines.

Saint Luke's total occupancy in 1972 was 85.4 percent (the board had budgeted for an even higher 88 percent), with med-surg at 84.7 percent, obstetrical at 73.5 percent, pediatric at 50.1 percent and ICU at 84.9 percent. For 1973, occupancy at 84 percent was budgeted.

Charles H. Price II was elected to the Saint Luke's board in January, 1973. He brought distinction to the hospital by remaining a director while serving as U.S. Ambassador to Belgium and later Great Britain.

The prohibition against tobacco's use in the hospital had long since been lifted. However, it was reported at the February, 1973, meeting of the board that the Executive Committee recommended banning the sale of cigarettes on hospital premises, based upon medical-staff condemnation of smoking. There was considerable concern expressed over the effect of this on hospital patients addicted to nicotine, but the ban was approved as consistent with the hospital's goal of providing good patient care. Smoking was not yet prohibited, but patients would have to find some off-campus source of tobacco. They did not have to go far, however ... cigarette machines were installed in the medical office building across the street!

Occupancy in early 1973 was much above the budgeted 84 percent. If it continued at that level, the hospital's financial performance might exceed price-control limitations. Accordingly, a scheduled room-rate increase was limited to $4, even though Blue Cross already had approved a $5 raise. Meanwhile, the federal guidelines' restrictions were of great concern, and both the KCAHA and the Missouri Hospital Association were developing recommendations for transmittal to Washington. Another concern: reduced federal support of nurses' training, including scholarship loans ... private financing would have to compensate.

The medical staff reviewed the hospital's system for prevention of Medicare abuse. Any possibility of Medicare disallowance of payments for unwarranted care or excessive hospital stay had serious potential; approximately 42 percent of Saint Luke's medical-surgical patients and one-third of its revenues were generated by Medicare.

The staff also investigated the reasons for the long waiting lists for hospital admission, noting an increasing number of emergencies that avoided the regular admission procedure ... in January, 1973, 70 percent of all admissions were on an emergency basis, reflecting large-scale circumvention of the normal admission process.

A new interdenominational chaplaincy training program involving three students under the directorship of Chaplain Jerry Kolb was approved.

Some comparative fifty-year statistics for Saint Luke's were compiled in March of 1973, reflecting a bed increase from 150 in 1923 to 634 in 1973; annual admissions up from 2,872 to 25,135; births from 306 to 2,284; total days' treatment from 28,980 to 202,471; average length of stay reduced from 11 to 8.1 days; and significant gains in the volume of surgical procedures, lab tests, and X ray examinations.

After long deliberation, the nursing school decided to change the freshman year's academic affiliation from suburban Avila College to the more accessible Penn Valley Junior College.

Coping with price controls was a complicated business. The IRS had approved the hospital's 1973 price structure, including the anticipated net gain. An April change in price-control regulations enabled the hospital to redesignate the base years used to compute its allowable net gain, permitting a bottom-line increase to 3.93 percent from 2.98 percent.

An audit of charges for laboratory services by the nation's hospitals was conducted by the Government Accounting Office. The GAO was critical of pathologists' compensation in particular. Chief radiologist Gerhard Schottman cited the criticism as a good example of increased pressure on health care providers to control costs. He reviewed the various methods of reimbursing hospital-based physicians and stressed the importance for all segments of the health care industry to carefully monitor costs and revise cost-accounting procedures to reflect in patients' charges the true costs of the services rendered. But he also acknowledged that health care costs would continue to escalate despite economies because of specialized medical training, increased public demands and expectations, automation, and improved medical technology.

The Florence Crittenton Home contemplated relocation, and Saint Luke's was assured the first opportunity to purchase the Home's existing facility on the hospital campus.

Because of Saint Luke's Hill-Burton participation some eighteen years earlier, the Missouri Division of Health reminded the hospital of an obligation to provide "a reasonable volume of free care" under revised Hill-Burton regulations. Elsewhere, attorneys for the poor sought to enforce that right to free care. There were three options available under the guidelines. The one chosen by Saint Luke's: to provide annually until March 7, 1976, uncompensated care for persons unable to pay, equivalent to at least 10 percent of the sum of all Hill-Burton grant support received within the past twenty years. For Saint Luke's, this amounted to $115,829.17 annually—a level of charity care regularly exceeded by the hospital.

Patients began to insist that doctors and hospitals share more information with them before accepting treatment, and there evolved the doctrine of "informed consent." At its May meeting, the board was advised of a legal obligation to advise patients, especially those undergoing surgery, of the risks and the alternatives to their proposed care. Because of the loss of hospital charitable immunity to malpractice suits, this informed-consent issue had financial implications; the legal liability of directors was undergoing review. The medical staff also was discussing the issue thoroughly. A disclosure requirement was adopted, and it is now an uncontroversial and accepted practice, but at the time of implementation it caused some consternation among Saint Luke's doctors. Surgeons in particular were reluctant to unnecessarily alarm their patients.

• • • • •

Competition among hospitals grew more intense. Shawnee Mission, St. Joseph, and Olathe hospitals opposed construction of a 400-bed hospital in suburban Overland Park, Kansas, by for-profit Extendicare Corporation. The local planning agency, MACHPA, refused to approve the project but was overruled by a Kansas appeals panel. Extendicare then filed a retaliatory suit to halt proposed expansion by Shawnee Mission Hospital. Both cases were pending in Johnson County District Court. Saint Luke's was supportive of Shawnee Mission (hoping for reciprocal support of its own expansion plans), but not to the extent of intervention in the litigation. Kansas had no certificate of need requirement, and the new hospital was subsequently allowed.

A representative of MACHPA, in response to an inquiry regarding conflicts of interest by MACHPA members, acknowledged:

> "There are probably 50 vested interests in MACHPA ... In some of those meetings there are issues that some of those folks shouldn't be voting on. But the bylaws don't control that. Some new bylaws might remove some of the problems if they are approved."

• • • • •

Ernst & Ernst, a national accounting firm, conducted a study for Connecticut's Hartford Hospital of the financial impact of medical education and concluded that it would cost a teaching hospital more to pay for the services provided by the students than the cost of the medical education program. But there was a serious flaw: the study did not include the considerable expense of teaching beds.

The Long-Range Planning Committee reviewed studies by Midwest Research Institute and James A. Hamilton & Associates. One thousand beds now seemed indicated for Saint Luke's at its present location. An existing need was seen for specialized beds rather than for general medical-surgical beds. There was also an immediate need to expand ER services.

The studies noted various trends and methods in health care delivery, including comprehensive, prepaid health care plans such as Kaiser-Permanente and the Harvard Community Health plan. There also was increasing affiliation and networking among health care providers.

Pickets posted by the Communications Workers of America, seeking recognition at Menorah Hospital, were withdrawn by the union, but the organizational effort continued. Meanwhile, the National Nurses' Association was considering a campaign to represent area nurses. Charles Lindstrom advised that the hospital had a plan to combat such activity but predicted that in the next five years all Kansas City hospitals would probably be at the bargaining table despite their resistance to union organization. His pessimism was misguided, however—union attempts to organize hospital employees in Kansas City were unsuccessful.

Mr. Barnes Romine had acquired control of part of the parking lot on Wornall Road across from the hospital's main entrance, and announced plans to build a "Don's World of Beef" fast-food restaurant at that location. It was Mr. Romine's contention that hospital employees should be offered a convenient fast-food alternative to the fare available in the hospital cafeteria or the auxiliary's coffee shop … he told Robert Wagstaff that he was doing him a "huge favor." Romine appeared undeterred by the facts that the property's existing zoning did not permit this enterprise, the hospital was strongly opposed, and the Medical Plaza Corporation was equally adamant. After a stormy meeting with Romine, in which an irate Robert Wagstaff was supported by the Medical Plaza's Dr. Arthur W. Robinson, Wagstaff was able to advise the board that "Mr. Romine was now aware of the difficulties of pursuing the proposed restaurant construction." That brought the matter to an end.

Dr. E. Grey Dimond suggested a novel system of area-wide residency for the UMKC medical school—with residents visiting a consortium of several different hospitals for their training. Saint Luke's agreed to participate in this educational experiment but also maintained its own independent residency programs.

For many months, plans for expansion of obstetrics, pediatrics, the cardiovascular lab, and ER were discussed at Saint Luke's. The medical staff was fully supportive, and a presentation was prepared for MACHPA. The cost: almost $6 million. Dr. Schottman stated that if these improvements could not be effected, programs in cardiology and renal dialysis might have to be curtailed for lack of space. Letters of support were promised by Children's Mercy, the UMKC medical school, and the Jackson County Medical Society. The Kidder, Peabody investment banking house believed that the project was financially feasible, but the hospital's ability to support a construction loan was clouded by the government's economic-stabilization program. New federal guidelines on hospital pricing were in the offing, and once these were issued Kidder could determine whether or not the loan was feasible.

• • • • •

The success of the heart program introduced additional pressures on Saint Luke's facilities and resources. There was "a delicate and difficult problem" in scheduling cardiac surgery because of other demands on the operating rooms. The new CV lab would increase even further the demand for heart operations, and it might be necessary to place a limit on those procedures or lose the support of other surgeons at Saint Luke's.

Dr. Maxwell Berry stated that there appeared to be two problems: "One is that Saint Luke's has a very good general-surgical staff, and the other is that we also have one of the best cardiovascular teams in the country." Dr. Berry added that he "hoped we don't upset the balance of the surgical service."

The pressures to accommodate the rapidly expanding cardiac-surgery and cardiology programs at the hospital would in a few years lead to development of Saint Luke's Mid America Heart Institute.

In early November, the federal Cost of Living Council announced further price-control regulations tailored specifically for the health care industry. These were scheduled to take effect January 1, 1974. Hospitals would be allowed a 7-percent increase per year in charges for each admission if the number of admissions remained the same and an increase of 6 percent for overall outpatient charges. Employees remained subject to a 5.5-percent limitation on salary increases, plus .7 percent on fringe benefits. Charles Lindstrom described these as "very prohibitive guidelines" that favored outpatient care. The American Protestant Hospital Association and the American Catholic Hospital Association joined to fight the restrictions. The two associations represented 57 percent of the hospital beds in America.

• • • • •

An editorial in the November 19, 1973, issue of the *Journal of the American Medical Association* suggested that a trend toward training additional physicians more quickly might produce inferior doctors. This was of considerable local interest because an accelerated program combining the B.A. and M.D. degrees was the novel premise upon which the new UMKC School of Medicine rested, accepting students directly from high school. UMKC's vice chancellor for health affairs said the current criticism was based more on emotion than fact. "These programs are all so new it is difficult to evaluate their value yet," he said. He also noted that most students accepted by UMKC actually had completed college.

The accelerated programs originally were seen as a way to meet what had been billed by the government as a shortage of physicians. But now the pendulum had swung the other way. The Graduate Medical Education National Advisory Committee predicted a surplus of physicians and recommended that medical schools downsize and reduce class numbers. HEW's Assistant Secretary for Health suggested that the Nixon Administration might reduce or even terminate federal aid for health-manpower education in order to avert a possible surplus of physicians.

In an interview, the president of the American Academy of Family Physicians strongly disagreed about physician surplus, saying that in fact there was a shortage—at least in rural and ghetto areas and in the ranks of family physicians. He noted an urgent need for programs to train family physicians to provide primary care, and he stated that the federal government should prepare "to use its financial muscle to pressure medical schools to produce more generalists, such as the family physician."

Congressional action, to subject hospitals to the provisions of the Taft-Hartley labor law, was deferred in reaction to New York strikes that left patients in that city abandoned by a walkout of hospital employees despite a restraining order prohibiting such action.

The Budget Committee struggled to formulate a 1974 budget conforming to federal guidelines. In past years, the budget received board approval in October and was submitted to Blue Cross for acceptance in November, but now a final budget would not be ready until December. Meanwhile, despite increased occupancy, net gain for the year was lower than anticipated. The Finance Committee was unable to address possible financing of future expansion until a budget was developed and the impact of economic controls better understood.

A national "energy crisis" was declared in Washington and was closely watched for its possible effect on the hospital. Saint Luke's administration was looking at structural and operational modifications as ways to conserve.

One-third of the Saint Luke's nursing students were from the metropolitan area and two-thirds from rural areas.

The operating rooms' scheduling problems continued to receive a great deal of attention. Only two rooms were big enough for cardiac surgery, and there were limits on the use of one of these. There were eighty cardiac-surgery cases in October, when a load of sixty per month was anticipated. While existing problems could be handled, there was a much bigger question concerning how Saint Luke's would meet future demands for cardiac surgery.

· · · · ·

When Saint Luke's declined to join St. Joseph Hospital in building a hospital to the south of Kansas City, the Saint Louis-based Sisters of Saint Joseph of Carondelet decided to go it alone. The move had an adverse impact on Kansas City's Linwood and Prospect area, from the standpoint of adequate health services as well as economic loss. But St. Joseph could no longer afford to remain at its inner-city location. Saint Luke's Dr. Charles B. Wheeler Jr., now Kansas City's mayor, declared: "I am not in a position to block a move I consider inevitable." However Mayor Wheeler did say that a health czar should be sought from outside the city to deal with the proliferation of hospital beds in the community:

> "The inability to control the proliferation of beds in Kansas City has been demonstrated over the years and calls for the entrance into Kansas City of a very renowned professional whose reputation can prevent it from continuing into the indefinite future. None of us has faced up to this problem in a realistic fashion, and in my opinion it's time to do so."

At a meeting the end of November, the MACHPA board approved the relocation of St. Joseph Hospital as proposed. There was opposition from the city health director as well as from a consumer representative on the board. Also opposed was the chairman of a MACHPA committee that had drawn up an area master plan for health care services. They all objected to investing $26 million in a new 300-bed hospital on the city's outskirts.

In December, 1973, Saint Luke's Budget Committee presented a proposed operating budget and also an interim budget. The latter, reflecting the uncertainties facing the health care industry under the Economic Stabilization Act, would be used until an exception was granted under new guidelines or until the hospital was given the option to use existing guidelines. The interim budget imposed drastic cuts in operation costs as well as a freeze on personnel and deletion of proposed salary increases scheduled for July, 1974.

TWENTY-SEVEN
1974-1975

PSRO ... Essie Souders ...
tax exemption revoked and restored ...
Rape Treatment Center ... 4400 Broadway ...
basic research ... hospital expansion ... high-risk maternity

As a result of Public Law 92-603, considerable impetus was given to the development of a nationwide system of professional standards-review organizations (PSROs) at local levels, to control abuse of Medicare and Medicaid and insure quality medical services in institutional settings. In January, 1974, Saint Luke's Dr. Fred Fowler, president of the Jackson County Medical Society, told his physician constituents that implementation of the program might reduce hospital admissions by up to 20 percent. Cases deviating from statistical norms (such as inordinately long hospital stays) would be identified, and the PSROs would have power to deny Medicare and Medicaid payments for improper or unnecessary treatment.

Doctors were given the first opportunity to form PSROs, and the Jackson County group organized a PSRO for thirty counties in Northwest Missouri. This initiative was the result of a task force organized in July, 1973, with Saint Luke's doctors Thomas, Fowler, and Blim as strong supporters. The Saint Luke's medical staff endorsed the concept, and Saint Luke's participation followed.

The Cost of Living Council published new regulations in February, but Saint Luke's exercised an option to use existing guidelines and budgeted accordingly. Meanwhile, national Protestant and Catholic hospital associations filed a lawsuit challenging the stringent regulations singling out the health care industry. The American Hospital Association took similar action, arguing that it was unwarranted discrimination to restrict the health care industry and leave other industries unregulated.

There was an altercation with Miss Essie Souders, one of the residents of an apartment building owned by the hospital. For thirty years she had fed birds and animals in neighboring Mill Creek Park from hundred-pound sacks of feed stored on her premises. The feed attracted rats, vermin and mice—a health hazard. Neighbors complained, and the hospital tried to evict her. Her plight attracted sympathetic media coverage. She also received a great deal of fan mail, including a letter from an inmate of the Missouri State Penitentiary. "If I have to move out of here, I'll just die," said Ms. Souders. In the face of hostile public sentiment, the hospital relented, helped to clean up the area, and built a fancy bird-feeding station for Souders. "I am so happy I don't have to move," she told reporters.

The nursing school worked out a new arrangement for the first-year academic program—students would take instruction at UMKC rather than at Penn Valley.

$$\bullet \quad \bullet \quad \bullet \quad \bullet \quad \bullet$$

Judicial review of the State Tax Commission's decision favoring the hospitals produced a decision in April. The Saint Luke's board was shocked when Judge Keith Bondurant of the Jackson County Circuit Court ordered the commission to revoke the hospital's tax-exempt status as well as that of Research and Baptist hospitals. Ironically, Bondurant had served a three-year term on the Saint Luke's board from 1961 to 1963.

The twenty-one-page decision had implications for all of Missouri's nonprofit hospitals. Bondurant's opinion concluded that the hospitals in question enjoyed a substantial profit from their patient services and erroneously charged that they had no programs to aid the needy, aged, or poor. According to the newspaper account, the crucial legal deficiency that condemned all three hospitals was their failure to operate "wholly" for charitable purposes. Bondurant's ruling was appealed to the Missouri Supreme Court.

Meanwhile the board's response to the tax decision was constructive. Bishop Vogel said that "we should be attentive to what the community is saying and examine our posture as well as defend ourselves" … Robert

Wagstaff agreed that "Saint Luke's must be as charitable as possible in providing services to the community."

· · · · ·

The Executive Committee favored establishing a Rape Treatment Center at Saint Luke's. The physicians were supportive. The matter was carefully considered—there were financial ramifications and need for support personnel. Recognizing that the program was "a major step in broad community involvement," the board approved the center. Similar centers existed in Philadelphia and Denver. A subsequent newspaper account said:

> "Saint Luke's was recommended as the site for the first center here by the Metropolitan Co-Ordinating Committee for the Treatment and Prevention of Rape because of its trained personnel, central location, willingness to accept such a responsibility, and a relatively low workload at the peak period of reported rapes ... "

National acclaim followed. A publication by the University of California noted:

> "A 24-hour rape treatment center that will offer care for the physical and psychological needs of rape victims will open soon at Saint Luke's Hospital, Kansas City, Missouri. Special educational training will be provided all nursing, medical and paramedical personnel involved with rape victims in order to help them assist victims with their unique pyschological and physical needs."

Saint Luke's officially opened the center on August 1, 1974, and continues to provide this important community service.

· · · · ·

Dr. Don Blim dreamed of a pediatric practice open seven days a week, with office hours from 8 a.m. to 10 p.m. However, the Medical Plaza management balked at keeping the building open for the additional time. So Doctor Blim, one of the first occupants of the Medical Plaza offices, joined pediatrician Dr. Dominic Tutera in adding another medical office building to the Saint Luke's campus ... at the west end of the campus, 4400 Broadway. The site was leased from Saint Luke's, with ownership, including all improvements, to revert to the hospital in the year 2116.

Hospital occupancy remained in the stratosphere: 92.4 percent in med-surg year to date, and 89.9 percent overall, year to date. Consequently, there was a critical shortage in support staff, to be partly alleviated when forty-two nursing school graduates joined the hospital. Meanwhile, the hospital's financial picture "looked good."

May, 1974, marked the end of the Economic Stabilization Act and its controls, greatly simplifying the budget committee's work. There were some "corrections" to the budget at the May board meeting.

In June, forty California hospitals were struck by the California Nurses' Association, supported by the Kansas City-based American Nurses' Association. At Saint Luke's, administration sought to identify and deal with areas of dissatisfaction. Approximately one-third of Saint Luke's registered nurses belonged to the ANA.

Saint Luke's offered treadmill testing, using an endless belt on which monitored patients walked or ran—a new procedure described to the board by a cardiologist.

There were further budget adjustments. While subject to the Economic Stabilization Act, local hospitals adopted minimal wage increases across the board of approximately 3 percent, as recommended by area guidelines. Now freed of the Act, area hospitals made up for lost time, granting general increases of 5.5 percent, with some going as high as 9 percent. The board approved 5.5 percent as well as a 10-cent-per-hour pay differential for evening and night shifts.

• • • • •

Dr. Kenneth L. Goetz, director of Saint Luke's Division of Experimental Medicine, received a prestigious grant from the National Institutes of Health to continue research on the role played by heart sensors in the regulation of blood volume and kidney function. This kind of basic research by a private, community hospital was unique. Before the arrival of Dr. Goetz, Saint Luke's boasted of a research department, but the hospital performed little if any basic research. The department's role largely was confined to the accumulation of published papers for the hospital library.

Hospital land at 4434 Broadway was sold to Dr. Keith Whitaker. The tract became the site of a small medical-office building occupied by a group of highly skilled neurosurgeons.

MACHPA approved the expanded Saint Luke's proposal for pediatric, obstetrical and CV facilities, and ER improvements. Once state approval was issued, Kidder Peabody would assist in seeking the financing that had to be in place within one year under conditions imposed by MACHPA.

• • • • •

The arrival of Dr. Thomas T. Crouch from the Mayo Clinic greatly enhanced nephrology expertise at Saint Luke's, where he organized an outstanding renal service. Dr. Crouch reported that the 1973 federal legislation, providing a new reimbursement mechanism for dialysis patients, had resulted in a steadily increasing demand for dialysis services. In response, a new seven-bed dialysis unit was added.

A budget for 1975 was adopted after much discussion of the special role of Saint Luke's as a teaching hospital offering tertiary care to very ill patients. Thirty-six percent of the patients were referral patients. Threatened union organizational efforts required that salaries and wages remain competitive. Increased expenses and provision for a small contribution to the reserve for growth and development would result in greater costs.

To defray these costs, increases in operating income amounting to $26.86 per patient day were necessary. Eighteen dollars of this additional revenue would be generated by patient charges. More cost shifting ensued, and pressure increased for future support of medical-education programs to come from outside sources such as the foundation.

However, there was no suggestion that medical education be abandoned. The quality of care at Saint Luke's would be altogether different without the medical-education program. Many of the special-care units would not exist, and many distinguished members of the medical staff would go elsewhere.

November, 1974, saw a continuation of union organizational activities and the hospital's efforts to combat them.

For the year, Saint Luke's recorded 740 open-heart operations with eight deaths for a mortality rate of 1.1 percent—one of the lowest in the country.

At year's end, new bylaws were adopted providing that the board would be self-perpetuating. No longer would there be the confusing and cumbersome procedure in which directors, wearing their members' hats, met annually to re-elect themselves. The first annual meeting of directors under the new, simplified format was held in January, 1975.

A flu epidemic in January further strained the hospital's capacity to care for all of the patients seeking admission.

President Nixon proposed a comprehensive health insurance program requiring employers to cover their employees. The proposal enjoyed the support of Senator Edward Kennedy of Massachusetts. However, it fell into limbo as the Watergate scandal accelerated. In his first message to Congress following Nixon's resignation, President Gerald Ford asked for passage of national health insurance but later withdrew his administration's plan because it would exacerbate inflation.

President Ford also pocket-vetoed renewal of the Nurse Training Act. The effect on Saint Luke's School of Nursing was substantial—half of the student body received federal aid. An article in *The Kansas City Times* quoted the school's director as saying, "There simply are no other adequate funding sources." The article also noted that a nursing shortage had existed for at least a decade and that "skyrocketing unemployment" in other industries did not affect the need for nurses. The executive director of the KCAHA said:

> "Spurring the demand for nurses … is the construction of more hospital rooms, the new fields opening to health care workers and the 'more intensive' services offered by hospitals."

The board continued the Clinical Pastoral Education Program and endorsed the idea of full accreditation of the hospital as a chaplains' training center.

A lease agreement with Hometels Corporation of America was approved … construction could go forward on the Granada Royale Hometel at 43rd and J.C. Nichols Parkway. The lease was for a term of fifty-one years, but Saint Luke's would have interim purchase options. Meanwhile, substantial rental would be paid to the hospital. A number of rooms would be held back daily until 3 p.m. to accommodate Saint Luke's patients and their friends and families. The hospital agreed to dedicate a strip of hospital land to widen Forty-third street.

Saint Luke's and the Florence Crittenton Center joined in a combined disaster plan, and Saint Luke's also assisted the center in obtaining accreditation by the Joint Commission on Accreditation of Hospitals … thereby gaining for Crittenton better reimbursement for its services.

The medical staff initiated preadmission screening of all Medicare patients, a program imposed by the Social Security Administration. Hospitals were required to establish admission criteria, the cost to be borne by their patients. Hospital audits also were required. Dr. Christopher Y. Thomas, now medical-staff president, viewed the expensive program as usurping the power of the Department of Health, Education, and Welfare. The latter's PSROs, introduced to control costs, were themselves costly—the PSRO to which Saint Luke's Hospital belonged incurred operational costs of $2.2 million per year. This experience by hospitals gave rise to a contention that the PSRO program cost more than it saved, but the program continued.

The Family-Centered Maternity Care Program enabled 80 to 85 percent of all maternity cases at Saint Luke's to avoid general anesthesia.

• • • • •

Judge Bondurant's tax decision, appealed to the Missouri Supreme Court, was overturned in March, 1975. The court restored the tax-exempt status of Saint Luke's and the other two hospitals involved in the case.

A Saint Luke's proposal to lease an EMI head scanner was approved by MACHPA. (EMI scanners were manufactured by British-owned Electronic Music, Inc., of Beatles' fame, and hence the "EMI" identification.) KU and Menorah already had acquired this expensive diagnostic tool. The agency then placed a moratorium on further scanners for the Kansas City area. Meanwhile, Saint Luke's submitted a proposal for a costly linear accelerator for treating cancer patients.

The Saint Luke's Articles of Incorporation required that the hospital's directors and officers be communicants of the Episcopal Church. Robert Wagstaff announced that Charles Lindstrom had joined the Church and proposed that, in recognition of his many years of service to the hospital, he be appointed to the board and elected the hospital's executive vice president. This was unanimously accomplished, and Lindstrom became the first Saint Luke's administrator to serve as a director and officer of the hospital.

Lindstrom reported in April that there was 103 percent medical-surgical occupancy "which reflects both the increasing demand for services at Saint Luke's Hospital and the seemingly recession-proof nature of the health care industry."

Dr. Robert Newman, chairman of the department of obstetrics/gynecology, presented a lengthy report on the hospital's Rape Treatment

Center. A newspaper article described the center as a five-county resource. There had been one male victim, a six-year-old boy. Only twenty-six victims had prosecuted their assailants. Relationships with the county prosecutor's office were strained because of the service of subpoenas on ER doctors, compelling court appearances on short notice.

· · · · ·

State approval was issued for the ER improvements and the expanded OB/Ped/CV facilities, and there was extensive board review of the financial implications of the project. Kidder studied available financing alternatives. Arthur Andersen, the hospital's auditors, prepared a feasibility study stating the requirements to fund the anticipated debt and how to support it from rate increases and other sources.

It was evident that many of the directors had qualms about the cost of such an undertaking in what were viewed as uncertain times. The financial impact of utilization-review legislation, PSRO requirements, and accompanying restrictions and charges could not yet be determined. The Finance Committee believed, in light of the Arthur Andersen study and conversations with Kidder, that the hospital could handle the additional debt, but many assumptions were made in the process, including: third-party payors would continue to reimburse on the same basis; various expenses in post-1975 years would be subject to no more than a 10-percent rate of inflation; Medicare utilization would remain constant at the present 32.8 percent, and no change would be made in the basis for its reimbursements; Blue Cross and other commercial insurers would continue to pay billed charges; construction-cost projections were realistic; occupancy would continue at its existing 87-percent level; and educational programs would not be expanded. The possibility of national health insurance and resulting government controls was another concern.

MACHPA approval was contingent upon commencement of the project by October, 1975. This exerted pressure to accelerate the board's painstaking authorization process. A motion to proceed with the plan as presented was introduced, debated, and withdrawn, to allow time to develop further information. The officers and Executive Committee were then authorized to negotiate for construction, financing, and preparation of working drawings and then resubmit the plan to the board. This passed with one opposing vote.

The Building Committee selected an architect and a general contractor for the new construction. Neville, Sharp and Simon would do the architectural work, and Universal Construction Company the construction work.

• • • • •

Saint Luke's open-heart surgery program boasted greater volume and lower mortality than the Mayo Clinic.

Health care providers were not immune to the cost of their own employees' health care. After a 33-percent increase in Blue Cross charges for insuring Saint Luke's employees, the Personnel Committee proposed a self-insured employee medical program for the hospital backed by a stop-loss policy with an insurance company. After discussion, a motion to that effect carried unanimously, ending a thirty-six-year contractual relationship.

Saint Luke's hired 60 percent of its nursing school's graduating seniors; most of the rest found employment elsewhere in Kansas City. Meanwhile, the school was compelled to turn away qualified applicants … there was no room for them.

A "conflict of interests" resolution was adopted by the Board at its June, 1975, meeting. It recognized that board positions did not disqualify directors from business relationships with the hospital but did require compliance with all legal and moral requirements where duality of interest existed, including disclosure and fair terms. Directors also were asked to abstain from voting on matters in which they had financial interests.

A revised utilization-review plan was adopted by the Executive Committee of the medical staff. Patients could remain in the hospital after reimbursement limits were reached as long as they were willing to undertake full payment of all hospital costs. Meanwhile, HEW and the Social Security Administration quarreled about jurisdiction over utilization review.

The ER was experiencing problems because of delays in treating emergency cases. Occasionally the delays were unnecessary, but usually they resulted from the volume of cases and the triage nature of ER activity. Those with the most serious needs were seen first. ER renovation and expansion under the pending construction project would triple capacity and eliminate much of the congestion.

The hospital withdrew from the KCAHA multi-employer bargaining unit and undertook independent negotiations with the Operating Engineers. A July 7 *Kansas City Star* article reported a strike deadline for the following day with the Operating Engineers. A federal mediator was involved. There had been an earlier strike threat affecting Menorah, Trinity, St. Joseph, and Research, but it was postponed when a two-month contract extension was offered. A July 8 article in *The Kansas City Times* reported approval of a new Saint Luke's contract by the union membership after a slight wording change. The vote was not without dissent, however, and union resistance was building.

$$\cdot\ \cdot\ \cdot\ \cdot\ \cdot$$

In July, a board Long-Range Planning Committee called for a change in the hospital board's composition—dilution of the required 100 percent Episcopal membership. As proposed, only forty-one of the fifty-one members would have to be communicants of the Diocese. The articles of agreement and bylaws of the hospital corporation later were amended to this effect. Bishop Vogel did not oppose the reduction of Episcopal representation:

> "Bishop Vogel presented a brief review of the history of the Episcopal Church's affiliation with Saint Luke's Hospital. He said that the Articles and By-Laws Committee's recommendations, which would be presented later in the meeting, have his support. He noted that Saint Luke's Hospital is truly a community institution and that while affiliation with the Episcopal Church should not be disrupted, input from others in the community is needed, and such input will not change the Christian mission of the hospital, that of providing care for the sick."

Under the bylaw revisions, the president of the medical staff became an ex-officio member of the board. The auxiliary president also was given board membership—fifty-seven years after that organization's initial request for such recognition.

The change also permitted the addition to the board of Henry W. Bloch, a prominent Jewish civic and business leader, Terrence P. Dunn, the Roman Catholic CEO of J.E. Dunn Construction Co., and John H. Robinson, Presbyterian managing partner of Black and Veatch, consulting engineers.

$$\cdot\ \cdot\ \cdot\ \cdot\ \cdot$$

The revocation of Missouri's charitable-immunity doctrine had the anticipated impact. Many insurance carriers deserted the malpractice field, due to very bad experience with losses.

Argonaut Insurance Company, the hospital's carrier, increased its premium substantially; other national companies declined to bid at all for the hospital's liability insurance. Local companies were solicited.

The hospital anticipated further increases in premium expense during the next two years despite its excellent record.

Two self-insurance proposals were considered and discarded. Finally, after inconclusive discussion, the hospital's officers were authorized to purchase the insurance for the ensuing year "upon terms which appear to them to be in the best interests of the hospital."

The hospital was not alone in its insurance predicament. Its physicians also experienced unprecedented difficulties in purchasing malpractice coverage at reasonable rates. Charles Lindstrom was appointed to a committee of the Jackson County Medical Society investigating long-range industry solutions.

Financing arrangements were completed for the new construction, and a $9.2 million insurance companies' loan was approved, as were the construction contracts. The interest rate was a whopping 10.5 percent, but the project could now proceed.

· · · · ·

The board accepted a $1.5 million grant from the McWilliams Trust for a proposed high-risk maternity center. Such centers were recommended by the American College of Obstetricians and Gynecologists. A Saint Luke's *Intercom* article in December described the "Regional Center for High-Risk Maternal and Infant Care" that would result from the grant. A goal of the project was to reduce the number of infant deaths and the number of children born handicapped or mentally retarded because of inadequate medical attention.

Saint Luke's already had one of the nation's leading high-risk maternity programs. Now several hundred additional patients could be treated, and the residency programs in obstetrics/gynecology would be strengthened. There was expansion of facilities and personnel at Saint Luke's to meet the increased patient load.

Nationally, the traditional rotating internship was discontinued by medical educators. Instead, residency programs added another year. Future Saint Luke's house staff would consist of residents only—no more interns.

MACHPA approved the linear accelerator for treatment of deep-seated lesions; arrangements were made to lease the equipment.

• • • • •

In December, 1975, Drs. William Reed and James Crockett presented a proposal for the establishment of a "Heart Institute" as a part of the hospital. Following discussion, a resolution was adopted:

> "RESOLVED, That the board of directors of Saint Luke's Hospital enthusiastically supports in principle the concept of a Heart Institute as presented to the board by Drs. Reed and Crockett, to be situated on the Saint Luke's campus, administered as an integral part of Saint Luke's Hospital, and providing cardiac surgery and care on a regional basis."

The KU Medical Center suspended its cardiac-surgery program that same month as a result of the departure of two heart surgeons. There was a dispute at the medical center over whether or not "some conditions of the operating unit posed unnecessary dangers to patients." (A replacement heart surgeon from Saint Luke's would be hired the following March, and in April, 1976, KU would resume open-heart surgery.)

TWENTY-EIGHT
1976-1979

"The Presence of Care" ... MAHSA ... "C.A.T. fever"
... VHA ... Heart Institute ... strikes ...
sports medicine ... ambulatory surgery

A February, 1976, article in *The Kansas City Star* concluded:

> "Four of the six hospitals here performing open-heart surgery on adults fail
> to meet 'a carefully considered guideline' of operating on a minimum of
> 200 patients a year ... "

This conclusion was the result of a MACHPA study. Saint Luke's was
one of the two that met the 200-patient minimum.

The 200-case guideline was suggested by The Inter-Society
Commission for Heart Disease Resources. Their statement:

> "For purposes of intelligent planning, hospitals should not give serious con-
> sideration to establishing a cardiac surgical service unless there are reason-
> able prospects of generating this caseload (of 200 patients a year) ... High-
> volume programs with a broad mix of patients are, in the judgment of our
> authors, more likely to assure development and maintenance of this ability
> to decisively intervene when emergencies and complications occur."

The situation has changed little in the intervening years—the difference being that Saint Luke's volume has increased even more while the
nonqualifying local programs have greatly proliferated.

In March, 1976, the medical staff approved prohibition of smoking in
all patient areas. This would later be expanded to cover the entire hospi-

tal—recognition of the harmful effects of tobacco and the incongruity of a health care provider permitting the use of tobacco on its premises. The prohibition generated less protest than anticipated.

• • • • •

An issue arose over termination of unwanted pregnancies. Bishop Vogel advised the board of the policy of the Episcopal Church recognizing "the sanctity and quality" of human life and urged the hospital to witness to society its position in the matter. A resolution adopted by the diocesan convention the previous year on that subject was proposed as hospital policy. The policy rejected the practice of induced abortion, which involved the killing of a life already conceived "save at the dictate of strict and undeniable medical necessity." The policy called for nonlethal solutions, including financial, medical, and social support during pregnancy, efficient adoption procedures, quality day care nurseries, training and education for the handicapped, and education in the responsible practice of human sexuality. After medical-staff input, the policy was adopted.

At his first meeting of the board as chairman, in June, 1972, Bishop Vogel had praised Saint Luke's as a "hospital that cares." Now he proposed that "The Presence of Care" be adopted as the motto of Saint Luke's Hospital. He declared:

> "Reference is frequently made today to the 'health industry'; the product of hospitals is said to be 'the delivery of care.' We at Saint Luke's want to disassociate ourselves from the factory concept of medicine."

The new motto, an inspired proposal, was unanimously approved.

• • • • •

An April article in *The Kansas City Star* reported that the highest daily room rate in the area was $81.50 a day … at Saint Luke's Hospital. Nonetheless, the hospital continued to experience "extremely high occupancy," a situation that required patients to be admitted to recovery-room hallways and examining rooms.

A proposed name for the anticipated Heart Institute—"Mid-America Heart Institute"—was reserved with the Missouri Secretary of State, and a feasibility study by Booze, Allen, and Hamilton was authorized.

An organization called "Mid-America Health Systems Agency, Inc."

(MAHSA) was designated by HEW as the federally funded health planning body for the eight-county metropolitan area, succeeding MACHPA.

Medicare continued its parsimonious ways. A Budget Committee recommendation to increase the Medicare contractual allowance adjustment reserve by $200,000 was adopted in May. During the summer interim, the Executive Committee of the board approved a further increase—$300,000—in the hospital's reserve for Medicare adjustment.

The Lee's Summit Journal announced that Longview Community College now was offering Saint Luke's peripatetic first-year nursing school program on the Longview campus.

In October, Blue Cross implemented premium increases for its 29,000 non-group policy holders. It cited hikes in hospital and physician charges and increased use of both by subscribers as the reasons.

The recently developed computerized axial tomography scanner (C.A.T.) was an expensive but highly effective diagnostic tool. Hospitals coveted it, and physicians wanted to install it in their own imaging centers.

An October article in *The Star* noted the advent of "C.A.T. fever" in Kansas City:

> "The ailment affects the judgment and pocketbook most seriously, but it has been known to cause bureaucratic pains as well."

There was no official way at the time to control the proliferation of physician-owned C.A.T.s in Missouri—the state's certificate-of-need law was not passed until 1979. Meanwhile, Blue Cross stepped into the regulatory breach, warning area physicians that it would disallow claims made for body scans performed on equipment not approved by the area health-planning agency. Hospitals already were required by an agreement with Blue Cross to seek agency approval for any capital expenditure in excess of $350,000.

A November article in *The Kansas City Star* noted that the Institute of Medicine, a branch of the National Academy of Sciences, called for new controls over hospitals in an effort to reduce the number of beds by 10 percent in five years. They recommended that the government and third-party payors mandate review of hospital costs and services before bills were paid and that health-insurance programs not require policyholders to check into a hospital for services that could be provided on an outpatient basis.

A letter agreement was executed by the hospital with Prime Health, the pioneer Kansas City health maintenance organization (HMO). Prime Health subscribers were limited to doctors on the HMO's staff or, in the case of specialists, those selected by a Prime Health staff physician.

Contractual discounts exacted by Prime Health and others placed a premium on cost containment. A Cost Containment Committee was appointed by the board at its October meeting to study internal hospital operations, with the first meeting focusing on control over utilization of hospital services.

Charles Lindstrom showed slides of the hospital's expanded, improved ER at the December board meeting. He discussed the triage nursing concept, the ER's physician complement, and the hospital's relationship with them.

Fred Fink, a hospital consultant with Booze, Allen, and Hamilton, reviewed the results of his firm's feasibility study—concluding that it was in the hospital's best interest to establish the proposed Heart Institute in order to meet patient demand. He recommended a fund drive to finance the institute. Drs. Crockett and McCallister urged the board to establish the institute and affirmed that it would be an integral part of Saint Luke's.

The hospital was authorized to purchase malpractice insurance for 1977; meanwhile, the board continued its pursuit of a self-insurance program to be effective no later than January 1, 1978.

• • • • •

A report by the president of the auxiliary, Mrs. Frank Koger, in January, 1977, described the multitude of services performed for the hospital by that organization. Eighteen thousand hours in volunteer time were invested annually, with areas of service including the chapel, the library cart program, and the surgical waiting room. Money-making projects included the coffee, gift, and Nearly New shops and the sale of baby pictures. Financial support resulted in five nursing scholarships, the salary for Sister Angela (a chaplain), support for the clinical pastoral-education program, scholarships for foundation and hospital employees, and redecoration of the radiology waiting area and the surgical waiting area. The auxiliary's Holly Ball continued to provide handsomely for the foundation … in February, the Holly Ball chairman presented the foundation with a check for more than $22,500 in ball proceeds.

Among the labor-union issues of the day was one raised by efforts to organize medical residents. The threshold question was whether medical-school graduates pursuing advanced training programs were students or hospital employees. If employees, they were subject to the provisions of the National Labor Relations Act and could be organized into unions. This issue was debated in March at the annual meeting in Kansas City of the American Society of Internal Medicine. The president of an organization representing 6,000 young doctors in New York City argued that his constituents were hospital employees. Edward T. Matheny, Jr., a lawyer and Saint Luke's director, argued that they were not. While this was a hotly debated matter at the time, it has since disappeared as a concern to hospitals. There has never been any such organization at Saint Luke's.

The pressure from professionals in nursing education to require a B.S. in nursing was increasing. The Hospital might have to establish a four-year college of nursing or discontinue its school.

The board authorized construction of an ambulatory surgery center on the hospital campus and submitted an application to MAHSA for approval. A May 27 article in *The Star* reported that approval had been granted. The center was expected to cost about $1,667,500, be housed in a separate building, and be staffed with eighteen full-time personnel operating a day shift for five days a week.

There was concern over the potential effect on the health care industry of controls proposed by President Carter. However, this legislation got nowhere in Washington in 1977 ... although the measure passed the Senate, a massive lobbying effort by health care providers killed it in the House.

Saint Luke's continued its humanitarian mission ... providing expert neonatal care for high-risk cases, acute care for Medicare and other elderly patients, and an inordinate amount of charity care.

Former Vice President Hubert H. Humphrey stated:

> "It was once said that the moral test of government is how that government treats those who are in the dawn of life, the children; those who are in the twilight of life, the elderly; and those who are in the shadows of life—the sick, the needy, and the handicapped."

It was the conviction of Saint Luke's directors that nonprofit hospitals should meet the same moral test.

An August 18 article in *The Kansas City Times* reported remarks by Dr. Fred Fowler, Saint Luke's physician now serving as president of the Northwest Missouri PSRO, describing the growth of medical peer-review systems. Fowler said: "We see ourselves more as a technical assistance group than as a new army telling people how things should be done." The PSRO medical director declared that neither saving money nor shortening hospital stays was a purpose. However, a recently published book, *Sample Criteria for Short-Stay Hospital Review*, outlined standard dispositions for many of the problems requiring medical treatment. Data generated by the system would be fed into a computer to provide a basis for later review of medical practices.

• • • • •

Voluntary Hospitals of America (VHA) was formed in September 1977. This corporation was organized by some of the nation's largest, nonprofit, private hospitals to increase efficiency, engage in large-scale, group purchasing, and provide other benefits for member hospitals. Saint Luke's signed on as a founding member, and Charles Lindstrom became an active VHA supporter and a member of its board of directors. Saint Luke's participation in the organization (where it joined other elite hospitals in the country) provided many significant cost-saving benefits as well as access to other resources.

• • • • •

The board approved a presentation to MAHSA requesting approval for a free-standing Heart Institute with approximately 160 beds. There was no comprehension at the time of the struggle that was being launched. When Saint Luke's sent its Heart Institute proposal to MAHSA, objections immediately began to surface.

MAHSA's current health plan for the eight-county area prohibited any new beds until 1982, whereas the Heart Institute beds would increase Saint Luke's acute-care bed complement by 24 percent. Saint Luke's urged that the cardiovascular program be viewed from a regional perspective; the proposed institute would provide area heart patients with an alternative to the Mayo Clinic or the Texas Heart Institute.

MAHSA held hearings starting in September with respect to the proposal. A September 23 article in *The Star* reported that opposition was expressed in the five or six introductory meetings that preceded the first formal hearing.

The first formal hearing was held September 28 at the Hilton Plaza Inn, to elicit comments from the community. Twenty-three people spoke for the proposal, and four spoke against it. Among those supporting the project was Dr. Arthur W. Robinson, president-elect of the Saint Luke's medical staff. Opponents expressed concern over the effect on other hospitals. Research Hospital feared that Saint Luke's would "corner the market" on open-heart surgery. Other hospital letters to MAHSA expressed similar views, from the Kansas City College of Osteopathic Medicine, Baptist, Menorah, Providence-St. Margaret, Trinity, and Research. The only supportive hospital letter came from Medical Center of Independence.

Robert Wagstaff, although disappointed, was not surprised by the opposition of other hospitals. A major Coca Cola bottler, he said that if he were asked if there should be another bottling plant in Kansas City he would be opposed.

Several reasons were cited for Saint Luke's success in developing the largest heart-surgery program in Missouri, Kansas, Iowa, and Nebraska. One was the excellent patient outcomes—Saint Luke's mortality rate was the lowest in the country. As a result, the program was now the only one in the metropolitan area to perform the minimum number of open-heart procedures recommended to maintain the optimum level of skills.

In the first eight months of 1977, Saint Luke's performed 659 of Kansas City's 1,138 open-heart cases; Trinity was second with 139. The *Star* reporter who covered the hearing wrote:

> "The message one gets from talking to proponents of the heart institute is that other hospitals are envious of the success of the Saint Luke's program."

Saint Luke's proposal was supported by Dr. Charles N. Kimball, distinguished board chairman of the Midwest Research Institute, himself equipped with a Saint Luke's-installed pacemaker to regulate his heartbeats. He argued in an interview that the Heart Institute would be the catalyst for Kansas City to become a medical center rivaling Boston and Houston.

Dr. James Crockett said that what was being proposed was not a centralization of facilities in the metropolitan area but regionalization involving referral of outside patients.

The project was dealt a blow when a special MAHSA task force failed to capture the vision and recommended unanimously that "based on the capacity for such services already existing in the region, a need for such an institution in this community is not found." That negative recommendation went to MAHSA's Resources Development Committee, which predictably rejected the Heart Institute proposal, by a vote of eight to two. Hospital representatives immediately announced their intention to appeal to the full MAHSA board. In the interim there were conversations with Blue Cross and political representatives, as well as letters from the community directed to MAHSA. Support on both sides was being marshaled and expressed.

Meanwhile, Mr. and Mrs. Robert W. Wagstaff made a gift of $1.5 million to Saint Luke's, expressing the wish that their contribution be used to house the proposed Heart Institute.

The Heart Institute cause was further damaged when application of HEW standards demonstrated that there were already too many hospital beds in Missouri and Kansas. This excess was the subject of a November 7 article in *The Kansas City Times.* And a November 13 *Star* article discussed a MAHSA health-planning document opposing new construction by area hospitals. The agency's executive director said that the cost for the extra beds and support facilities would be borne by the consumers who used the hospitals. "We don't want to replace, expand, or renovate anything for a year."

The week before, Blue Cross and Blue Shield had blamed excessive hospital construction and underutilization of hospital beds for recent insurance-rate increases. And shortly thereafter, the Blues' two boards approved a statement calling for a two-year moratorium on any hospital capital expenditures that would either increase the number of beds or add services. In the process they expressed concern over "the rapidly rising health care costs and their impact on our subscribers and the community as a whole."

At a special December meeting of the Saint Luke's board, Robert Wagstaff reported on a session with the executive director of MAHSA. The conference had not been encouraging. Wagstaff warned that "further continuance or even withdrawal of the Heart Institute proposal presently before the planning agency might be required." The board authorized Wagstaff, Charles Lindstrom, and legal counsel for Saint Luke's to take such action "if they so deem necessary." Saint Luke's representatives later in December, reading the handwriting on the wall, requested that the MAHSA board postpone indefinitely its consideration of the Heart Institute proposal, explaining that Saint Luke's was "exploring other alternatives."

So the first campaign was lost. But not the war.

• • • • •

On November 2, 1977, Saint Luke's presented to the Kidney Foundation of Kansas and Western Missouri the pioneer artificial-kidney machine that it had first used in October, 1956, bearing serial number 0002.

• • • • •

Also in November, Kansas City's first HMO, Prime Health, completed its initial year of operation—a milestone whose significance was not generally recognized at the time.

Federal legislation had been enacted in 1973 to aid the formation and development of HMOs. The new law required businesses with more than twenty-five employees to offer at least one qualifying HMO as an alternative to conventional insurance. Grants and loans were provided to develop new HMOs. To qualify, HMOs had to offer a broad range of services and open enrollment as well as undertake difficult new administrative tasks.

As a result of these complexities, HMOs took several years to gain momentum. But now Prime Health was a going concern. It was aided by further congressional legislation, reducing some of the inhibiting requirements for HMOs and increasing federal aid.

Prime Health opened its own care center for outpatient services, developed a medical staff of twenty physicians, served twenty patients a day, and delivered its hundredth baby. Members were referred to Baptist, Menorah, and Swope Ridge Health Center. In addition, high-risk ob/gyn patients were referred to Saint Luke's specialists.

• • • • •

The Budget Committee projected slightly lower occupancy for 1978, reflecting the anticipated opening of more than 500 new beds in the community in the coming year and the completion of the Saint Luke's ambulatory surgical facility.

Increases in the minimum wage under federal law continued to affect hospitals. An increase of 35 cents—from $2.30 to $2.65 per hour—effective January 1, 1978, had a substantial adverse impact on hospital costs in neighboring Kansas. The Kansas Hospital Association president lamented:

> "Hospitals are in a no-win situation in the cost dilemma. We have pressures by the federal government to contain cost increases while at the same time are faced with increased costs, over which we have no control, which are legislated by the federal government."

The new year began for Saint Luke's with the Operating Engineers Union setting a strike deadline for January 4. When the hospital and the union were unable to reach agreement in the interim, the union struck. It was the hospital's first work stoppage.

Dissatisfied with earlier negotiating results, the hospital had withdrawn from a multi-hospital bargaining unit including Menorah, St. Joseph's, Research, and Trinity. The union maintained that the Saint Luke's offer was inferior to the wages and benefits prevailing at those other hospitals.

Other employees filled in for the striking union members, and the strike was ineffectual; according to the hospital it was "business as usual." The strike continued for eighteen days, ending when the union accepted a new three-year contract. The final stumbling block was Saint Luke's merit-pay plan, which the union accepted "under protest."

• • • • •

A January, 1978, issue of *The Kansas City Star* noted that social trends had spelled an end to some Kansas City institutions; one of those identified was the Florence Crittenton Home. At an earlier location it had been the "Florence Crittenton Home for Colored Girls." It was desegregated and moved to the Saint Luke's campus as a home for unwed mothers. The number of single girls who wanted to give up their babies for adoption and in the meantime keep their pregnancies secret was dwindling, and so the institution switched its emphasis to treatment of emotionally disturbed girls. Now it was building a new, suburban "Crittenton Center" at 109th and Elm, to serve children and adolescents of both sexes. Agreement was reached with Crittenton Center for purchase of its property on the Saint Luke's campus for $350,000.

A *Kansas City Times* article advised that bills submitted to Blue Cross the previous year reflected a further sharp increase in area hospital costs. Hospital and Blue Cross officials cautioned against comparing costs in various hospitals, however. "Saint Luke's and the University of Kansas Medical Center, which had some of the highest cost-per-case figures, both perform highly specialized and sophisticated procedures that inflate average costs." Also, "at Saint Luke's, patients help pay for a $5 million education program that another hospital may not have to figure into its charges."

Illustrative of the sophisticated procedures at Saint Luke's, a *Kansas City Star* article the next day described nuclear cardiology at the hospital—a new application of "nuclear" medicine in use for only four or five years and still not widely available. Also Saint Luke's had contracted C.A.T. fever … a MAHSA C.A.T.-scanner proposal was in preparation. Meanwhile, hospital occupancy was extremely high.

In May, the Saint Luke's Foundation celebrated its fifteenth anniversary. At that organization's annual meeting an endowment was announced for a visiting-professor lectureship honoring Dr. Mark Dodge, former president of the foundation and of the medical staff. There have been annual Mark Dodge Lectures since then, bringing to Kansas City distinguished endocrinologists who present lectures to physicians and students at Saint Luke's, KU and UMKC-Truman Medical Center.

On May 23, a local hospital filed a lawsuit against Blue Cross challenging the insurer's mandate that all projects in the Kansas City metropolitan area not reviewed and approved by MAHSA be denied Blue Cross reimbursement. The complaint alleged that this requirement violated the federal antitrust laws. Saint Luke's continued to seek MAHSA review and approval, but application of antitrust laws to health care providers would be a specter that haunted future hospital activities on a variety of fronts.

The Missouri Kidney Program, a state-financed organization, issued a grant of $229,492 to Saint Luke's for kidney-dialysis patients.

In July, 1978, the School of Nursing held its seventy-fifth anniversary celebration. Attending was Miss Cecelia (Callie) French, now ninety-two years old. (In September, 1942, Miss French had resigned her position as director of nurses and superintendent of the School of Nursing because of ill health and moved to the Southwest, where she lingered for thirty-six years.) Also present at the celebration was Miss Florence Parsons, now age 83.

The earlier failure of price controls under Nixon did not deter President Carter's administration from imposing voluntary price restraints in mid-1978. Saint Luke's would again have to cope with this complication until January, 1981.

In his presidential campaign, Carter had renewed the call for comprehensive national health insurance. However, as president he was reluctant to go forward with it because of the possible effect on his efforts to combat inflation.

Carter did release the general principles for a national health insurance plan in July, 1978, but his pace was too slow to satisfy Senator Edward Kennedy and other advocates, who fashioned a proposal of their own. Neither program was adopted.

Dr. James J. Mongan, then associate director of the White House domestic-policy staff and later executive director of Truman Medical Center and UMKC medical-school dean, afterward commented with respect to the Carter plan:

> "The proposal died quietly, with little attention from the media, after a two-year 'wasting illness' during which it shrank from a large, relatively robust proposal to a small, anemic shadow of its former self." (*Washington Post*, 11/9/93)

• • • • •

Early in September, Saint Luke's announced the creation of a division of sports medicine to help instruct local physicians and coaches in the avoidance of athletic injuries. The expertise of Saint Luke's physicians and technicians in the sports arena culminated in hospital physicians serving as doctors for Kansas City's professional athletic teams. This resulted in high visibility for the doctors and for Saint Luke's as well, as the media responded to the increased popularity of professional sports stars with increased coverage of the ailments that affected their performance.

When Saint Luke's opened its new ambulatory surgery center, it encouraged community use by making the cost-effective center available to any doctor licensed to practice in Missouri and in good standing on the staff of an area hospital. The auxiliary's Nearly New Shop, which had relocated on the surgery center site when the Granada Royale was built on the Sweet property, had to move again.

• • • • •

Saint Luke's yet-unauthorized new heart facility was officially named "The Mid America Heart Institute at Saint Luke's Hospital." Robert Wagstaff stated, in a *Times* interview, that this did not mean that Saint Luke's was going forward without MAHSA approval. "Instead, he said, his board was preparing a scaled-down version of the application for later submission to MAHSA."

The new Heart Institute proposal was submitted to Blue Cross for review prior to delivery to MAHSA. It sought approval of a smaller structure than the original project envisioned.

MAHSA hearings regarding the diminished Heart Institute proposal began September 20. It continued to be a controversial project. A *Kansas City Times* article described one tumultuous session at the Granada Royale across 43rd Street to the north of Saint Luke's. In the course of that proceeding, Mayor Charles Wheeler testified in favor of the scaled-down, thirty-nine-bed proposal. The MAHSA task-force chairman then suggested that because of the presence of Wheeler Laboratories in the Medical Plaza building, Dr. Wheeler had a financial interest in the project. An outraged Wheeler responded: "Sir, I would question your ability to judge quality medical care." However, it developed during their heated exchange that the chairman was a constituent of Mayor Wheeler's, and the nimble mayor ended his testimony by soliciting the chairman's vote in future political campaigns.

The Saint Luke's presentation included earnest testimonials from more than a dozen heart patients. MRI's Dr. Kimball continued to champion the cause, pleading:

> "I beg of you not to look at this enterprise in a limited way. I beg of you not to penalize competence. I'm simply saying to you that you can't have a half dozen institutions in this town that are equally good or equally bad. You end up having a common denominator ... and you need to have one or two that are eminent. There's an old analogy that says all the boats rise as the lake fills up with water. These people from Saint Luke's are proposing to fill up the lake."

The MAHSA task force unanimously determined that there was community need for the Mid America Heart Institute. And in November the directors were advised that the Resources Development Committee of MAHSA had approved the Heart Institute proposal. So there was shock and anger on the part of Saint Luke's supporters when later, after a marathon session, the MAHSA board again denied the Heart Institute request.

The MAHSA directors conceded that the concept was good and necessary but recommended resubmission without asking for additional beds. At one point in their deliberations the vote was eleven against, ten in favor, with one abstention. However the final vote was sixteen to three against the proposal. Wagstaff described the result of the hearing as "absolutely outrageous" but said the hospital still would explore all of the possible ways to comply.

In December Saint Luke's directors approved yet another Heart Institute proposal, deleting the additional acute-care beds. However, the price tag was not reduced—further modifications actually increased the cost of the project from $11.6 million to $13.5 million.

In January 1979, Wagstaff advised the Saint Luke's board that the MAHSA Resource Development Committee would review the latest Heart Institute proposal on February 8. It would go to the MAHSA board on February 22.

The MAHSA Committee recommended MAHSA approval, with only one person speaking in opposition—a Research Hospital doctor who complained that the Heart Institute could draw potential patients away from other hospitals. The Saint Luke's presentation was accompanied by a financial-feasibility study which MAHSA had requested, explaining the cost increase. And when once again the proposal reached the MAHSA board, it was finally approved.

Again Research Hospital representatives, with highly respected former mayor Ilus Davis acting as legal counsel, opposed the Heart Institute on the ground that the quality of patient care and of the cardiovascular program at Research would be adversely affected. The war was finally won, but not without an unfortunate legacy … impairment for many years of collegiality between Saint Luke's and the opposing hospitals, particularly Research Hospital.

• • • • •

In January, 1979, Saint Luke's Dr. Ed Slentz retired from the Richard Cabot Clinic staff. He began visiting the Clinic on Friday mornings in 1953, a brand new internist. He was one of many doctors who then paid visits to the Clinic, but as the West Side institution acquired regular staff members, the volunteer M.D.s disappeared. Slentz was the last holdover from the original group. He recalled:

> "We started with our hands and eyes and stethoscopes, and now we're pretty well equipped ... We've got a good working relationship with Saint Luke's Hospital. They do our lab work and X ray work. All in all, this is a good service for people on this side of town, something that they've needed."

A February, 1979, a *Kansas City Times* article reported on an examination of the right thumb of George Brett, the Kansas City Royals' stellar third baseman, by Saint Luke's orthopaedic specialist Dr. William M. Benson. Brett flew home for the examination from the Royals' spring training camp in Ft. Myers, Florida.

In April, there was a proposal to change the name of the hospital to the more grandiose "Saint Luke's Center for Health Sciences." The suggestion was discarded by the board.

A May, 1979, article in *The Kansas City Times* described the cost savings resulting from use of the ambulatory surgery center at Saint Luke's "where patients walk in, slip into anesthesia-induced sleep prior to the methodically swift operation, then walk out again" ... "We want you to sleep in the best bed in town ... your own," said Ruth Ronfeld, associate director of administration at Saint Luke's.

• • • • •

A lengthy article appeared in *The Kansas City Times*, quoting MAHSA's executive director as saying, "We're not at war with the hospitals; it's more of a pitched battle."

Saint Luke's rheumatologist John K. Layle accused MAHSA of "stifling the innovation and creativity" going on in health care to the detriment of patients:

> "I recently had to admit a patient to the hospital who was put in a closet. All the beds were filled. So she had to wait in what was essentially a storage room until a bed opened up."

Dr. Layle blamed a "maldistribution of beds," resulting in empty beds in unpopular hospitals and popular hospitals being overcrowded but not allowed by MAHSA to expand. "The law tries to solve the problem by forcing patients from popular hospitals to unpopular ones," he said.

Aware of Saint Luke's exhaustive effort, finally successful, to secure

Heart Institute approval, Layle argued that MAHSA had created an adversarial system which increased squabbling among the hospitals:

"The agency has increased the feeling of competition between hospitals, and that's to all our detriment."

Layle also said that up to 25 percent of a patient's hospital bill went to satisfy requirements imposed by federal regulations. "And MAHSA is just another example of that sort of thing."

Dr. Layle was echoed by the speaker at the annual banquet of the Saint Luke's Hospital Foundation, a past president of the American College of Surgeons. He said the Carter administration and the public had singled out hospitals and the medical profession as primary targets in the fight against inflation. Since the passage of the Medicare Act in 1965, controls and regulations imposed by the federal government had driven up the cost of medical care and made it less efficient.

The Heart Institute structure was named "The Robert Wilson Wagstaff Building" in honor of the president of the hospital, whose philanthropy and other support were so instrumental to the successful completion of the institute project.

The chairman of the economic-policy committee of Citibank, the nation's second-largest banking institution, predicted to an assembly of Kansas City bankers that President Carter's voluntary wage and price guidelines were doomed to failure.

In June, the KCAHA published wage and benefit recommendations as guidelines for the member hospitals' next fiscal year. Noting the possibility of price-fixing sanctions, Saint Luke's urged legal review of the recommendations. Revised recommendations emphasized that only minimum standards were involved, disseminated for informational purposes only, to help hospitals avoid substandard conditions of employment.

• • • • •

Like a bad penny, Miss Essie Souders—now 84 years old—turned up again in June, 1979. The cause was another attempted eviction, this time prompted by the space needs of the hospital. Her apartment building occupied part of the site of the planned Robert Wilson Wagstaff Building. Again she resisted evacuation, and once more her plight attracted the attention of television commentators and the print media—where she was gleefully described as "the last of the big-time bird lovers." Again the hospital capitulated, agreeing in exchange for her vacation of the premises to pay for up to thirty days' temporary lodging and also to cover the charge for boarding her cats at the Small Animal Hospital. In addition, Saint Luke's would pay for moving and storing her belongings and contribute up to $300 toward a security deposit and her first month's rent when she found a permanent residence.

As the *Kansas City Times* account began:

> "With a menagerie of cats, several antique armchairs, and one elaborate bird feeder in tow, Miss Essie Souders will move today from her home of 30 years with a light heart."

The board continued to struggle with the expense of various insurance programs. At its September meeting, the board decided to discontinue an experience-rated arrangement for dental insurance with Equitable Life Assurance Society and to self-fund that program.

A September article in *The Kansas City Times* reported that the area hospitals were competing for nurses without precipitating a bidding war. The "philosophy" of a hospital's doctors and administrators was said to be more important to prospective nursing employees than monetary considerations. A director of nursing stated the issue thus:

> "Is she viewed as a bedpan carrier or is she considered to be a partner, a significant contributor to a patient's well-being?"

Hospitals that continued to run their own schools of nursing had the edge in the rivalry for nurses, but they paid a high price for that advantage. At Saint Luke's, in addition to the expense of the nursing school, there was pressure from the nursing profession to offer a four-year program that culminated in a bachelor's degree and "professional" nurses.

• • • • •

A draft of national health planning goals was published for comment in the Federal Register. After analyzing responses, HEW would publish its National Goals for Health Planning. Many of the goals of particular interest to hospitals would be repeated under various auspices in the years to come: regionalization of care with formal linkages among institutions, creation of competing forms of health care systems within the community, shared support services, use of quality of care as a factor in determining a facility's need for capital expenditures, uniform cost-accounting and utilization-reporting systems, access for everyone to the full range of health care services, and determination of the effectiveness of new technology prior to placement on the open market.

In December, 1979, the board adopted a resolution requiring all members of the medical staff to carry professional liability insurance.

Saint Luke's completed 1979 well within the top 1 percent in size of the 4,700 private hospitals in the country. The year's contribution to the reserve for growth and development was $1,493,477—a very modest 2.4 percent of gross patient revenue. This "profit" was $205,936 under budget, with the underage due primarily to larger-than-anticipated Medicare contractual allowances and teaching-care expense.

The hospital's 1980 operating budget projected gross revenues of approximately $73 million. 85.9-percent occupancy was anticipated.

TWENTY-NINE
1980-1981

*Edward T. Matheny Jr. ... liver transplant ... George Brett ...
Dr. Geoffrey O. Hartzler and balloon angioplasty ...
Lifewise ... Hyatt skywalk collapse ...
Level One trauma center ... Medical Plaza II*

*M*AHSA and local elected officials feuded over rival candidates for the MAHSA board. The Jackson County executive threatened litigation if MAHSA failed to seat the county's candidate. The county executive declared:

> "MAHSA has said they want to keep health planning out of politics and therefore out of the hands of elected officials. But there is nothing short of pure politics in what they have been doing all along."

The dispute was largely academic. Missouri had adopted a certificate-of-need law effective January 1, 1982, and would replace MAHSA with the Mid-America Regional Council (MARC) as the local planning body.

• • • • •

On January 21, 1980, attorney Edward T. Matheny Jr. succeeded Robert W. Wagstaff as president of Saint Luke's Hospital. Wagstaff became vice chairman of the board.

A January 31 article in *The Kansas City Times* reported the results of its survey of local hospitals, indicating that they were following a nationwide trend toward concentrating high-risk surgery in a few hospitals. And this would mean improvement, according to the newspaper:

"A recent national study suggested that hospitals which do more high-risk surgery—mostly heart operations—have a much better record of patient survival than hospitals handling fewer high-risk surgical cases."

The study, published in *The New England Journal of Medicine,* showed increased mortality rates in hospitals performing fewer than 200 each of several major operations, including coronary artery bypass, open heart, major vascular surgery, and complicated prostate operations. Of the hospitals surveyed locally, only Saint Luke's reported doing more than 200 cases of each procedure annually.

There was disagreement with the IRS over whether revenues from pathology services provided by the hospital for the medical staff were subject to federal income tax. This resulted in litigation, with a Federal District Court decision issuing in June in favor of the hospital. The court's opinion depended to a considerable extent upon Saint Luke's involvement in medical education and in particular the participation of the pathology residents in the procedures that produced the income. The government filed an appeal but later withdrew it. The case attracted national attention.

There also continued to be considerable controversy over college degrees for nursing students, fueled by a national nursing organization's proposal that bachelor's degrees be the minimum educational requirement for new registered nurses after 1985. As a precaution, the board approved an agreement that would provide an option for graduates of the Saint Luke's School of Nursing to obtain a baccalaureate degree through Webster College.

• • • • •

On April 1, the first liver-transplant operation at Saint Luke's was undertaken by Dr. Thomas Helling. Liver transplants at that time were performed at only two other locations in the world—Cambridge, England, and Denver, Colorado—and were extraordinary, last-ditch efforts to save lives. Dr. Joseph G. Fortner, a New York transplant surgeon lecturing at Saint Luke's, described liver transplantation as "so difficult several surgeons had discontinued their attempts."

At first report, Dr. Helling's patient was doing well, but the next few months would be crucial from the standpoint of organ rejection and infection. On May 8, the patient died after developing an infection.

The board adopted a resolution authorizing the Missouri Health and Educational Facilities Authority to finance the Heart Institute project with its tax-exempt securities. This was the first such project and a learning experience for the new authority. In May, $14,800,000 in revenue notes were sold to Aetna Life & Casualty Co., bearing interest at 10 percent and purchased at 96.705 percent of par.

· · · · ·

As the Kansas City Royals' fortunes improved on the baseball diamond, interest in their physical condition mounted. It was noted in May that catcher Darrell Porter was admitted to Saint Luke's after complaining of chest pains, and in June George Brett hobbled into the hospital with a torn ligament in his ankle, sustained when he attempted to steal second base in a game against the Cleveland Indians. Brett was injury-prone because of his headlong style of play and was a frequent patient at Saint Luke's.

Brett's most famous medical emergency occurred during the World Series in October, 1980, when he entered Saint Luke's for treatment of what sports writer Joe McGuff described as "the world's most widely covered case of hemorrhoids." The pain forced Brett to leave the Royals' line-up in the middle of the second game of the Series. Brett said: "I'm going back to the same room I always have at the hospital. I've had it five years in a row." No one at the hospital was permitted to relay information about the Royals' third baseman, but Saint Luke's officials fielded a huge number of telephone calls, cards, flowers, and get-well posters. Fans all over the world suggested remedies.

· · · · ·

Dr. Geoffrey Hartzler, a recent addition to the Saint Luke's medical staff, introduced a new procedure to the Kansas City medical community—balloon angioplasty. The technical name was a mouthful: "percutaneous coronary transluminal angioplasty," or PCTA. A June 25 article in *The Kansas City Times* reported that Dr. Hartzler performed twenty-three angioplasties at the Mayo Clinic between October, 1979, and June, 1980, before moving to Saint Luke's, where he had done three to date.

Only about 500 angioplasties had been done in the world since the technique was developed by Dr. Andreas R. Gruentzig in Zurich three years earlier. Saint Luke's was the twenty-ninth institution to perform the operation, and Hartzler expected to do three a week once the procedure gained wider acceptance. There was some risk involved in PCTAs. "A catheterization lab has no business doing them unless they have a high volume of experience," said Hartzler, observing that Saint Luke's did more than 2,500 catheterizations a year.

In July, there was another visit by Chinese physicians when a team of mainland China doctors watched angioplasty at Saint Luke's.

A heat wave in the Kansas City area resulted in July occupancy exceeding budget expectations. Advice was published in the media for avoiding heatstroke, together with the telephone number of the Saint Luke's emergency room.

The Eighth Circuit Court of Appeals decided the Blue Cross case in July, ruling that there had been no violation of the antitrust laws in Blue Cross' enforcement of MAHSA planning efforts, because federal legislation encouraged such cooperation. However, hospital lawyers continued to counsel care in other areas posing possible antitrust problems, including restricted staffing, price-fixing, monopolies, division of markets, and exclusive contracts with specialists.

Although there had been doubt about the application of antitrust laws to nonprofit health care institutions, this no longer was open to question. The U.S. Supreme Court held that health care was a business, in commerce, and conducted for economic benefit. Anticompetitive conduct by hospitals and doctors was subject to antitrust sanctions. This new concern further complicated a field of endeavor that was already highly complex.

C.A.T. fever had not abated in Kansas City. An August, 1980, article in *The Kansas City Times* discussed C.A.T. scanners, their cost, and overabundance in the Kansas City area. They were described as "a metaphor for modern medicine out of control." Kansas City reportedly had more C.A.T. scanners than all of Sweden, and this was said to be one field in which America's private system of health care was less efficient than the typical European brand of socialized medicine.

Government authorities maintained that C.A.T. scanners didn't break even unless they performed 2,000 scans a year and recommended 2,500 scans as a minimum figure to justify investment in expensive equipment. There were seventeen Kansas City area scanners, and only four of these met the government volume criteria. One of the four was at Saint Luke's, which leased a scanner from General Electric after receiving planning-agency approval.

Dr. Rex L. Diveley died in November, 1980. The Rex L. Diveley, M.D., Memorial Lectureship was established in his honor.

At its November meeting, the board voted to place the hospital's professional-liability insurance coverage with the Missouri Professional Liability Insurance Association, as the search for a good, long-term solution to liability-insurance protection continued.

· · · · ·

Articles in *The Kansas City Star* the latter part of November, 1980, discussed the history, successes, and failures of health planning. At that time, the nation had a network of 204 health systems agencies charged with holding the line on health costs while insuring that quality care would be available in rural and urban areas alike. In Missouri more than eighty different agencies monitored health care. One of these agencies was lame-duck MAHSA, which had received about $2 million in funding since its formation in 1976.

A New York study determined that 25 percent of all hospital bills in that state went to pay for government regulation of some kind.

Dr. John Layle, now editor of the monthly *Jackson County Medical Society Bulletin,* was especially biting in his editorial criticism of health planners. He argued that "the sick people" were lost in the planning process and once denounced a visiting health planner from California as a "demagogue." However, he did agree that the system of third-party payors was largely responsible for health costs careening out of control. Other factors he cited were more patients, medical "magic," and waste. In the latter category, he lumped health systems agencies together with fraud and abuse, hypochondriacs, and malpractice insurance.

President-elect Ronald Reagan promised to "get government off the backs" of citizens, and this crusade represented a further threat to the planning agencies' continued existence. But even before the 1980 presidential election, President Carter decided that many health agencies were not performing a useful function; his 1981 budget reduced their financial support considerably.

· · · · ·

On February 8, 1981, following expiration of the contract ending the 1978 strike, the thirty-one Saint Luke's members of the Operating Engineers' Union went out on strike once more. Supervisory personnel handled maintenance and boiler-room duties, and the hospital announced that it was providing "patient care as usual." The memory of the three-week strike in 1978 was still fresh, and a merit-pay issue was left over from that earlier dispute. Also in 1978, the hospital tried unsuccessfully to switch union employees to its pension plan and in the intervening three years had not increased contributions to the union's plan.

The impact of the 1981 strike on the hospital again was minimal, and at the end of April the dispute was settled for no more than Saint Luke's pre-strike offer. This was the last strike by the Engineers' Union.

On February 27, future Hall of Famer George Brett was back in the hospital—his hemorrhoids again. This time surgery was performed, and a four-day hospital stay ensued.

Shortly after Brett's release, Clint Hurdle, Royals' right fielder, was admitted to Saint Luke's with a strained lower back. Unlike Brett, Hurdle hadn't been in a hospital since fifth grade. *The Star* reported that the son of the Royals' groundskeeper was occupying a room in the hospital directly below Hurdle's, the result of a broken bone in his neck suffered in an auto accident.

Dr. Paul Koontz of the Saint Luke's staff was chairman of the board of Hospice Care of Mid-America as well as chairman of Saint Luke's patient-care committee. While hospice did not promise cures or entirely relieve families from suffering, it allowed the dying to remain part of the world for as long as they lived. The program would increase in importance in the years to come, and Saint Luke's relationship with the Mid-America organization was a significant part of the hospital's mission.

The hospital leased property located on the southern edge of the Kansas City metropolitan area. Investment in this facility, named "Horizons" for its far-flung vistas, including a view of distant downtown Kansas City, marked the beginning of a major commitment by Saint Luke's to the prevention of illness through healthy living.

In April, 1981, Saint Luke's announced that a new enterprise, "Lifewise," would be housed at Horizons. Lifewise participants learned to avoid self-induced health problems through programs available to business, professional, and social organizations and to the community at large.

The facility also complemented the hospital's sports-medicine program.

The first corporate Lifewise program was installed for the U.S. Department of Energy at Kansas City's Bendix plant. And the first sports-medicine Lifewise program was initiated with the Rockhurst College women's basketball team.

In May, George Brett returned to Saint Luke's for an X ray of his right ankle, injured while sliding home in a ball game.

Saint Luke's established a for-profit organization that provided other hospitals with biomedical engineering, dialysis training, pharmaceuticals, remote pulmonary function and respiratory contracts, and laboratory and microfilming services.

Joseph A. Califano Jr., former Secretary of Health, Education, and Welfare, addressed the annual Saint Luke's Foundation Banquet in May. Before HEW was split in 1980 into two separate Cabinet departments—Health and Human Services, and Education—it administered a gigantic budget of $200 billion, much of it in the health care arena. Califano presided over this vast empire. In his address, the Secretary called attention to the rapidly rising cost of health care and warned that President Reagan would never balance the federal budget in the 1980s without controlling that cost. He suggested limiting annual increases in hospital costs to 30 percent of cost-of-living increases. Although other speeches and published materials by Califano reflected strong views that might have been offensive to hospitals, he courteously refrained from expressing these at the banquet.

Area hospital utilization was scrutinized by a committee of Kansas City's prestigious Civic Council, which proposed a review of privately insured patients comparable to the PSRO program for Medicare/Medicaid patients.

A KCAHA recommendation of patient utilization review by area hospitals also surfaced. It proposed a one-year trial program with results to be informational only and payment made to the hospitals regardless of outcome. Blue Cross endorsed the KCAHA recommendation but objected to the "informational-only" limitation. It also insisted on the right to make its own decisions in certain areas—for example pre-existing conditions and exclusions such as diagnostic admissions. And it wanted to provide the management and individual review associated with such a program.

The KCAHA supported community health-planning programs that

were locally controlled and the establishment of certificate-of-need programs in Missouri and Kansas with parallel provisions, recognizing that the Kansas City market area embraced both states. However the association's own "planning principles" were innocuous—leaving it to the boards of individual hospitals to develop their own master plans and determine how those plans should address "the needs of the community."

Elizabeth Nave Flarsheim, a communicant of St. Paul's Episcopal Church, bequeathed approximately $400,000 to Saint Luke's in June—one-third for nursing-student loans, one-third for the construction and equipping of the Heart Institute, and one-third for study opportunities for resident physicians.

The auxiliary continued its financial support of nursing education, with a $60,000 contribution to the Nursing Student Grant Fund.

$$\bullet \ \bullet \ \bullet \ \bullet \ \bullet$$

On July 17, the emergency preparedness of area hospitals was tragically tested with the collapse of skywalks during a tea dance at the Hyatt Regency Hotel. One hundred twelve people died, and another 200 were injured. By chance, Saint Luke's radiologists were present in the hotel for a dinner meeting and served as litter bearers. Dr. Keith Ashcraft, a Saint Luke's/Children's Mercy pediatric surgeon, was also on the premises and was one of the medical heroes, performing emergency surgery and amputations to free trapped victims. A Saint Luke's employee was the triage officer and afterward received many accolades from the policemen and firemen who provided emergency services.

A number of the victims were brought to Saint Luke's with varying degrees of injury. Some were released promptly; others remained for months. Newspaper accounts ran updates of the condition of the hospitalized victims from time to time over an extended period.

The Kansas City Health Department appointed a task force to review the response to the emergency by area ambulances, hospitals, and doctors. A forty-page report was published in *The Journal of Emergency Medical Services*. The report said: "How good was the response in Kansas City? It was damn near perfect." Subsequently the KCAHA presented programs around the country on the design and development of disaster-preparedness plans, and the National Safety Board adopted the Kansas City plan as a model.

As of August 1, 1981, Saint Luke's had transplanted 212 kidneys.

On August 12, a challenge grant was announced by the Kresge Foundation of Troy, Michigan, of $150,000 for constructing and equipping the Heart Institute.

A 1928 plaque in the hospital memorializes "A Thank Offering from Bishop and Mrs. Partridge for the Recovery of their Daughter Amalia ... ." Amalia (now Amalia Partridge Ingham) wrote from Seattle, Washington, that she planned to visit Saint Luke's and was looking forward to viewing the hospital portrait of her illustrious father. This prompted a search for the bishop's portrait, finally located hanging in the medical library. Following Mrs. Ingham's visit, it was rehung with suitable ceremony in the boardroom, where Bishop Partridge later was joined by Bishops Robert Nelson Spencer and Edward Randolph Welles.

In September, the X ray Department was pressed into service after Brett injured his rib cage while "barreling" into second base to break up a double play.

• • • • •

Saint Luke's was designated a Level One trauma center by the State of Missouri, one of two in the area to be so recognized. The other was a joint designation of Truman Medical Center and Children's Mercy Hospital, two Hospital Hill neighbors comprising a single center for trauma purposes. The KU Medical Center, located just across the state line, also met the requirements for a Level One center, but the state of Kansas did not provide formal trauma-center designations.

The Level One identification helps paramedics to more quickly determine where to take critically injured patients, since Level One hospitals have specialists and equipment on hand around the clock. Only a major teaching hospital can guarantee such resources, and there are but a handful of Level One institutions in the State of Missouri.

• • • • •

A November, 1981, article in the Sunday *Star* described the progress of construction work on a second Medical Plaza building, Medical Plaza II. Occupancy of the new medical office building was expected in mid-March, 1982. Two-thirds of the space already was leased. The owners were the same physician/dentist shareholders who owned the original

Medical Plaza building. This investment by and proximity of key medical specialists would continue to be a source of strength and stability for Saint Luke's.

The other construction project with long-term implications for Saint Luke's was the Heart Institute facility. The Heart Institute building was dedicated on December 15, 1981, with the principal address offered by famed Houston pioneer heart surgeon Dr. Michael DeBakey. He was an appropriate participant, because early encouragement for the project was supplied by Dr. DeBakey when Saint Luke's representatives traveled to Houston to meet him and discuss their Heart Institute dream. While there, three queasy directors watched DeBakey perform open-heart surgery.

The heart program at Saint Luke's had achieved a status deserving of the magnificent new Robert Wilson Wagstaff Building. Under a decade of leadership by Dr. William Reed, open-heart surgery increased from 286 in 1971—the first year of those procedures—to an estimated 1,050 in 1981. In the process, Saint Luke's consistently reported some of the lowest mortality rates in the nation. Demonstrating support for Children's Mercy Hospital, Saint Luke's refrained from expanding its heart surgery into the pediatric area.

Of the cardiac catheterizations performed by Saint Luke's cardiologists, only three-tenths of 1 percent developed potentially life-threatening complications. Saint Luke's cardiologists were acknowledged to be world leaders in balloon dilatation. Dr. Geoffrey Hartzler alone worked his wizardry on some 250 people after joining the hospital's medical staff the previous June, with a better-than 85 percent success rate. And cardiologists also monitored and corrected heart-rhythm disorders using complex electrophysiology technology.

THIRTY
1982

Dr. Ben D. McCallister ... streptokinase ...
neonatal intensive care ... Dr. Dennis O'Leary ...
Centennial ... Spelman

*A*January, 1982, article in the *Star* noted the expected
demise of MAHSA on March 31. MAHSA's executive
director predicted that the result of the agency's departure would be further hospital growth, but there were no lamentations at Saint Luke's,
where the prevailing view was "good riddance."

The president of the KCAHA remarked: "The whole health care system is in ferment, and where it settles out, no one knows."

The Heart Institute admitted its first patients on January 1, and its first
heart operation was performed on January 4.

Also in January, 1982, a columnist of *The Kansas City Star* paid a visit
to the Saint Luke's emergency room. He subsequently wrote about his
experience:

> "The cost of medical care goes always up, but it might be argued that care
> costs more because, as in the place I've described, it has gotten vastly abler
> and easier to get. And that is not regrettable."

Saint Luke's leadership role in disease prevention through healthy living
styles was noted in a February, 1982, issue of *Kansas City Magazine,* pro-
filing the hospital's Lifewise program at its Horizons facility. Prevention of
disease was said to be vastly preferable to painful, expensive cures.
Corporations were expected to be major participants in Lifewise, whose

physical-fitness programs already had met with success. These programs were supervised by doctors and designed to satisfy individual needs.

The medical-staff president, Dr. Fred D. Fowler, announced physician support for the addition of a radiation oncologist to the staff. Dr. Arthur J. Elman, a product of Harvard and Massachusetts General Hospital, added another dimension to cancer treatment at Saint Luke's.

Prime Health had celebrated its fifth anniversary the previous November, and now Blue Cross/Blue Shield (the two Blues merged in 1982) began to compete with the pioneer HMO, utilizing something the Blues called "Total Health Care." Under either plan, subscribers paid a single set fee for access to a broad range of medical services, from physical examinations to open-heart surgery.

The hospital continued to experience a high census. However, volume did not insure financial success. Blue Cross sustained a $2 million net operating loss and reverted to withholding hospital payments. It introduced a 3-percent "retention"—deferred payment that threatened to become a discount—from the amounts owing area hospitals. Insurance premiums for Blue Cross policyholders also would go up significantly.

The culprits were said to be spiraling health care expenses, demand for full range of medical services, and inaccurate projections of hospital costs. The chief financial officer for Blue Cross/Blue Shield said: "We've got a problem in Kansas City. The use of health care services in this community is among the highest in the nation." He blamed an excess of hospital beds and physicians.

Saint Luke's advised that it did not plan to pass on to consumers its increased costs from the Blue Cross action, but the hospital would have to compensate somehow.

The board heard from cardiologist Ben D. McCallister in February about the use of streptokinase, a clot-dissolving drug, in the treatment of cardiac disease. This was followed by a March 5 *Star* article, quoting Dr. Hartzler at length on the same subject. The Food and Drug Administration had not yet approved the use of the drug, and the work at Saint Luke's was characterized as "investigational." Only a dozen institutions in the world were using streptokinase, and Saint Luke's was one of the first to combine it with balloon angioplasty.

The medical staff supported the development of a sophisticated Level III neonatal intensive-care unit at Saint Luke's. This became a reality July

1, 1982, by means of a contract with Children's Mercy Hospital, thanks in large part to the evangelism of Dr. Robert Hall of Children's Mercy and to a $25,000 commitment by the Saint Luke's Hospital Foundation.

Despite critical acclaim, efforts to promote the use of the Horizons facility were not succeeding. Part of the problem was the inconvenient location and part was its ambitious, expensive program. A Board committee examined the goals and objectives of the enterprise.

The academic arrangement with Webster College resulted in baccalaureate degrees for twelve Saint Luke's nursing graduates. More than 100 registered nurses were enrolled in Webster's fourth-year program. Meanwhile, Saint Luke's School of Nursing received an eight-year accreditation from the National League of Nursing. Tuition and room rates, unchanged since 1975, were increased effective in the fall of 1982.

In May, Saint Luke's opened a new child care center. Initially it would operate from 6 a.m. to midnight and would facilitate recruiting and retaining employees—nurses in particular. This enterprise was highly successful from the outset. By September, twenty pre-schoolers and fifty infants would be enrolled, and there would be a waiting list of forty-five.

• • • • •

Dr. Dennis O'Leary, dean of clinical affairs at George Washington Medical Center, Washington, D.C., spoke at the foundation banquet on May 12. He praised the foundation, stating that it was increasingly difficult to offset the expense of medical education and research with patient-care dollars, and he predicted that supporting organizations such as the Saint Luke's Hospital Foundation would be the salvation of such programs. Dr. O'Leary maintained that excellence in medical care and education "absolutely go hand in hand:"

> "An inquisitive resident keeps you on your toes. In my view, it is the most important aspect of continuing medical education. That's where we really educate our people—by the dynamics of this interaction between physician and student or resident. The absence of that stimulation, I think, would be a great loss to the hospital setting and would result in the reduction of the quality of medicine practiced in that setting."

O'Leary also praised Saint Luke's trauma center, describing his own experience as spokesman for George Washington Hospital, where President Ronald Reagan was hospitalized following an assassination attempt ... a role that led to O'Leary's characterization as "the nation's handholder." He termed Saint Luke's Level One designation "a phenomenal accolade" for a private hospital.

Since its Level One designation, Saint Luke's has been placed on "standby" for presidential visits to Kansas City. Advance preparations include assuring that blood is available at the hospital's laboratory of the same type as the chief executive's. A Kansas City trip by Gerald Ford resulted in an appreciative letter to Charles Lindstrom from the United States Secret Service.

Saint Luke's care for professional athletes continued to enjoy a high profile. Veteran Royals pitcher Dennis Leonard was treated at the hospital in May after he suffered fractures of two fingers when struck by a line drive.

In remarks at the annual board/medical staff dinner in June, Edward Matheny noted challenges confronting Saint Luke's in its centennial year. Some of these were financial, resulting in large measure from continuing reduction of government reimbursement for Medicare and Medicaid patients, discounts for Blue Cross/Blue Shield patients, and growing resistance by commercial insurance companies to the resultant cost shifting to their own patients.

Matheny also commented that not only was Saint Luke's one of the most complex enterprises in town but also one of the largest ... an enterprise that did not engage in "the manufacture of widgets" but in "providing health care to many thousands of people each year and health education to new generations of doctors, nurses, and other health care professionals." He went on to state:

> "In 1981, Saint Luke's admitted 26,000 patients and had 194,714 patient days. In addition there were 3,000 cases in ambulatory surgery, 19,000 emergency room visits, and 10,160 outpatient visits. Within our hospital walls the following occurred: 2,472 babies were born, there were 12,700 inpatient surgical procedures, 840,000 laboratory procedures, 9,600 radiation-therapy procedures, 2,900 gastrointestinal procedures, 13,500 dialysis procedures, 2,900 cardiac-catheterization procedures, 193,000 respiratory-therapy treatments, 55,000 physical-therapy treatments, and 34,000 occupational-therapy treatments. And to top it off we processed 3,500,000 pounds of laundry."

• • • • •

Much of a June 7, 1982, *Medical World News* article was devoted to Dr.

Geoffrey Hartzler, referring to him as a "clinically zealous angiographer" who had bypassed angioplasty pioneers in his successful dilations of as many as five constricted coronary sites in a single session. Hartzler submitted a paper at an American College of Cardiology meeting asserting that angioplasty in many cases compared favorably with coronary-bypass operations in the results achieved. A second paper told of using the balloon technique to treat forty-one patients while they were actually experiencing heart attacks. In most of these cases, dilation was preceded by infusions of the clot-dissolving streptokinase.

In the words of the article's writer: "Heart-attack therapy is starting to shift away from the coronary-care unit to the cardiac-catheterization lab." However, a colleague warned that Dr. Hartzler's techniques "shouldn't be tried or even considered by beginners or even by angiographers with intermediate-level experience." Hartzler reported an 86-percent overall success rate in 444 dilation attempts and was described by the Swiss father of balloon dilation, Dr. Andreas R. Gruentzig, as "an artist—I've watched him work in Kansas City." Another colleague said:

> "Dr. Hartzler is a superb angiographer. What he's doing is admirable. I just wanted to add a caution for people sitting in this room who were deciding whether they want to do angioplasty. What they were hearing was not beginner talk. Only half a dozen people in the world have the experience to do what he is doing."

Harvard cardiologist Robert C. Leinbach called Hartzler's results "amazing." He said: "I think what shocked everyone is that Hartzler seems to do better than we all feel we can."

The article continued:

> "Contributing to Dr. Hartzler's success are his background—including three years of full-time angiography at the Mayo Clinic—patient volume (nine to fifteen angioplasties a week now), and backup. At the Mid America Heart Institute, located in Kansas City's Saint Luke's Hospital, seasoned personnel and operating rooms are always at the ready. Between 4,000 and 5,000 catheterizations and 1,000 bypass operations are done there annually."

The volume of angioplasties at Saint Luke's was noted in a subsequent report to the diocesan convention:

> "During the past year over 1,300 'balloon dilatations' were performed at Saint Luke's Hospital, placing it second in the world in number of dilata-

tion procedures performed. In addition, streptokinase, a drug used to dissolve blood clots as a means of intervening acute myocardial infarctions, was first used at Saint Luke's Hospital in September of 1981. Over 100 such procedures have since been performed."

• • • • •

A regional neuroscience center was opened at Saint Luke's, featuring the area's first laboratory equipped to record brain activity on a split screen coupled with a simultaneous telecast of the patient. Neuroscience was a rapidly evolving specialty ... only three years earlier, the department of neurology had been formed; before then, neurosurgery was a part of surgery, and neuroscience a part of medicine.

The Civic Council's Mid-America Committee on Health Care Costs continued its effort to obtain business support and health care providers' cooperation in cost containment. The stimulus was the ever-increasing financial burden on business of the cost of health care.

A column in *The Greater Kansas City Medical Bulletin* by the committee's chairman, John H. Kreamer, cited a variety of reasons for the cost escalation, including an insurance system that encouraged utilization of expensive in-hospital services instead of lower-cost office or ambulatory care; cost-shifting as a result of under-reimbursement by Medicare and Medicaid; technology; and excessive resources. He announced that the program proposed earlier for utilization review of privately insured patients, to be called "Midlands Medical Review Plan," was about to become a reality. Also the Kansas City Area Health Planning Council would be formed to replace "the recently demised and little-lamented" MAHSA. Kreamer expressed the hope that the council would "operate free of the image of bureaucratic red tape and irrational regulators which the federally funded community health planning groups have created."

In August Dr. Clarke L. Henry and Dr. Patrick G. Graham, thoracic surgeons on the Saint Luke's medical staff, sued Dr. William A. Reed, claiming that he was monopolizing open-heart surgery at Saint Luke's. Dr. Henry had performed the first such procedure at Saint Luke's in 1958, using Dr. Kolff's heart-lung machine. A copy of a letter from the plaintiffs to their colleagues on the medical staff explaining their action was posted in the doctors' lounge at the hospital.

Efforts to mediate on the part of the hospital president and the president of the medical staff were to no avail. Because of the prominence of the heart program at the hospital, the litigation attracted considerable attention in the community.

Experience with the hyperbaric oxygen chamber was disappointing, and Saint Luke's doctors questioned the medical value of oxygen therapy. There were, however, a few illnesses where such treatment had shown positive results, to wit: osteomyelitis, anemia, carbon monoxide poisoning, decompression sickness, gas gangrene, skin grafts and acute cyanide poisoning. Saint Luke's used its chamber mainly to treat osteomyelitis of the face and spinal cord.

An adolescent care center opened in early September at Paseo High School with support services from Saint Luke's and Children's Mercy Hospital.

The Blood Gas Laboratory at Saint Luke's, one of the largest in the United States, was selected by a branch of the American Lung Association to serve as a national reference laboratory—only ten across the country were chosen.

In September, the board was apprised of the anticipated adverse effect upon hospital finances of the Tax Equity and Fiscal Responsibility Act (TEFRA) ... its Medicare and Medicaid spending reductions would become effective October 1. The latter included limits on hospital operating costs, prohibition against payments for certain anti-union activities, and lower reimbursement rate for inpatient radiology and pathology services.

• • • • •

A variety of observances in the fall of 1982 celebrated Saint Luke's Centennial. A special fried-chicken dinner was served to 3,200 Saint Luke's employees. Senator Jack Danforth of Missouri, an ordained Episcopal priest, congratulated the hospital in a speech on the floor of the Senate, which was published in the *Congressional Record*. Newborns on the maternity floor sported pink or blue shirts as appropriate, designating the wearer as a "Centennial Baby." And the Newcomen Society in North America honored the hospital at an October 12 dinner celebrating its 100 years of existence and achievement. The hospital also purchased a special multi-page insert in the October 3, 1982, issue of *The Kansas City Star*.

More tangible recognition of the Centennial came from the Saint Luke's Auxiliary, which gave the hospital $100,000 as an anniversary present. Of that amount, $60,000 was presented to the student-loan fund of the School of Nursing.

This was the year when Paul Starr published *The Social Transformation of American Medicine* (Basic Books, Inc., New York, 1982) providing the first authoritative account of how the American health care system evolved. A *New York Times* book review summarized some of Paul Starr's message as follows:

> "The national health care system is a part of a culture, a history, a political and economic order. It embodies our view of a basic social commitment to the care of the sick, the weak and the helpless. It speaks to issues of justice and equity and human rights. It expresses our belief in the power of science and our attitude toward physicians. It is the product of a century of political struggle."

Saint Luke's Hospital was a product of that same hundred-year span.

The Centennial year also saw the death of Callie French at the age of 90. She was a Saint Luke's patient at the time.

• • • • •

The effort continued to identify educational programs of mutual interest to UMKC and Saint Luke's. Representatives of the two institutions met to discuss a cooperative agreement between their respective nursing schools.

Saint Luke's outreach in the Northland area was extended when it sponsored Clay County's Spelman Memorial Hospital for affiliated membership in VHA. The relationship would be further strengthened a few months later when the hospital supported Spelman's application for a certificate of need to build a hospital near the busy intersection of I-29 and Barry Road, in neighboring Platte County.

The KCAHA endorsed the Civic Council's Midlands Medical Review Plan and encouraged efforts to develop a single utilization plan for all area hospitals. But the association let individual hospitals decide whether to participate in the Midlands Plan. The KCAHA itself declined to participate in the plan, a rejection that would hamper attempts to make the organization effective. However, antitrust concerns seemed to justify the decision.

The cost of Saint Luke's self-insured hospitalization/dental plan was discussed in November, resulting in greater employee contributions and a change in the administrative carrier. Like its counterparts in the business community, the hospital was experiencing ever-increasing expense in providing employee health care benefits.

In December, Dr. Kenneth L. Goetz, director of research at Saint Luke's, attended a conference in Vienna, Austria, sponsored by the Austrian Biophysical Society. He was one of nine research scientists who spoke and the only American—the others were Austrian or German. Goetz's investigation of sodium metabolism was financed by the Saint Luke's Hospital Foundation and grants from the prestigious National Institutes of Health and the American Heart Association. Joining him in research efforts had been Dr. Martti Hukimaki of Kuopio, Finland, who, as the foundation's first International Research Fellow, spent nineteen months at Saint Luke's.

The auxiliary held its tenth biennial Holly Ball at the Westin Crown Center Hotel. Kitty Wagstaff was the honorary chairman.

Twenty-one of the hospital's beds were reclassified, bringing the total number of licensed beds to 686.

A December 26, 1982, article in *The Kansas City Star* discussed the Sleep Disorders Laboratory at Saint Luke's, noting that seventy-one such labs in the United States studied narcolepsy and other medical aspects of sleep. "Saint Luke's laboratory has machines that monitor a patient's eye movement, heart rate, muscle movement, brain waves and respiration. Other hospitals have less-sophisticated sleep labs … "

During 1982, fifty-two sets of twins and two sets of triplets were delivered at Saint Luke's.

THIRTY-ONE
1983

Life Flight ... perinatology ... Senator Kassebaum ...
PPOs and HMOs ... AIDS ... DRGs ...
cyclosporene ... for-profit hospitals

*T*he first noteworthy manned flight in Kansas City occurred on July 3, 1869, when a local balloonist ascended from the vicinity of Third and Grand Avenue and landed on a farm east of Independence. Aviation had made considerable progress by 1983 and was an important part of the trauma service at Saint Luke's.

Through the efforts of cardiologist Warren L. Johnson, a hospital fixed-wing aircraft (flying ambulance) occasionally brought patients from smaller communities several hundred miles distant. And for many years a "Life Flight" helicopter operating out of St. Joseph Hospital transported critically ill or injured patients to the Level One trauma center at Saint Luke's. The flights landed in nearby Mill Creek Park.

The helicopter landings were always dramatic, heralded by the arrival of fire engines and police cars as a precaution against an accident on park property. Once the flight was on the ground, policemen escorted the victim and accompanying medical attendants across busy J.C. Nichols Parkway.

In January, 1983, the hospital sought city approval for a helipad on the roof of the nine-story East Building. Preliminary approval was granted for the improvement, expected to cost $500,000 and be completed in a year. However, subsequent review by the Finance Committee of the board resulted in a postponement of the project until 1984. Meanwhile, the exciting helicopter traffic in Mill Creek Park went on unabated.

• • • • •

Blue Cross/Blue Shield instituted a 5.9-percent discount against the hospital's requested rate increase for 1983, in addition to the 3-percent across-the-board postponement of payment imposed on all area hospitals. Historically, Saint Luke's had enjoyed special consideration by Blue Cross because of its major commitment to medical education and related charity care, and the discount was later rescinded, but the relationship was beginning to suffer in a more competitive environment.

Saint Luke's treatment of professional athletes continued. Even minor procedures were deemed newsworthy. A January, 1983, newspaper account reported X rays of the foot of Larry Drew, a point guard on Kansas City's short-lived professional basketball team, the Kings.

A February 18 article in *The Kansas City Times* reported on the two-year-old Lifewise wellness program, still housed at the suburban Horizons facility. The struggling program had three facets: one for executives, one for corporations interested in improving employee health, and one for individuals.

The increasing importance of the heart program at Saint Luke's was underscored with the creation of rules and regulations for a separate Department of Cardiovascular Diseases.

The hospital's physicians, under the leadership of medical staff president John L. Barnard, increased their dues substantially; a major part of the additional funds would be donated to the foundation to help pay for medical-education programs. This generous act demonstrated the continuing loyalty of the hospital's excellent medical staff and their commitment to medical education.

March was observed as National Hemophilia Month across the country. A comprehensive hemophilia center for children had been instituted at Children's Mercy in 1980, and the treatment was expanded to adults in 1982 through a cooperative effort with Saint Luke's, supported by federal funds. The joint service, entitled "Midwest Comprehensive Hemophilia Diagnostic and Treatment Center," served hemophilia sufferers in Kansas and Western Missouri. This was one of many partnership efforts by Children's Mercy and Saint Luke's over the years.

The Spelman/Saint Luke's attempt to obtain certificate-of-need approval for construction of Platte County's first hospital, in the vicinity of Interstate Highway 29 and Barry Road, was not initially successful. The Missouri Health Facilities Review Committee rejected the Spelman proposal as well as competing proposals by Research Medical Center and Qualicare—the latter a hospital-management company based in New Orleans.

Far from ending the matter, however, the committee's opposition led to appeals to the state by all three contenders. A fourth candidate, AHI Health Services Inc., an independent osteopathic hospital firm, entered the field, giving notice to state health planning officials that it, too, planned to apply for a permit to build in the same area.

•••••

Improved care for high-risk pregnancies was assured in the Kansas City area with the employment by Saint Luke's of Dr. Howard O. Grundy, the first perinatologist to practice in the vast area between St. Louis and Denver. Saint Luke's Center for Perinatal Medicine was the only local facility for treatment of high-risk pregnancies. An April 28, 1983, article in *The Kansas City Star* noted that "more than 200 babies had drawn their first feeble breath at the center … " Cost of treatment ranged from $15,000 to $55,000, depending on length of stay and extent of medical care.

Dr. Robert Hall, chief of neonatal medicine at Children's Mercy, and four of his neonatologists, worked part time at the center … characterized by Dr. Hall as "a milestone in cooperation." Dr. Hall attributed the relationship's success to avoidance of duplicated services.

•••••

Senator Nancy Landon Kassebaum spoke at the Saint Luke's Hospital Foundation Banquet on May 16, 1983. She noted with concern the rising cost of health care, while praising Saint Luke's for its long service to the community. But her prescient remarks were addressed primarily at the federal role in health care, particularly current efforts at cost containment and recent developments in ethical issues.

Concerning cost containment she said:

"At some point, and the point is not far away, we have to ask: When do we reach our limit on spending for health? And when we reach that limit, how will we ration the health care we can afford?"

Meanwhile, Senator Kassebaum noted that Congress would soon introduce a new payment methodology for Medicare:

> "The new system, under which Medicare will reimburse hospitals at a predetermined rate for specific medical procedures rather than basing reimbursement on actual costs, creates new challenges for hospital management. Administrators will have to maximize the efficiency of their operations while maintaining quality care."

Concerning ethical issues:

> "In spite of our stated intentions to remove government intrusion from the private sector, there is a developing trend in all three branches of government—executive, legislative, and judicial—toward more involvement in the loaded issue of medical ethics. As medical technology expands and the prolongation of life becomes easier, government is entering the debate over life and death."

The senator went on to note the contributions of private citizens to quality and equitable access, at Saint Luke's and elsewhere. And she concluded:

> "In reflecting on how each of us addresses our responsibilities, I would like to quote Alan Alda in his commencement address to graduates of Columbia University's School of Medicine: 'I hope you will always remember this: the headbone is connected to the heartbone. Don't let them come apart.' "

• • • • •

A certificate-of-need application was filed for construction of an outpatient center on the Saint Luke's campus to provide more cost-efficient care to ambulatory patients.

A May article in *Internal Medicine News* described a presentation by Dr. Ben D. McCallister at the Kansas regional meeting of the American Cardiology Association. The report focused on angioplasty treatment of septuagenarian patients. In 1975, Drs. McCallister and William A. Reed first disclosed the results at Saint Luke's of bypass surgery on patients over age 70 and had since maintained an active interest in the care of such elderly coronary patients. Statistics and study results were cited, enhancing the reputation of the Heart Institute as a quality institution for cardiac care and clinical research.

Dr. Max Berry, now a senior physician, also had an interest in aging patients … they comprised a large part of his practice. In the course of remarks at a Heart Institute Forum, Dr. Berry decried the efforts of 20-year-old dietitians to improve the eating habits of seniors who had already survived for three score and ten years. And he admitted that the first thing he did on examining his older patients was look to see if their socks matched.

A May 31 article in *The Kansas City Times* noted an increase in open-heart surgery units in Kansas City. More hospitals, pursuing prestige and income, were establishing their own units and competing for patients whom they previously had referred to other institutions. Saint Luke's accounted for nearly half of the 2,178 heart surgeries in the Kansas City area in 1982. After Saint Luke's, which drew patients from across the country, the number of cases ranged from 17 to 235 at the other area hospitals.

• • • • •

Another *Times* article of the same date criticized the increasing cost of health care, beginning:

> "This nation's rush for miracle cures, improved technical sophistication, and accessible medical care raises concerns that unchecked costs threaten to strangle the American economy."

While cost containment might be universally acclaimed in the abstract, like restricting pork-barrel politics it was painful to apply when Americans' own oxen were being gored. People were loath to confront their mortality. Comedian Woody Allen was quoted as saying:

> "It's not that I'm afraid to die. I just don't want to be there when it happens."

In a parking lot post-mortem that followed a cost-containment session, Truman Medical Center Chairman Donald H. Chisholm summed up the dilemma succinctly: "When it's you in the hospital I'm all for cost containment, but when I'm there I want everything you've got."

Noting the federal government's role in expanding the medical establishment, Saint Luke's Charles Lindstrom commented: "We were told 'Go out and build and get big.' Then we were told 'Go out and develop more services.' Now they're saying, 'We've created something too big, cut down.'"

One proposed remedy was direct competition among health care providers, and it was prophesied that in such an environment not all hospitals would survive. After Ronald Reagan was elected president in 1980, he chose two of the leading proponents of the strategy of competition in health care for top positions—the new director of the Office of Management and Budget and the new secretary of Health and Human Services. A shakeout period was forecast.

Another consequence noted in a *Times* article (June 1, 1983) was the development of PPOs and HMOs. Saint Luke's already had authorized the formation of a preferred provider organization, and the pioneer health maintenance organization, Prime Health, had been in existence for several years.

A characteristic of HMOs was their agreement to take patients at a competitive charge, gambling that they could keep them healthy and still make money. This led to a reduction of hospital stays and negotiation of discounted hospital rates. Moreover, physicians upon whom hospitals had formerly relied for patient referrals joined HMOs allied with a limited number of hospitals; these alliances intensified the competition for a dwindling pool of patients.

Unlike HMOs, PPOs simply offered discounts to businesses if they used particular hospitals or their physicians.

Blue Cross/Blue Shield had earlier entered the HMO fray with its "Total Health Plan." But it warned that it would not accept hospital cost-shifting that charged Blue Cross/Blue Shield patients more in order to compensate for revenue lost due to discounts or lower patient occupancy.

•••••

Saint Luke's was a tertiary-care hospital with highly trained specialists … the hospital attracted so many Mayo-trained doctors that it was referred to sometimes as "Mayo South" by Saint Luke's, and "the Kansas City Raiders" by Mayo executives. It continued to count heavily on a strategy that featured quality care, believing that a knowledgeable consumer would choose as much for quality as for price—particularly where his health or that of his family was at risk.

George Brett remained a regular at Saint Luke's, most recently when a fractured little toe put him out of action for fifteen days. Pitcher Dennis Leonard made a repeat visit to the hospital when he was treated for a torn tendon in a knee, an injury suffered during a June ball game with the Baltimore Orioles. The hospital was accustomed to hosting press conferences involving professional athletes and knew what the media expected in the way of facilities. When Leonard was confronted by the bright TV lights following his surgery he compared it to "the president coming into the oval room." A few weeks later the news media reported that right fielder Jerry Martin would require hand surgery after a Saint Luke's bone scan revealed a stress fracture in his left hand.

On June 12, 1983, a reunion was held for children who had been in the intensive-care nursery at Saint Luke's between January, 1980, and the end of 1982. According to *The Kansas City Times,* they came back with their parents "to praise the staff at Saint Luke's for their compassion and their lifesaving skills."

The third annual Mid America Heart Institute Symposium was attended by 245 physicians from around the world, and Geoff Hartzler and his colleagues traveled the globe preaching the gospel of angioplasty. Some 10,000 cardiac surgeries had been performed at Saint Luke's since 1971.

Later in June it was announced that a two-year study of diltiazem, a new medication for coronary artery disease, would be conducted at the Mid-America Heart Institute, funded by a research grant from Marion Laboratories. Dr. McCallister advised that 600 patients would take part, with half receiving the new drug and half receiving placebos. In ensuing years, the partnership between the Heart Institute and Marion would be very productive in terms of clinical research.

In July, 1983, anxiety was rising over the mysterious and deadly disease called AIDS, which recently had made its appearance in Kansas City. Dr. Joseph Brewer, a Saint Luke's specialist in infectious diseases, treated a half dozen AIDS patients, most of whom were in the early stages of the disease. Men and women called Brewer's office daily, worried that their various symptoms might be signs of AIDS.

Dr. Thomas Helling performed another liver transplant, three years after his initial effort. No transplants had been attempted in the interim because of a lack of appropriate candidates for the difficult and expensive procedure. Financial arrangements for the new patient were left to be "worked out later." He survived the surgery, only to succumb ten months later to pneumonia.

• • • • •

In August, Blue Cross/Blue Shield embarked upon a further aggressive program with its "Preferred Care" plan, expected to reduce health care costs by requiring discounts from participating doctors and hospitals. The plan was described as a PPO, and only certain hospitals were to be invited to participate.

Blue Cross was one of the biggest area sources of hospital income, second only to the federal government. Following years of serving mainly as a financing agency, the organization was now assuming a greater role in controlling hospital care while reducing the number of its hospital providers. Concern was expressed that subscribers to other insurance plans would end up subsidizing the discounts provided to Blue Cross members. The question being asked was: "Could this result in more cost shifting?" Twenty-eight hospitals bid to be included in the plan; twelve were chosen, including Saint Luke's. Meanwhile Saint Luke's invited other hospitals to join its evolving PPO, now called HealthNet.

In the aftermath of the Blue Cross announcement, health care consultants predicted that hospitals excluded from the Preferred Care plan could lose 10-15 percent of their patient-care revenue and find themselves struggling to survive. Blue Cross expected to sign up as many as 2,500 doctors, which could mean that nonparticipating hospitals would lose patients. However, the price of participation was steep—as much as a 45-percent discount for some institutions—and concern was expressed that "hospitals that bid discounts to be a part of the Blue Cross plan might have overreached, especially considering developments in government payments for health care for the needy."

Despite Saint Luke's financial strength, discounts were a problem. The hospital's charges already were among the lowest in the area, and its medical-education and charity commitments to the community were expensive and unique among Kansas City's private hospitals.

· · · · ·

All of the attention focused on the increasingly commercial aspects of health care prompted a great deal of soul-searching within the nation's medical community. An article in the September 1, 1983, issue of *Hospitals* magazine reflected this. It quoted the chancellor of Memorial Sloan-Kettering Cancer Center in New York:

"The close-up, reassuring, warm touch of the physician, the comfort and concern, the long, leisurely discussions in which everything including the dog can be worked into the conversation, are disappearing from the practice of medicine, and this may turn out to be too great a loss for the doctor as well as for the patient."

However, the article also noted:

"Hundreds of hospitals, notably including many if not most of the very best, together with thousands of physicians, notably including the best, are doing what they have always done, going about their business of caring for their patients as best they can day after day, worried about the changes in the economy that keep making their tasks more difficult but don't necessarily shake their faith in the ideals of professionalism and volunteerism."

The medical staff donated $50,000 to the Foundation in September, 1983, largess made possible by the recent dues increase. The Speas Foundation provided a $60,000 grant for design of a joint curriculum for the Saint Luke's School of Nursing and UMKC.

• • • • •

Medicare introduced a revolutionary change in its formula for payment of hospital billings, imposing prospective payment regulations based upon "diagnostic related groups" or DRGs. This was the "new system" predicted at the foundation banquet the previous May by Senator Kassebaum.

Medicare payments to hospitals were fixed according to prices established for 468 different DRGs, without regard to total charges, costs or length of stay. Exceptions: capital-related costs, outpatient costs, and direct medical-education costs would—for the present—continue to be paid based on retrospective reasonable costs. There was also a lump-sum payment for indirect medical-education costs. The hospital had to establish a methodology that took these changes into account when budgeting contractual allowances (discounts) for the following year (1984).

Informational programs were planned for the board and the medical staff to educate them on new procedures.

• • • • •

The Saint Luke's board was advised of a possible affiliation with a Kansas group of hospitals known as "Health Frontiers, Inc." This opportunity was pursued, in an investigation that included meetings in Kansas City and in Hays, Kansas, with Health Frontier principals. The proposed affiliation was reviewed by several board and medical staff committees; all favored affiliation. Following discussion of organizational structure, autonomy of individual hospitals, potential joint ventures, preservation of referral bases, and the financial stability of Health Frontiers, the board voted to pursue membership. Saint Luke's would be the first Missouri hospital to join.

In a subsequent announcement, hospital president Edward Matheny stressed that Saint Luke's would retain its identity and autonomy. The world's eighth-largest multi-hospital system, Health Frontiers explained that it had sought Saint Luke's because it was a "very prestigious institution" and would be a major resource in terms of medical education and specialty areas such as cardiac treatment.

At a September meeting of the Kansas City Board of Parks and Recreation commissioners, the hospital unveiled preliminary plans for a neighborhood fitness park. The required funding, an estimated $1 million, would be raised by hospital officials who expected the proposal to be welcomed by residents and businesses in the Plaza vicinity. The site was Mill Creek Park, near the Country Club Plaza and directly east of Saint Luke's across J.C. Nichols Parkway. Initial plans were quite ambitious, including a fitness-screening station with blood-pressure checks and other modest but thorough health evaluations.

Cyclosporine, a dramatic new drug for combatting rejection problems in transplant patients, soon would be available. This would be a boon for kidney-transplant candidates and also would lead Saint Luke's to consider seriously plans for a heart-transplant program.

Kansas City's Martin Luther King Jr. Memorial Hospital closed its doors in October, 1983. A black-owned and -operated institution that had been a source of pride for Kansas City's African Americans, King Hospital was forced to close primarily because of lack of general community support—particularly its failure to win the confidence of physicians. It filed for reorganization under federal bankruptcy laws in 1982, but the plan adopted did not stave off foreclosure.

In October, two Kansas City hospital consortia were among fifty-nine groups selected by the National Cancer Institute to be part of the nationwide Community Clinical Oncology Program. Saint Luke's was a member of one consortium, together with Children's Mercy, Bethany Medical Center, and University Hospital. The program brought the latest in cancer research to more patients; forty-five new cancer treatments were available as a result.

$$\bullet \ \bullet \ \bullet \ \bullet \ \bullet$$

An October article in *The New England Journal of Medicine* compared for-profit hospitals with nonprofit institutions with respect to costs. In the past, for-profit hospitals had not been much of a factor in Kansas City. But that was about to change. Public financing of patient care, with the enactment of Medicare and Medicaid in 1965, made health care attractive for investors. This led to the growth and geographic expansion of shareholder-owned hospitals, with their focus on the bottom line.

The article reported that a detailed study comparing hospitals in California, Florida and Texas found charges per admission for patient care to be 17 percent higher in the investor-owned hospitals. The differences were due largely to substantially higher revenues from ancillary services such as laboratory tests and radiologic procedures, and supplies. Total operating expenses per admission (excluding professional services) were 4 percent higher in investor-owned hospitals, but the latter managed to generate a greater net income by virtue of their higher charges. Two other sources reached the same conclusions. The article concluded:

> "What these reports seem to boil down to is this: As businesses, the investor-owned chain hospitals may have been more successful at generating net income (before taxes) for their owners, but only by virtue of charging more per admission, not by operating less expensively. Judged not as businesses but as hospitals, which are supposed to serve the public interest, they have been less cost-effective than their not-for-profit counterparts."

Profit-making enterprises understandably had little enthusiasm for treating those who could not pay; nonprofit hospitals uniformly treated the poor and usually treated them well. Humana, a Louisville-based, investor-owned hospital chain, had succeeded Extendicare in ownership of the 400-bed hospital in affluent Johnson County, Kansas, and was becoming an increasingly formidable competitor for the health care dollar. However, there were fewer poor among its patients.

$$\bullet \ \bullet \ \bullet \ \bullet \ \bullet$$

The medical-staff president, Dr. John Barnard, advised the board in October that the staff recommended Saint Luke's participation in the Civic Council's Midlands Medical Review Plan. The board approved hospital membership in the Plan.

A December article in *The Kansas City Business Journal* stated:

> "Surgeons at the Mid America Heart Institute of Saint Luke's Hospital, already the busiest heart doctors in town, may begin performing heart transplants within the next two years."

Such operations were being performed at only a limited number of American and foreign hospitals; the leader in the field was then Stanford University Medical Center, and Saint Luke's heart patients were being flown to Palo Alto for transplants. Cyclosporine had greatly improved the success rate for these operations.

Formal membership in Health Frontiers was deferred pending the necessary legal agreements, including in particular those affecting Saint Luke's autonomy. The autonomy issues never were satisfactorily resolved, however, and at its December, 1983, meeting the board reversed its earlier decision and voted against membership "at this time," ending that attempt at regional networking on the part of Saint Luke's.

Dr. Joseph Brewer continued to work with AIDS patients, numbering among his appreciative patients activists who were leaders in helping the Kansas City homosexual population cope with the disease.

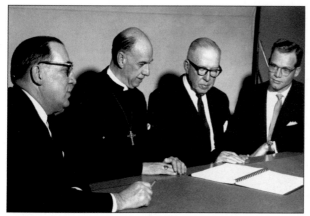

With occupancy exceeding 100 percent, Saint Luke's studied its growth options in 1960. Consultant James A. Hamilton, left, presented a master plan to Bishop Edward R. Welles II, David T. Beals Jr., lay leader of the hospital, and administrator Robert Molgren.

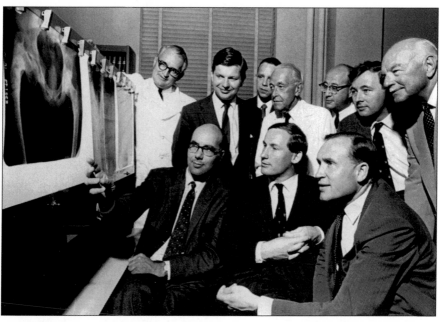

Saint Luke's orthopaedic specialists shared their expertise with physicians from around the globe, including this group from England and New Zealand in 1962. Seated from left: Dr. Anthony Harrold of Harrow, Dr. John Morris of Aukland, and Dr. Alan Murley of Cambridge. Standing, from left: Dr. Richard H. Kiene, chief of orthopaedics at Saint Luke's; Dr. John Wilkinson of London; Drs. John L. Barnard, Frank D. Dickson and Paul D. Meyer, all of Saint Luke's; Dr. David Evans of Sheffield; and Dr. Rex L. Diveley of Saint Luke's.

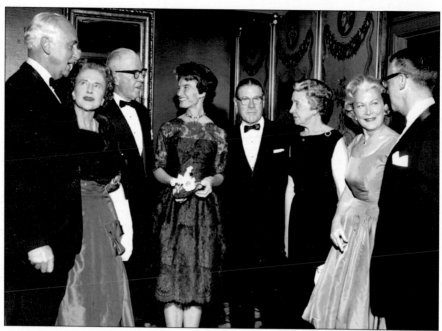

Saint Luke's has enjoyed support from the business and social elite of Kansas City since its early days. Shown here at a 1962 Building Fund Banquet are civic leaders and their wives, from left: Herbert O. Peet, lay leader of the hospital from 1963 to 1965; Mrs. David T. (Helen) Beals Jr. and her husband, who served as lay leader from 1952 to 1963; Mrs. Robert (Kitty) Wagstaff; Mr. and Mrs. Charles McArthur, Mrs. H.O. (Marguerite) Peet; and Robert Wagstaff, the lay leader of the hospital from 1965 to 1980.

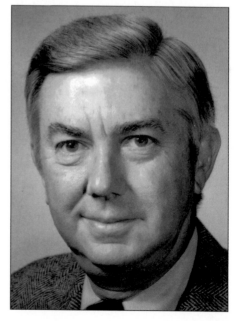

Dr. Christopher Thomas led Saint Luke's down several new medical avenues. In 1956, he helped the hospital acquire the second kidney dialysis machine ever made and the first used in a hospital setting. The next year he helped bring the first heart-lung machine to Kansas City, and in 1966, he performed the first successful kidney transplant at Saint Luke's.

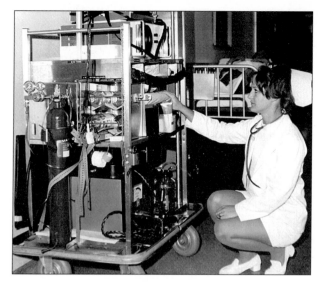

The makeshift Code Blue cart, containing electronic heart stimulating equipment, special drugs and supplies, was credited with saving many lives at Saint Luke's.

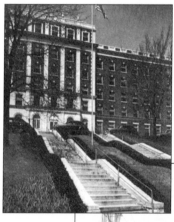

Construction of the east wing, below, in 1964 changed the eastern face, left, of Saint Luke's Hospital and what had come to be known as "cardiac hill."

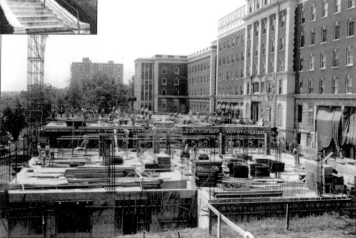

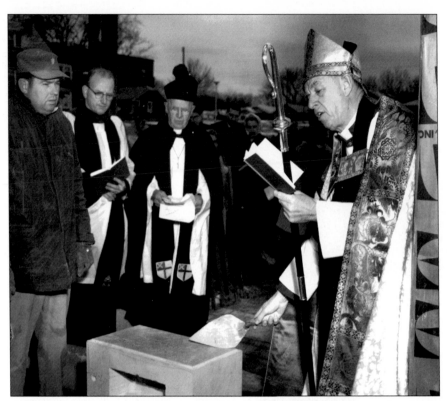

Bishop Welles presided over a ceremony in 1964 to place the cornerstone of a new chapel, to be built adjacent to the main hospital entry on Wornall Road. Also attending were, from left, administrator L. George Yeckel, Dr. William Beachy, an Episcopal prient, and the Reverend Thomas Simpson, hospital chaplain.

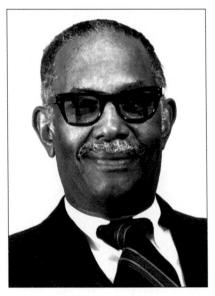

Integration was a slow but steady process throughout the 1950s and 1960s at Saint Luke's. Black patients were first admitted, without notoriety, sometime between 1954 and 1956. In 1963, Bishop Welles made an impassioned plea to add minority doctors to the medical staff, and subsequently a recruitment effort was launched. In 1964, the School of Nursing changed its policy to accept black applicants, and the first minorities enrolled in 1965. Everett P. O'Neal, right, was the first black elected to the board of directors, in 1969.

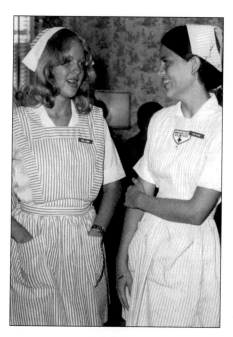

Candy Stripers— high school girls who volunteered their summers to work at the hospital—provided occupational therapy and other types of patient care throughout the 1960s and '70s.

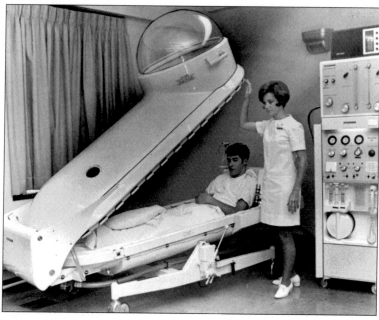

Amazing new medical equipment had become the norm at Saint Luke's during the 1950s and '60s, so the hospital was proud to acquire Kansas City's first hyperbaric bed. This machine, however, yielded rather disappointing dividends compared to groundbreaking devices Saint Luke's had introduced to the city in the past, such as the kidney dialysis machine and the heart-lung machine.

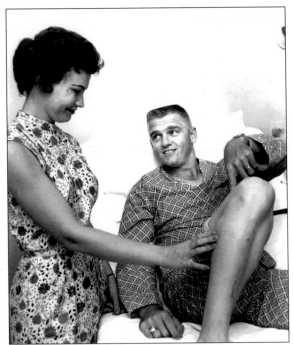

Princes and presidents, athletes and entertainers, chose Saint Luke's for their medical care while in Kansas City. Mrs. Whitey Herzog, right, inspects her husband's baseball injury during a 1960 hospitalization. Herzog later returned to Kansas City to manage the Kansas City Royals.

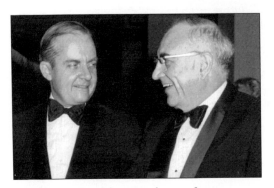

Saint Luke's Hospital generated some of its own notables. Dr. Charles Wheeler, above left with Dr. Arnold Arms, served as mayor of Kansas City, Missouri, from 1974 to 1982, while a member of the medical staff.

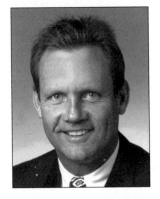

Perhaps the hospital's most famous patient—locally at least—was Kansas City Royals baseball star George Brett, who visited so often during his career that he joked about having his own peronal room.

Photograph of George Brett by permission of the Kansas City Royals

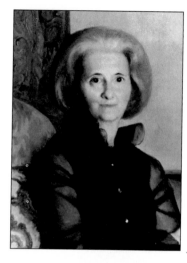

A gift from the Kenneth A. & Helen F. Spencer Foundation in 1970 allowed Saint Luke's to build the library and auditorium that bears Mrs. Spencer's name. Her portrait hangs in the lobby area on the second floor.

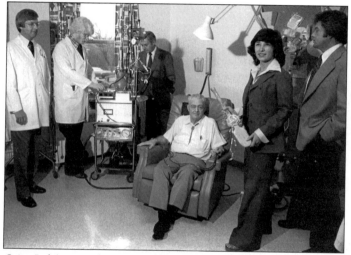

Saint Luke's received a grant for more than $200,000 from the State of Missouri in 1977 to expand its kidney dialysis services. From left, Dr. Thomas Crouch, technician Karl Hirsh and Dr. Chris Thomas monitor patient Burl Slates' dialysis with Kidney Foundation representatives Gloria Cooledge and Larry Kist.

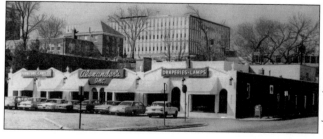

The Auxiliary's Nearly New Shop, foreground, survived for twenty years, despite being uprooted several times for Saint Luke's expansion projects.

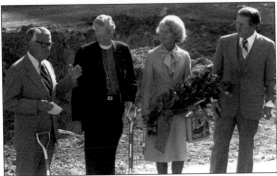

Robert Wagstaff, left, championed the Heart Institute project and donated $1 million to see it built. He is pictured at the ground-breaking with Bishop Arthur A. Vogel; his wife, Kitty; and Charles Lindstrom, Saint Luke's executive director from 1966 to 1995. Bishop Vogel served as hospital chairman for 17 years and provided Saint Luke's with its motto, "The Presence of Care."

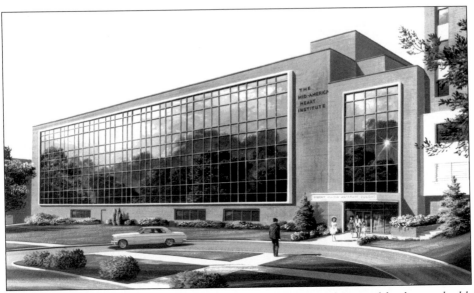

First proposed in 1977, the Mid America Heart Institute was denied approval by the area health planning agency for "lack of need." After much effort, this scaled-down version was approved in 1979 and opened in 1982. The Heart Institute was more than doubled in size through a 1991 expansion.

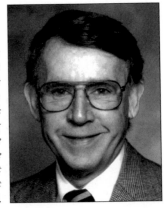

Dr. William Reed, a thoracic surgeon who came to Saint Luke's in 1970, was instrumental in recruiting new doctors for the hospital's cardiac programs and pushing the Heart Institute to the forefront of cardiac care. He performed the first heart transplant operation at Saint Luke's in 1985.

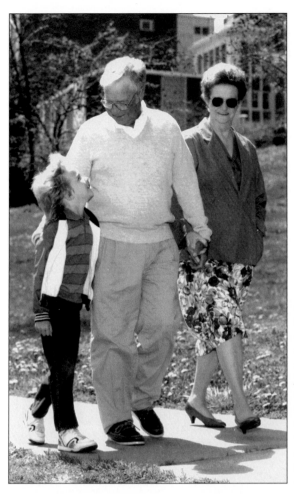

Saint Luke's first heart transplant recipient, Sam Harrison of Grandview, Missouri, was featured in a hospital publication five years after his historic operation. He was active and in good health, though struggling, he admitted, to control his weight, per doctor's orders. Harrison is pictured with his wife and grandson.

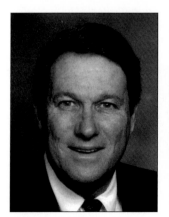
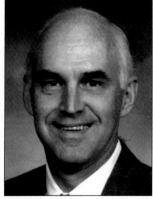

Dr. Ben McCallister, left, pioneered the use of streptokinase, a clot disolving drug, with angioplasty, while Dr. Joseph Pinkerton, right, was instrumental in the development of the hospital's Stroke Center and Blood and Marrow Transplant Center.

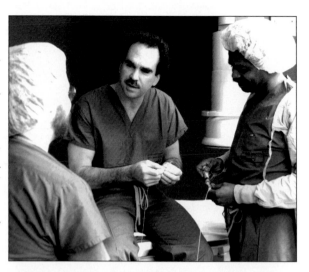

Dr. Geoffrey Hartzler, center, gained international acclaim for himself and the Mid America Heart Institute with his skill in performing percutaneous coronary transluminal angioplasty, also known as PCTA or balloon angioplasty. One esteemed colleague described Hartzler's early results as "amazing," and the inventor of the procedure, Dr. Andreas R. Gruentzig, proclaimed him "an artist," after having watched him operate in Kansas City.

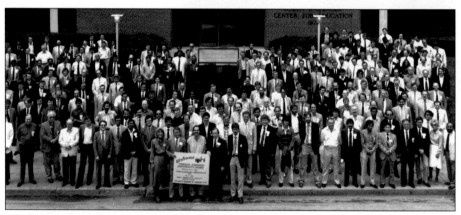

The Mid America Heart Institute began "training the competition" in the life-saving technique of balloon angioplasty. Physicians from around the world attended PCTA Conferences at Saint Luke's, featuring Dr. Hartzler and his Heart Institute colleagues.

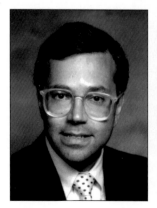

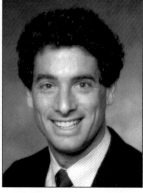

Heart Institute physicians continued to make history: In 1986, Dr. Loren Berenbom, left, was the first Kansas City cardiologist to implant an automatic defibrillator in a patient, while in 1993, Dr. David Steinhouse, right, implanted the first heart monitoring device for patients with congestive heart failure.

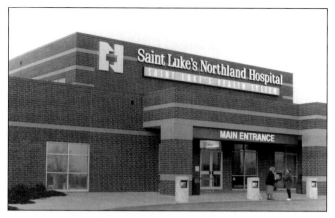

Saint Luke's first venture beyond the central campus was the development of Spelman/St. Luke's Hospital in Kansas City, North. The hospital, which opened in 1989, was a joint venture with Spelman Memorial Hospital in nearby Smithville, Missouri.

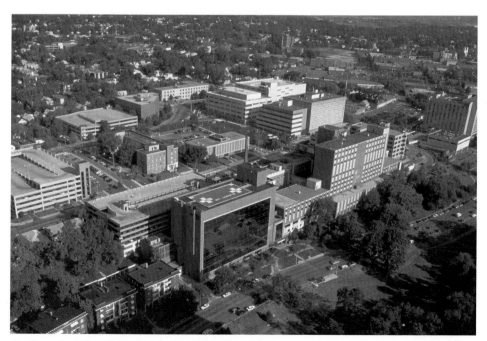

By the early 1990s, Saint Luke's Hospital had solidified its stature as a major regional medical center. The campus, covering more than eight city blocks, featured educational and research facilities, two outpatient centers, four physician office buildings, ample parking, and a hospital licensed for more than 600 beds.

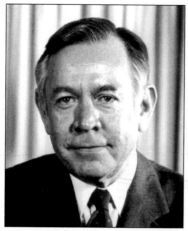

Kansas Citian Charles H. Price II was elected to the Saint Luke's board in 1973 and continued to serve while U.S. Ambassador to Belgium and to Great Britian in the 1980s.

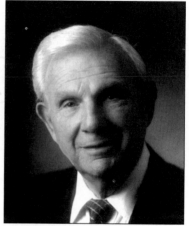

Prominent Jewish civic leader Henry W. Bloch, CEO of H&R Block, Inc., was elected to the board in 1975 after bylaw changes allowed non-Episcopalians to serve.

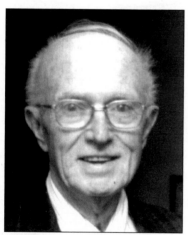

Dr. Charles Kimball, Ph.D., a respected scientist and head of the Midwest Research Institute, was a vocal proponent of the Heart Institute. He served as a hospital board member from 1980 to 1984 and as a foundation director from 1985 until his death in 1994.

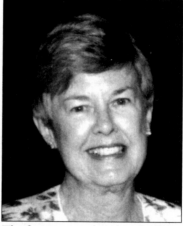

The first women elected to the Saint Luke's Hospital board were Marilyn McMullen, a past president of the hospital auxiliary, and civic leader Ellen Hockaday (not pictured). They joined the board in 1989.

As the metropolitan area grew and managed care required new distribution channels and expanded services, Saint Luke's grew through various means. It acquired Spelman Memorial Hospital, right, in Smithville, Missouri, in 1992 ...

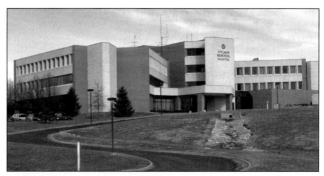

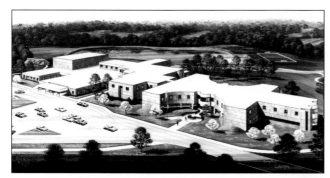

... Crittenton, left, a children's psychiatric hospital in South Kansas City (it had at one time been located on the Saint Luke's campus) in 1992 ...

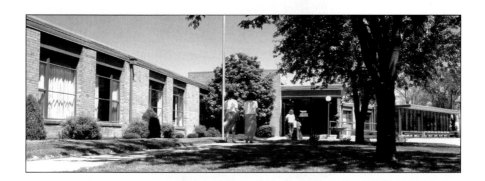

... signed a lease agreement to operate Wright Memorial Hospital, above, in Trenton, Missouri, in 1994 ... and agreed to lease and operate Anderson County Hospital, right, in Garnett, Kansas, in 1995.

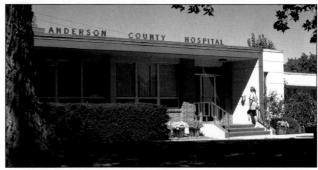

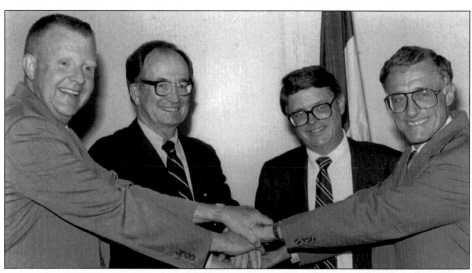

Saint Luke's Hospital and University of Missouri officials who celebrated the signing of a medical education affiliation agreement in 1989 included, from left, M.U curator Edwin M. Turner, hospital president Edward T. Matheny Jr., James Mongan, dean of the medical school, and C. Peter McGrath, president of the University of Missouri System.

Saint Luke's became a partner with Saint Joseph Health Center in operating the Life Flight air ambulances in 1985. The helicopters had been bringing patients to Saint Luke's for many years, landing across from the hospital in Mill Creek Park. A helipad was created atop the expanded Mid America Heart Institute in 1991.

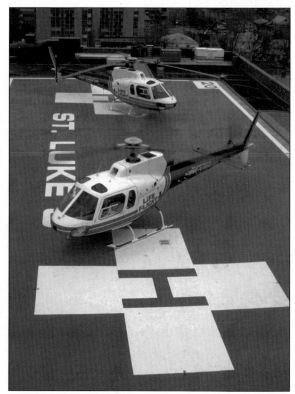

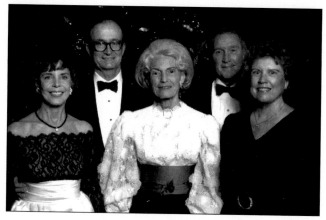

The Holly Ball, a holiday fund-raising gala established in 1964 by Mrs. Robert (Kitty) Wagstaff, center, raised more than $400,000 for medical education at Saint Luke's through 1996. Pictured with Mrs. Wagstaff at the 1988 Holly Ball are Mr. and Mrs. Edward T. Matheny Jr. on the left and Mrs. and Mrs. Charles Lindstrom to the right.

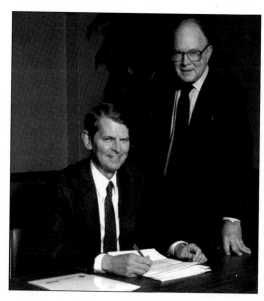

Robert H. West, left, the Chairman and CEO of Butler Manufacturing Company, became the thirteenth lay leader of Saint Luke's Hospital in 1995. He is pictured with David H. Hughes, who served as the first lay president of the Saint Luke's Foundation, from 1985 to 1990.

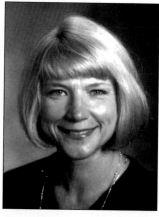

Dr. Marilyn Rymer, who helped establish the Saint Luke's Stroke Center, became the first woman to head the medical staff in 1996.

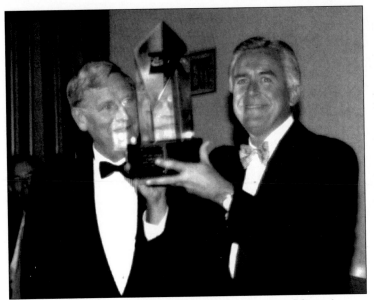

Saint Luke's became the first hospital to win the prestigious Missouri Quality Award in 1996. CEO G. Richard Hastings accepted the award from Gov. Mel Carnahan on behalf of the hospital staff.

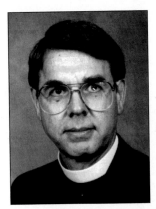

The Right Reverend John C. Buchanan, who was named Bishop of the Diocese of West Missouri in 1989, presided over Saint Luke's development into a health system with multiple locations.

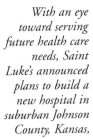

With an eye toward serving future health care needs, Saint Luke's announced plans to build a new hospital in suburban Johnson County, Kansas,

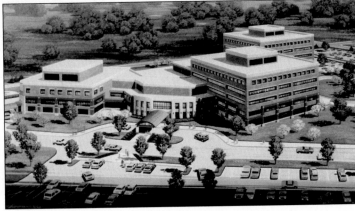

THIRTY-TWO
1984-1985

discounts ... outpatients ... Mill Creek Park ... HealthNet ...
David H. Hughes ... Dr. John L. Barnard ... MRI ...
heart transplants ... bonanza ... occupational medicine

*I*ntensified demands for discounts by various organizations led to the creation of an ad hoc pricing committee of the board under the chairmanship of Stephen C. Higinbotham. In January, 1984, a pricing-policy statement was adopted prohibiting contractual discounts unless patient volume was enhanced; in no event would the 2.1-percent Blue Cross discount be exceeded (preference accorded the Blues by contract, characterized as "favored nation" treatment).

A resolution was adopted at the January, 1984, meeting mourning the death of Herbert O. Peet on January 7. A *Kansas City Times* article noted his civic contributions, including his role at Saint Luke's as First and Executive Vice President and Chairman of the Executive Committee ... "a position held for many years by his father, A.W. Peet." The hospital board attended the funeral service in a body.

A January 19, 1984, article in *The Wall Street Journal* commented on the friction generated in some parts of the country between doctors and hospitals, the result of Medicare's DRG system. Hospital cost-monitoring of doctors to identify "overusers" angered some physicians, and clashes over malpractice liability were predicted as well. Doctors maintained that the government created the Medicare problem by overpromising and underfunding and now was trying to blame them. Administrators were unhappy to be cast as policemen, even though the AHA supported prospective payment on the ground that under the old system there had been excessive testing of patients.

Doctors' fees were not governed by the new system, and it appeared that the incentive for limiting the cost of patient care lay entirely with hospitals. However, administrators pointed out to physicians that new equipment could not be purchased if hospitals were financially strapped, that certain expensive procedures might be eliminated, and that staff privileges of overusers might be at risk. At Saint Luke's, the medical staff was cooperative for the most part. Joint educational efforts were advanced by a board-medical staff retreat on the subject of DRGs, held at the Elms Hotel in Excelsior Springs, Missouri.

A February, 1984, issue of *The Town Squire* magazine published the results of a poll among Kansas City's physicians, naming those regarded by their peers as the "best doctors" among the city's various specialists. There had been a similar poll in 1979. In both instances an overwhelming number of "winners" were to be found on the staff of Saint Luke's, the city's largest hospital. The magazine's editor responded to criticism by noting that few doctors voted "the straight hospital ticket"; rather, nearly every ballot showed a wide representation of hospitals, staffs, and practice groups.

• • • • •

An architectural consortium designed Saint Luke's proposed outpatient center, now approved for a certificate of need. To pay for the new facility, the Board authorized additional indebtedness of $18 million. The new building would provide the community with a full spectrum of comprehensive cancer treatment, including state-of-the-art technology; permit continued delivery of regional dialysis services; and—in anticipation of future emphasis on ambulatory treatment—focus on less-expensive outpatient care.

The costly new technology, including linear accelerators, was necessary to a major teaching hospital. And the dialysis investment was warranted because of Saint Luke's volume—the hospital performed about half of those treatments administered in the area.

The center would include a room specially insulated to house a Magnetic Resonance Imager, the latest highly effective but very expensive diagnostic tool. The noninvasive MRI machines use a strong magnetic field and computer technology to produce detailed cross-sectional images of the body without exposure to X rays. Approval of the center, clearly spelling out the MRI component, augured well for later approval of a separate certificate of need required for the MRI itself.

The Mid-America Coalition on Health Care urged area hospitals to join in setting up free-standing regional facilities to house the costly MRIs rather than go it alone. Saint Luke's declined to participate, correctly anticipating that its volume of procedures would warrant a separate center.

· · · · ·

Acting on a Finance Committee recommendation, the board elected not to purchase and further develop the leased Horizon facility at 146th and Holmes. That suburban enterprise was a disappointment, and its future prospects were not bright enough to justify greater investment in light of other priorities and the financial imponderables of the fledgling DRG system. However, the Lifewise program survived in a different setting ... Saint Luke's was chosen to manage the fitness center at the Vista International Hotel in downtown Kansas City, and Lifewise was offered there.

The end of an era occurred in March, when the auxiliary voted to close its Nearly New Shop, now located at 4137 Pennsylvania Avenue in the Westport area. The secondhand store was a stalwart source of funds for hospital support for two decades, but the auxiliary found it increasingly difficult to provide inventory and volunteer workers.

In April, development of a Mid-America VHA organization was announced. Charles Lindstrom played an important part in this enterprise, exercising his influence as a national leader among health care professionals. Lindstrom's title at the hospital was now "chief executive officer" (CEO), recognition of his role as the head of Saint Luke's management team.

The auxiliary president, Mrs. Carter Kokjer, advised of a gift of $50,000 to the nursing school's scholarship fund as well as other monetary contributions to the hospital.

Infrequently, the medical staff recommended that the board deny staff privileges to a doctor. The April board meeting was one of those unhappy occasions when it was reported that, after following the appropriate procedures to insure fairness and due process, Saint Luke's physicians had determined that a particular doctor should not be reappointed. The board thereupon voted to reject the doctor's application, recognizing their personal legal exposure but relying on the medical staff's assessment.

Construction of an additional hospital parking garage was approved at a cost of $2,562,000, which amounted to $4,362 per car.

The diocese continued its spasmodic efforts to establish a retirement facility with hospital involvement. It now had a name—"Bishop Spencer Place"—and Dr. Charles B. Wheeler was a tenacious supporter. But hospital sponsorship was refused on recommendation of the Finance Committee because of potential negative impact upon the hospital's bond ratings.

A newspaper account of the death of a Saint Luke's oral surgeon, Dr. Farrell Webb, recalled that President Harry S Truman was among his patients. Webb's widow remembered that once, when Truman woke up after having anesthesia, Webb asked him whether he would like tea or coffee. "Hell, no. Bourbon's just fine," said the president. Webb, who could take a hint, went out and bought a bottle.

The nation's hospital inpatient populations declined as physicians used less-costly alternatives such as outpatient surgery centers and home health nursing services. *The Kansas City Business Journal* noted that ten Kansas City hospitals reported declines in patient days between 1982 and 1983. Saint Luke's census dipped to 83.3 percent in 1983, from 86.2 percent the year before. However, Dr. Chris Thomas remained confident of Saint Luke's future. He told Ferne Welles, hospital archivist:

> "Medical care will be done more on an outpatient basis. There will be a lot of care given in the suburbs rather than centrally. As we get into the medical competition a little bit more, the hospital will suffer temporarily but in the long run ... a hospital that has had itself dedicated to education and to the furtherance of patient care as this hospital ... will develop in such a way that there will be no way for it to fail. I'll tell you what the key word is ... it's 'programs.' The thing that separates the major medical institutions from just a good private hospital is programs."

• • • • •

In May, efforts to establish the Mill Creek Park fitness trail went forward, due in large measure to determined support and energetic fundraising on the part of Dr. Ben McCallister and Miller Nichols, chairman of the J.C. Nichols Company. The anticipated universal acclaim for the project had not materialized, however, and the original, major physical-fitness proposal was scaled down in the face of opposition by neighbors and the editorial board of the influential *Kansas City Star.*

The revised plan was submitted to the Park Board for approval despite newspaper editorials vehemently denouncing the project. *Star* writers disregarded the fact that sparkling Mill Creek had long since disappeared underground, encased in subterranean sewer pipe; that the park's rank ground cover of grass and weeds was infrequently mowed; and that the trees and bushes flourished untrimmed and untamed. One editorial, entitled "Leave Mill Creek Alone," declared that "the best thing that could happen to this ill-advised scheme to rip up Mill Creek Park would be to file it at City Hall to gather dust. That's all it deserves."

Another editorial argued:

"Kansas City has gotten along quite nicely with Mill Creek Park virtually as it is since the property was acquired. The landscaping has been upgraded and the lovely Nichols Fountain added. Otherwise it is pretty much as it always has been and we see no overriding reason to change it."

A third editorial lectured the Park Board on its civic duty, warning:

"If the park board decides to permit exercise walkways in Mill Creek Park across from Saint Luke's Hospital, it should be only with the ironclad guarantee that no structure—shelter or whatever—will ever rise to mar the profile of that grassy strip. If clients and patients from the hospital and its satellites jam the small park with joggers and demon walkers, that will not be a signal to put up a building but to cut back on the traffic and try to undo a mistake."

Final approval was obtained from the Board of Parks and Recreation Commissioners on July 3, 1984.

The newspaper's misgivings were misplaced. A much improved park, maintained largely through an endowment fund contributed by the hospital and other neighbors (including local merchants and apartment dwellers), and replete with well-behaved "joggers and demon walkers," is a real jewel of the park system. The park's gnarled old locust trees, migrants from Isaac McCoy's "Locust Hill," are a link with the past.

• • • • •

By mid-May, HealthNet had enlisted seven hospitals and 300 doctors in its preferred-provider organization. It held a press conference to announce its success and incidentally to promote the reduced-rate services available to companies contracting with HealthNet for their employees' medical care.

Many of the Medical Plaza Corporation's original physician shareholders were reaching retirement age and wanted to liquidate their investment. In June, 1984, the hospital board authorized purchase of the corporation's office buildings by a newly formed partnership, Medical Plaza Partners. Saint Luke's, acting through its for-profit subsidiary, became the general partner, and Saint Luke's doctors were offered limited partnerships.

Preparations for heart transplants at the Mid America Heart Institute proceeded. Protocols for the program were submitted to Blue Cross, which announced that it would pay for such operations for its policy holders as long as the program met the insurer's medical criteria. Board approval was given for initial hospital funding of $250,000.

Meanwhile, the University of Kansas Medical Center performed the area's first heart transplant and now questioned whether or not Kansas City could support multiple programs. The implication was that KU had preempted the field and Saint Luke's should gracefully withdraw.

The executive vice chancellor for the KU Center said:

> "It is the job of a first-class university medical center to do the most modern medicine in the world ... The real issue is whether or not a transplant program should be housed in a major academic medical center or in the private sector."

But Saint Luke's forged ahead, obtaining a ruling from the Missouri Health Facilities Review Committee that a certificate of need would not be required for the program because the hospital already was offering kidney and liver transplants ... consequently, this was not a new service.

A new HMO, a modified version called an "independent practice association" (IPA), appeared in Kansas City. "Health Plan of Mid-America" (HPMA) was the project of Saint Luke's pediatrician Don Blim. It was an organization owned by the physicians themselves, and each doctor-owner invested $2,000 in capital. HPMA was designed to preserve the doctors' private practice of medicine, with members consulting their own physician in the private office setting. The doctor-owners would participate in setting the IPA's policy for quality assurance, peer review, and pre-admission certification. HPMA became operational September 1, 1984, as Kansas City's fourth HMO after becoming federally qualified, a significant accomplishment. Within a month after inception the new HMO was adding some of the community's major employers to its membership roster, attracted by the medical luminaries who owned it.

There was an appeal of the Saint Luke's board's earlier decision to reject reappointment of a physician to the medical staff. After a hearing, a board panel recommended that the application for reappointment be denied. The full board adopted that recommendation—reappointment was rejected despite continuing concerns over possible litigation.

The Vista International Hotel fitness center operation was assumed by the Hospital's for-profit SLH Management, Inc. The board authorized the transfer of $452,437 to SLH for implementation of the project. It was not the relatively risk-free managerial role originally proposed for the Vista site; instead, Saint Luke's leased the entire top floor of the new hotel for a medically directed fitness and health management center. The hospital also invested in significant leasehold improvements, including an eighteen-meter swimming pool.

The 18,000-square-foot facility was a major commitment to downtown Kansas City, available for business executives as well as hotel guests. Fitness center members received a health assessment, including various evaluations and analyses, and information regarding physical fitness, nutrition, and stress management.

In October, the chairman of the Budget Committee, Roger Ewing, remarked upon the recent impressive financial performance of the hospital. 1983—and 1984 to date—produced outstanding financial results, with the threat of the DRGs and the need for cost containment providing the incentive. Moreover, the 1985 budget anticipated a contribution to the bottom-line reserve for growth and development of $15 million—even more than the expected results for 1984.

A committee was formed to review and recommend an appropriate policy concerning open versus closed medical staffing at Saint Luke's. This was a sensitive issue because of the obvious antitrust implications. The committee retained the services of Peat Marwick Mitchell & Co. as consultants, and a report was expected by October 1, 1985.

The Saint Luke's cardiology connection with Marion Laboratories continued to be mutually beneficial, with Dr. Lee Georgi conducting clinical research as the first Marion Laboratories Fellow.

Fred Lyons, President of Marion Laboratories, was added to the Heart Institute Committee as a community representative.

By December, 1984, more than 97,000 babies had been born at Saint Luke's—2,606 of them that year. The hospital organized a Saint Luke's Hospital Baby Alumni Club and issued honorary diplomas. Some 1,500 mothers had gone through the hospital's Lamaze classes, a series designed to prepare mothers and their "coaches" for labor and delivery.

Wesley Medical Center, a nonprofit institution in Wichita, Kansas, was lead hospital in Health Frontiers. The medical community was shocked when informed in December, 1984, of the proposed sale of Wesley to for-profit Hospital Corporation of America. This threatened the continued viability of Health Frontiers and confirmed the wisdom of Saint Luke's decision to decline membership in that group.

Christmas continued to be observed at the hospital. In 1984, the School of Nursing held its annual childrens' party in the school's auditorium. Youngsters from the hospital's day care center caroled in several departments and the choir of Grace & Holy Trinity Cathedral sang in designated patient areas. Santa Claus (who beneath his beard looked remarkably like Charles Lindstrom) made a cheery visit to patients and on-duty personnel on Christmas morning.

• • • • •

At its January 9, 1985, meeting, the Saint Luke's Hospital Foundation approved an organizational change permitting a lay person to serve as the foundation president—an office previously reserved for a physician. David H. Hughes, president of Hallmark Cards, Inc., became the foundation's head. The president of Saint Luke's Hospital continued to serve as ex-officio foundation board chairman.

Also in January, the hospital board approved purchase of the small Plaza Hospital property to the north of Saint Luke's. The building became the site of administrative offices.

Dr. John L. Barnard was appointed to fill the position of director of medical affairs at the hospital, a post he occupied with distinction after withdrawing from the Dickson-Diveley partnership.

The Saint Luke's Hospital Foundation in February received a $50,000 grant from the John W. and Effie Speas Foundation, through Boatmen's First National Bank, for use in developing the new outpatient center under construction.

Stanley Ladley, a Saint Luke's director serving as chairman of the

KCAHA, irately responded on the KCAHA letterhead to allegations of local hospital billing errors appearing in a March 5 article of *The Kansas City Times*. The article was fraught with errors of its own—some of the incidents it cited had not even occurred in Kansas City.

An April, 1985, *Kansas City Times* article described the care provided at Saint Luke's developmental preschool, where disabled infants were referred for treatment and therapy. The death rate during the neonatal period of high-risk children had dropped significantly, but survivors included a number of disabled or handicapped children requiring special care.

Nine Kansas City hospitals joined together to use a lithotripter, a $1.7 million machine using sound waves to shatter kidney stones and eliminate surgery. The machine was located at the KU Medical Center, but urologists from other hospitals were assured ready access to the machine. Saint Luke's was one of the nine participants in the consortium, but scheduling problems caused the experience with the cooperative arrangement to be disappointing.

Sale of the Medical Plaza office-building complex to Medical Plaza Partners proceeded. A preliminary prospectus filed with the Securities & Exchange Commission provided that all ownership units were to be sold by May 20—with an option to Saint Luke's to thereafter acquire unsold units.

As anticipated, 1984 was a very good year financially. Net revenue from operations increased 68 percent. Cost containment and favorable payment rates under Medicare's prospective payment system (DRGs) were largely responsible for this outstanding result.

Blue Cross/Blue Shield amended its bylaws to remove area hospital representatives from its board of directors ... the Blues were distancing themselves from hospitals in general. Physicians were retained on the Blues' board, however.

Seminars sponsored by members of the Cardiology Department continued to attract physicians from many nations. Saint Luke's cardiologists were sharing their expertise and, incidentally, training their competition worldwide.

The certificate of need was issued permitting Saint Luke's to purchase a magnetic resonance imager (MRI) ... the first Kansas City hospital to receive such approval. Upon completion of the outpatient center, the

MRI would be installed there. Meanwhile it occupied a temporary home in two leased trailers, where technicians and physicians were trained in its operation.

• • • • •

The hospital's first heart transplant was successfully completed on June 7, 1985. Cardiologist Ben McCallister described the thrill and excitement of seeing Sam C. Harrison of Grandview, Missouri, transformed by the insertion of a donated heart into an empty chest cavity. A July 10 *Kansas City Star* article described the patient's departure from Saint Luke's just seventeen days after the operation. He had beaten the expected release date by two to four weeks and "all but skipped out of Saint Luke's Hospital."

The Saint Luke's operation was followed by a *Kansas City Star* article (July 21, 1985) discussing area heart transplants and speculating whether the region could provide enough donors and candidates for all existing programs to be conducted at a safe and efficient level. The greatest danger was said to be in postoperative care, and experts expressed concern over lack of sufficient experience to deal with complications such as heart rejection.

Saint Luke's argued that the transplant programs that survived would be those with a complete spectrum of heart care and a good referral network—a description of the Saint Luke's program—while KU continued to maintain that it should have the only program in the area. Dr. Kay Clawson declared:

> "We've had a public stance since the very beginning that we think there's room for only one heart-transplant program for this region. As the major academic health center in this area, we felt a need and responsibility to develop the capability to perform heart transplants. We think our program is enough."

In ensuing years, the Saint Luke's program has predominated in the region, aided by Bill Reed's recruitment of transplant specialist Dr. A. Michael Borkon from Johns Hopkins Hospital. The addition of Dr. Jeffrey M. Piehler, a thoracic surgeon from the Mayo Clinic, further strengthened the program.

These personnel improvements were due in large measure to the initiative of Dr. Reed; they were expensive additions to his private practice group, not subsidized by the hospital. The group practices of Saint Luke's doctors recruited specialists from time to time to fill gaps on the medical staff, entrepreneurial efforts that benefited their groups and the hospital.

Reed considered employment of the Jarvik artificial heart as a "bridge" to sustain transplant candidates awaiting precious donor hearts, but this measure was subsequently rejected.

• • • • •

The School of Nursing continued to provide a significant nucleus of Saint Luke's nurses; thirty-six spring graduates were hired.

A July 11 *Kansas City Times* article reported that Saint Luke's had joined St. Joseph Hospital as a partner in the Life Flight helicopter operation. Saint Luke's would build a helipad as part of its new outpatient center; a second helicopter was later added by the two partners. The choppers carried critically ill patients from as far as 150 miles away and operated around the clock.

A July 19 article in *The Kansas City Times* discussed infertility clinics in the Kansas City area. Dr. John Betts, a specialist at Saint Luke's, conducted about 100 laser surgeries at the hospital each year to correct infertility. Later developments in the specialty compelled the hospital to re-examine its role in light of the provision in the Articles of Incorporation that Saint Luke's would adhere to the doctrines of the Episcopal Church, and Dr. Betts removed his practice to Humana Hospital. Meanwhile, Saint Luke's pediatrician Don Blim was assaulted by an abortion protester when Blim removed anti-abortion signs attached to a tree outside his office at 4400 Broadway. The reproduction battle was heating up on several fronts.

The AIDS epidemic was expanding, and a *Star Magazine* article of August 4 noted community apathy and denial. Dr. Joseph Brewer continued his valiant efforts to combat the disease at Saint Luke's, saying that there were hundreds of pre-AIDS cases in the area, with all local hospitals seeing more of them. Meanwhile, patients were concerned about the possibility of blood transfusions using tainted blood drawn from infected donors. Many who anticipated blood loss in surgery were engaging in autologous blood-banking—storing their own blood in advance of their operations.

In September, the state approved a certificate of need for renovation of Saint Luke's second-floor obstetrical/gynecological facilities. In the previous year, the hospital had experienced a 40-percent growth in admissions for high-risk mothers-to-be. The Homer McWilliams Trust continued its support of the high-risk neonatal and perinatal programs at the hospital, delivering a Boatmen's Bank check to Saint Luke's in the amount of $600,000.

Reaction to a penicillin shot administered to Royals outfielder Willie Wilson necessitated surgery on his left buttock at Saint Luke's, to relieve swelling. As a result of this indignity, he was out of action for two weeks.

Also in September, the press discovered the bonanza reaped by Saint Luke's and other area hospitals from the new Medicare reimbursement formula. *The Kansas City Business Journal* reported that in 1984 Saint Luke's produced "an astounding $20.2 million in profits" ... a 9-percent profit margin on total operations. The big winner was coronary angioplasty, where Saint Luke's was a world champion; Medicare paid $12,990 for each procedure, 165 percent above Saint Luke's average cost for the operation. But the article went on to note:

> "Now, with the government wise, paradise may soon be lost. Reimbursement for coronary angioplasty is being lowered to $6,674."

Among the hospitals prospering was the area's for-profit hospital, Humana, which experienced an $8,251,000 profit despite a modest 35-percent occupancy rate.

• • • • •

A medical-staff survey identified oncology as the specialty offering the greatest opportunity for further development at the hospital. A Cancer Advisory Committee was now active, adding business leader and cancer survivor Joe Jack Merriman to its membership as community representative. It endorsed a multidisciplinary-team approach to cancer diagnosis and treatment and recognized the need for an oncology program director. Subsequently a search was initiated for a director, a project that proved to be more complex and time consuming than anticipated.

The Public Relations Committee of the board, chaired by industrialist Albert C. Bean, Jr., endorsed television marketing for Saint Luke's. This reflected a change in attitude on the part of nonprofit hospitals toward advertising. Whereas six years earlier no Kansas City hospitals had engaged in advertising, ten of the thirty-four area hospitals now ran TV commercials to enhance their image and promote their services. There was some criticism, but in general the public accepted hospital advertising. Saint Luke's expenditures were modest compared to the advertising budgets of several rival Kansas City institutions.

Not surprisingly, the 1986 operating budget, approved by the board at its October, 1985, meeting, required no price increases for hospital services.

October also saw the Royals win a World Championship. Dickson-Diveley's Dr. Paul Meyer was awarded a World Series ring for his role as team physician.

A November article in *The Kansas City Business Journal* listed Saint Luke's as twenty-first among the top fifty area employers, with 2,964 employees and a payroll of $55 million.

Nationwide, jobs in the health care field during this period were on the rise—increasing 26.6 percent between 1981 and 1987. But pay rates continued to be relatively low.

Saint Luke's persisted in providing unique services to the community as a Level One trauma center. The newspapers were full of references to automobile-accident cases and victims of shootings taken to Saint Luke's for emergency care. Drama and tragedy were commonplace in the trauma center, particularly on Saturday nights. Emergency medicine was now a specialty. The board approved the development of a separate Department of Emergency Services at the hospital under Dr. Michael Weaver, a reflection of the trauma center's activity and importance. The Rape Treatment Center also continued to serve as a great community resource.

Forty-year-old Industrial Clinic North, Inc., was acquired at a cost of $858,000. Between 700 and 800 companies used the clinic, one of the largest occupational-medicine centers in the region. The transaction marked Saint Luke's initial venture into occupational medicine. The clinic, located in North Kansas City, was Saint Luke's first satellite facility.

A joint Saint Luke's/UMKC Nursing Committee for various collaborative programs in nursing education was established.

Another *Town Squire* list of "Top Kansas City Physicians" appeared, again heavily laced with Saint Luke's medical-staff members.

The Spelman/Saint Luke's application was still pending to construct Platte County's first hospital. In aid of that effort, Saint Luke's provided $400,000 in development funds, to be applied as part of Saint Luke's equity contribution if a certificate of need was issued or to be refunded to Saint Luke's if the state rejected the CON application.

At the December board meeting, a transfer was approved to the Saint Luke's Hospital Foundation of $5 million in hospital funds, for medical-education endowment. The transaction demonstrated to the community the hospital's commitment to medical education and defused possible criticism of hospital "profits." The funds were used to defray direct expense of medical education and teaching-patient write-offs.

Blue Cross/Blue Shield adopted the DRG system employed by Medicare for its policyholders. The hospital's administration continued to wrestle with requests by third-party payors for hospital discounts, offering policy recommendations to the board's pricing committee.

· · · · ·

In December, the board received the long-awaited report from the ad hoc committee reviewing medical-staff-structure issues. A consultant from Peat Marwick Mitchell & Co. made the presentation.

The report reaffirmed the board's ultimate responsibility for medical staff appointments but noted that most credentialing and privileging matters were routinely delegated to the medical staff. Now there should be increased board control, for reasons including quality, malpractice concerns, physician oversupply, resource constraints, needs in specific practice areas, desire for teaching and research commitments, and concerns about physicians' "excessive use" practice patterns. Also, inappropriate physician involvement in staff appointments could cause exposure to conflict-of-interest and restraint-of-trade problems.

The days were long gone when an influential Ferd Helwig could interview medical-staff applicants and rely to a considerable extent on a young doctor's genealogy in recommending appointment or rejection.

After considering various alternatives, the committee urged the relatively new approach of "selective staffing," with staff appointments based on the hospital's strategic plan and the board's assessment of specialty-by-specialty needs. Specialties would be open or closed at a given time, with any closure subject to periodic review.

The cardiovascular program, with its regional and national reputation for excellence, warranted immediate attention. An exclusive contractual arrangement with Saint Luke's cardiologists for the performance of cardiology procedures was proposed, based on need to control quality and cost effectiveness. Cardiovascular surgery would be considered for a similar arrangement.

An important step in implementing this innovative program was the appointment of a Medical Staff Development Committee of the board to provide the framework for staff development. The hospital continued to conduct the credentialing/privileging process, primarily through its medical staff, pursuant to their bylaws.

THIRTY-THREE
1986-1988

selective staffing ... Branton lecture ...
Children's Mercy Hospital ... Dick Howser ...
ethical concerns ... Platte County ... self-insurance ...
capital campaign ... rehabilitation hospital ...
Center for Health Enhancement

*T*he competition over a CON to build the first Platte County hospital intensified. A January, 1986, article in *The Kansas City Business Journal* noted that in the near future the Missouri Health Facilities Review Committee would consider the AHI application. Meanwhile the Spelman/Saint Luke's proposal and a Research Health Services proposal were tabled by the committee until their previous applications—now four years old, and ensnared in appeals and red tape—were resolved. The committee offered to hear the new proposals in March if the applicants would drop their appeals.

Spelman Memorial Hospital entered into an agreement to purchase AHI's stock. It also offered to close thirty-six of its acute-care beds in an effort to mollify those concerned about overbedding in the Kansas City metropolitan area. Saint Luke's supported the AHI maneuver and agreed with Spelman to drop the joint Spelman/Saint Luke's proposal if a CON was issued to AHI. These changes led the legislature's committee to further postpone its decision.

In February, 1986, the Lois Cooper Nursing Scholarship fund was established following the death of Lois Bryan Cooper. Longevity was a characteristic of the nursing leadership at Saint Luke's. Miss Cooper, who died at the age of 91, was a graduate of the School of Nursing and for thirty years served as director of student health at the school.

• • • • •

In March, 1986, the chairman of the Medical Staff Development Committee reported efforts to formulate a medical-staff plan, including review of various issues surrounding the heart-transplant program. Responding to a Development Committee recommendation, the board voted to accept no new Cardiovascular Department applications until it addressed staffing issues involving that specialty. In meetings with members of the Cardiovascular Department, open versus closed staffing was discussed as well as exclusive contractual arrangements with both of the hospital's cardiovascular groups and with Bill Reed's cardiac-surgery group.

A March, 1986, *Kansas City Star* article described the pioneering work of Dr. Geoffrey Hartzler in curing ventricular tachycardia by electrocuting an area of heart muscle that caused the runaway heartbeat. A July, 1986, article in *Forbes* magazine recognized Dr. Hartzler as one of "cardiology's current A-team members."

A cardiologist from the Mayo Clinic—the chairman of its Division of Cardiovascular Diseases—spoke at the first annual William Coleman Branton Lecture, named for the longtime director and officer of Saint Luke's. Dr. Charles Kimball, director Charles Horner, and Dr. Ben D. McCallister were organizers and supporters of the popular lecture series.

Saint Luke's cardiology groups shared their expertise with the world through coronary-angioplasty conferences. The highlight of a Cardiology Consultants, Inc., meeting was a live, televised angioplasty procedure telecast from a Saint Luke's clinical laboratory. The telecast was viewed from nearby Spencer Auditorium by surgeons from several countries, including France, Japan, Belgium, the Netherlands, and South Africa. Dr. Hartzler, with his colleagues Dr. Barry D. Rutherford and Dr. David R. McConahay, presented eleven such courses at various sites, with more than 3,500 cardiologists worldwide attending; 2,000 of these specialists were drawn to the Saint Luke's campus.

At an April meeting, the Development Committee recommended a staffing policy providing for a single heart-transplant program and team at Saint Luke's, with only one heart-transplant protocol. The board adopted this policy in May and appointed Dr. William Reed as director of the Heart Transplant Program.

• • • • •

Research Medical Center outbid Saint Luke's for management of the physician-owned Health Plan of Mid-America, supplying a much needed $1.5-million capital infusion in the process. Saint Luke's doctors were the backbone of HPMA, and the hospital was dismayed at this development.

Another IPA was formed, solely by Saint Luke's physicians, called Saint Luke's Medical Group. It, too, permitted individual doctors and small medical groups to contract with HMOs, PPOs, and other large users of medical services while maintaining independent medical practices.

HPMA would subsequently fail, a victim of undercapitalization and lack of commitment by the participating physicians.

At its May, 1986, meeting, the board approved another joint program with Children's Mercy Hospital (a research project involving low-birth-weight babies) and transferred $86,000 to the Saint Luke's Hospital Foundation to fund the project. In June, Saint Luke's entered into an agreement to provide kidney-transplantation services to Children's Mercy. Agreement was reached in August between the two institutions for an experiment dealing with the oxygenation of blood, and that same month Saint Luke's agreed to serve as the Children's Mercy back-up for dialysis services. In October, Saint Luke's agreed to serve as a preceptor site for the training of neonatal nurse clinicians. These projects were the latest in a series of cooperative efforts between the two hospitals.

The two hospitals' joint regional perinatal center for high-risk mothers and infants was highly successful. Children's Mercy provided physicians and follow-up nurse practitioners at Saint Luke's, with hospital nursing care, equipment, and other support furnished by Saint Luke's. Most of the critical neonatal surgical cases were referred to Children's Mercy.

In 1985, Saint Luke's Level III intensive-care nursery experienced a 95-percent occupancy, with 2,082 patient days; the less-intensive Level II and Level I nurseries were also quite busy—Level II had 78-percent occupancy with 3,427 patient days, and Level I overflowed—141 percent occupancy with 5,175 patient days.

Saint Luke's involvement in pediatric medicine had reached its zenith with the opening of its Children's Hospital in 1925. Later, in the mid-

1960s, there were discussions, which came to naught, of moving Children's Mercy to the Saint Luke's campus.

In June, 1986, the two institutions formed a task force to study the feasibility and desirability of establishing an expanded regional facility, located on the Saint Luke's campus but identified with both hospitals by appropriate name. Considerable time and effort were devoted by the task force to this proposal over the next several months.

• • • • •

The Mill Creek Park Fitness Trail was completed in June, 1986. One of the volunteers putting the finishing touches on the path was Sam C. Harrison, the Grandview, Missouri, man who had been Saint Luke's first heart-transplant patient.

Occasionally the work of the trauma center resulted in patients under police arrest being confined to a hospital bed with a police guard outside in the hall to prevent escape. Despite these precautions, a wounded patient escaped in June wearing only his hospital gown. His attire provoked whistles and cheers ("Look at those pretty legs") from workers at a nearby construction site but did not impede his getaway. He later was recaptured in Oklahoma, having acquired shirt, trousers, and shoes in the meantime.

On July 22, 1986, the Royals' popular manager Dick Howser underwent brain surgery at Saint Luke's to remove a malignant tumor. Neurosurgeon Charles A. Clough was able to remove only part of the growth; severe brain damage would result from more extensive surgery. Press coverage was intense, and the Royals received hundreds of cards and letters wishing Howser a speedy recovery. Among them was a message from President Ronald Reagan.

Several weeks of outpatient radiation therapy at the hospital followed the operation. In December, 1986, Howser underwent experimental immunotherapy at a California hospital in a desperate effort to destroy or shrink the remainder of the tumor, using interleukin-2. Dick Howser subsequently lost his gallant fight for life, but his memory—and recollection of the tender care he received from Saint Luke's nurses in the course of that battle—are perpetuated by the Dick Howser Nursing Scholarship, funded primarily by the Royals organization. Nancy Howser takes a particular interest in this project.

Effective in April, Medicare reduced its reimbursement for balloon-angioplasty procedures by 50 percent. However, hospital profits from operations for the preceding year permitted Saint Luke's to transfer another $5 million to the recently established endowment fund at the Foundation, to defray medical-education expenses, including teaching-patient write-offs. The profits for 1985 were even greater than the record numbers posted in 1984: $34.9 million—the second highest in the nation. Approximately one-half of this was generated by Medicare patients. Medicare's DRG system placed a premium on efficiency, and Saint Luke's administration responded. This financial success benefitted the community in many ways ... hospital profits did not become stock-holder dividends. Unfortunately, not every service was financially rewarding; some of the programs of greatest value to the community were bottom-line losers.

Humana, the area's only for-profit hospital, realized a profit of $5,337,000 after taxes despite only 33-percent occupancy.

An Ethical Concerns Committee with membership composed of directors, clergy, medical staff and nursing representatives, and administrators was created at the hospital. The purpose was to grapple with some of the ethical problems in medicine running the gamut of human existence from revolutionary techniques inducing life, to its prolongation.

• • • • •

AHI Health Services, Inc., despite its late entry into the field, was awarded the certificate of need for the Platte County hospital. This was followed by Spelman's acquisition of AHI's outstanding stock. Saint Luke's and Spelman then negotiated a joint-venture arrangement for the construction of the hospital, to be called Spelman/Saint Luke's Hospital.

The Spelman effort to build a Platte County hospital was enthusiastically supported by Northland residents. Spelman Memorial Hospital had its origin in 1938, during the depths of the Depression, when the visionary Dr. Arch Spelman raised $11,000 from Clay County farmers and merchants to establish a new hospital in Smithville that would serve the health care needs of the people in Clay, Platte, and Clinton counties. A humanitarian who was also a true agent of change, Dr. Spelman determined at age 19 to become a physician and "with the help of men with the same moral convictions, to build a haven for suffering mankind." He not only realized that dream, but now his hospital—in partnership with Saint Luke's—was about to spawn another such haven.

• • • • •

On September 27, 1986, the Richard Cabot Clinic celebrated its eightieth anniversary. The clinic now offered a full range of health and dental care to residents of Kansas City's largely Hispanic West Side—about 1,600 patients a month who could not afford to pay for such services.

The Heart Institute continued to make news. Dr. Paul Kramer of Mid America Cardiology Associates was the first Kansas City physician to perform balloon valvoplasty on adults with obstructed aortic valves. His colleague Dr. Loren Berenbom became the first cardiologist in the area to implant an automatic defibrillator that detected rapid heart rhythm and corrected it through an electric discharge. Meanwhile, Saint Luke's was still training its competition; the latest instance involved staff who would work in a new open-heart surgery unit at Independence Regional Health Center.

In November, 1986, former Kansas City mayor Ilus W. Davis, who had opposed the Heart Institute proposal as legal counsel for Research Hospital, underwent heart bypass surgery at the institute.

Also in November, Saint Luke's joined more than fifty other Missouri hospitals in a lawsuit to recover funds denied by the U.S. Department of Health and Human Services in the early 1980s for treatment of certain obstetrical cases. The suit was part of a nationwide challenge by hospitals to withholding by Medicare. Subsequently, Saint Luke's received $138,000 in settlement of its 1979-1980 claims, plus interest of $81,000. As the hospital's chief financial officer, Ronald K. Bremer, observed, "Occasionally it pays to take on the government."

For years the Insurance Committee of the board had struggled with increasing liability-insurance costs and was easing into a self-insured program. Now the hospital's insurer announced termination of operations, a development that compelled further consideration of self-insurance. The board took the plunge at its December, 1986, meeting, self-insuring for its primary coverage and purchasing excess coverage from a reinsurance company ... an investment that now pays significant dividends.

In December, the troubling lawsuit between Drs. Henry and Graham on the one hand, and Dr. Reed on the other, was disposed of by a mutual stipulation of dismissal which provided:

"The undersigned parties to this suit, having duly considered the request of Saint Luke's Hospital to close this case, and having in mind the best interests of said hospital, do hereby dismiss, with prejudice, all claims and counterclaims made herein, and the same are hereby fully dismissed."

• • • • •

The board's Medical Staff Development Committee, chaired by director and board Secretary Kenneth Fligg, held a series of meetings that produced recommendations for staffing the cardiovascular-surgery section of the Department of Cardiovascular Diseases. The board held a special meeting on January 21, 1987, to consider these recommendations and their antitrust implications. The meeting resulted in approval of an exclusive contractual arrangement with Dr. William Reed's group—MidAmerica Thoracic and Cardiovascular Surgeons, Inc.—to provide for the hospital's cardiovascular-surgery physician staffing needs. Other currently credentialed cardiac surgeons were "grandfathered."

Physicians in the Cardiology Department spearheaded clinical research using the enormous database of 6,500 patients who had undergone balloon angioplasty at Saint Luke's. This represented the largest PCTA database in the world, a benefit of Saint Luke's worldwide stature within the cardiology community. Also involved were a senior project director, clinical-research nurses, and a data-entry technician. Funding all of this was a problem, and the assistance of the Saint Luke's Foundation was solicited. The latter responded with a supporting grant.

In April the board considered another sensitive proposal emanating from the Medical Staff Development Committee, to wit, that, subject to certain exceptions, all physicians engaging in cardiology work at Saint Luke's Hospital commit to full-time practice at Saint Luke's. A resolution was adopted implementing this recommendation.

There was a ripple effect from the cardiovascular staffing limitation, when the orthopaedic surgeons sought to restrict new membership in their department. A moratorium was placed on new orthopaedic appointments while a study was conducted of the department's needs. Upon completion of the study, however, the restriction was determined to be unnecessary.

• • • • •

At the hospital's invitation, the 1987 annual convention of the Diocese of West Missouri was held at Saint Luke's, utilizing—in addition to the Spencer Auditorium and other permanent hospital facilities—a large tent erected for a cardiology symposium.

Responding to a survey, 95 percent of Saint Luke's physicians favored restrictions on smoking in the hospital; one-third of those responding favored a total ban.

The Accreditation Council of Graduate Medical Education (ACGME) serves as the accrediting body for hospital residency programs. Although most of Saint Luke's residencies experienced little or no difficulty in obtaining ACGME approval, the internal-medicine residency was accepted on a probationary basis. The ostensible impediment to accrediting this, the hospital's largest residency program, was lack of ambulatory-care experience for residents. However, there were developing concerns over the survival of graduate medical education in private hospitals lacking formal medical-school affiliation and merged residency programs.

In September, the hospital leased a mobile mammography unit—a large, self-propelled clinic that could be parked in shopping centers and other easily accessible locations, offering inexpensive, convenient breast-cancer screenings.

A *Kansas City Star* editorial mourned the imminent closing of St. Mary's Hospital. It stated:

> "Because of the overhaul of Medicare, coverage restraints by private insurance carriers, and focus on corporate accountability rather than need, American hospitals have changed. Like other businesses now, they make profitability a priority. Those stubbornly holding to yesterday's mission of serving the sick, the poor, and marginally poor really can't compete as equals.
>
> "It is so unfortunate. They are needed. Their patients will turn to Truman Medical Center or the handful of other reachable clinics, further overburdening the last resorts.
>
> "Or they'll move away. Or do without."

President Edward Matheny responded with a letter to the editor published in *The Kansas City Star* on September 13, 1987:

> "Your editorial concerning the financial problems which beset St. Mary's Hospital appropriately praises the service rendered our community over the years by that remarkable institution and its caring sisters. The prospect of St. Mary's closing its doors is sad indeed and underscores the dilemma of acute-care hospitals today. But the mission of our community's other not-for-profit hospitals continues to be to serve the sick without regard to their

economic status. Not-for-profit institutions nationally deliver 73 percent of the indigent care. Locally, Saint Luke's Hospital alone provides charity and other forms of uncompensated care at a current rate of $8 million per year, in addition to other free or unprofitable but necessary community services.

"However, our hospital's constituency is the sick—not the poor exclusively. And while we do not make profitability a priority as an alternative to serving the poor, adequate net income is essential if we are to continue to serve. We are not tax-supported. Our revenues come basically from patient dollars, and to a lesser extent from philanthropy. But it should always be remembered that those revenues remain here in Kansas City and enable us to continue to furnish high-quality health care.

"It has been said that for-profit hospitals care for patients in order to make money, whereas not-for-profit hospitals make money in order to care for patients. If there is no profit margin, a hospital cannot for long carry out its healing mission. A Roman Catholic nun is credited with the truism: 'no margin, no mission.' That is what the present plight of St. Mary's Hospital demonstrates to us all."

The 1988 operating budget included provision for a $71-million payroll and an additional $8 million in other employee benefits.

With the endorsement of the Department of Medicine, a contractual arrangement was authorized at the October board meeting between Saint Luke's and the Kaiser Permanente Health Care Plan. Authorization was contingent upon a guaranteed financial commitment by Kaiser to medical education and satisfactory relationships between Kaiser and the Saint Luke's physician specialists. A managed-care contract later was signed with Kaiser.

The outpatient center was completed and dedicated in November 1987. The scheduled keynote speaker, the administrator of the Health Care Financing Administration (HCFA), was a "no show," as were a succession of last-minute Washington-based substitutes. President Matheny offered some impromptu remarks.

David H. Hughes, Saint Luke's Foundation president, advised the board in November that a foundation feasibility study supported a capital-fund campaign to finance the hospital's long-range strategic plan. Robert H. West, board member and CEO of Butler Manufacturing Co., agreed to head such an effort. The board then voted to proceed with the campaign— the hospital's first broad appeal for philanthropic support in many years.

A partnership was formed by a hospital for-profit subsidiary, Saint Luke's Health Ventures, with Continental Medical Systems, Inc., to develop and operate a rehabilitation hospital in Johnson County, Kansas.

Continental was a for-profit enterprise, and the venture was Saint Luke's first major collaborative effort of this nature. Bethany Medical Center of Kansas City, Kansas, also would be a partner.

Continental Medical was a strange bedfellow for Saint Luke's and Bethany. There seemed to be an inherent conflict between the goals of the for-profit Continental and the not-for-profit hospitals. However, the Mid-America Rehabilitation Hospital proved to be a good investment for Saint Luke's, while providing a needed service in a competent, highly professional manner.

The Cardiology Department's full-time Saint Luke's practice requirement was liberalized to permit Mid-America Cardiology Associates to develop a cardiac catheterization lab at Olathe Medical Center subject to certain limitations and protections. They later established a beachhead at Liberty Hospital with the same restrictions.

The Ethical Concerns Committee developed a "Do Not Resuscitate" policy required by the Joint Commission for the Accreditation of Hospitals. Code Blue miracles were not always appropriate.

•••••

The joint Children's Mercy/Saint Luke's task force, after several months' study, proposed that the two hospitals join in establishing a Kansas City regional perinatal center. The center would combine their considerable resources with those of Truman Medical Center and UMKC to meet the perinatal needs of Kansas City, eastern Kansas, and western Missouri. The task force recommended an "umbrella organization" to direct these perinatal services, with all hospitals in the Kansas City area invited to join, subject to conditions of membership that would meet the objectives of the new system. Saint Luke's and Children's Mercy would in turn develop a joint venture to contract for perinatal services with any institution joining the system.

However, by the end of 1987, it was clear that the Kansas City Regional Perinatal Center would not materialize. There was too much opposition within the hospital community, whose broad support the children's hospital needed. So the opportunity was lost, and perinatal and neonatal centers in the area proliferated.

•••••

In January, 1988, Saint Luke's was confronted with continuing pressures by third-party payors for discounted hospital services. The Board's Ad Hoc Pricing Committee adopted policies to promote consistency in contract negotiations, recognize a relationship between pricing and utilization, and provide flexibility to meet the challenges of the current environment. The committee also suggested that the hospital's marketing efforts emphasize that Saint Luke's prices before discount were already lower than other institutions that offered greater discounts. A subsequent publication of the KCAHA—*Acute Care Hospital Charges By Diagnosis-Related Groups*—confirmed this.

The hospital renewed managed-care contracts with Equicor, HealthNet, and PruCare, and approved agreements with Blue Cross, MetLife, Partners, and Principal.

Although official Washington was promoting the HMO concept as a panacea for health care economics, it did not escape notice that key administration officials and members of Congress did not themselves belong to HMOs. Several belonged to the Public Health Service Corps and were cared for by military hospitals and doctors; others chose the fee-for-service health insurance option offered by the Federal Employees Health Benefit Program; some were insured by Blue Cross; and more participated in private fee-for-service insurance plans.

• • • • •

Committees of Saint Luke's and Spelman Memorial met to consider bids for construction of the new Platte County hospital at I-29 and Barry Road. These meetings resulted in a construction contract with J.E. Dunn Construction Co. The Saint Luke's board at its January meeting approved resolutions authorizing $11,250,000 in financing for the new Spelman/Saint Luke's Hospital. Representing Saint Luke's on the Spelman/Saint Luke's board of directors: James P. Pace, William H. Shackelford III, and A.W. Zimmer III.

Also in January, Bishop Vogel, on behalf of the Ethical Concerns Committee, presented a proposed cryopreservation policy, which was adopted by the board. The policy first noted the hospital's affiliation with the Episcopal Church, and then went on to state:

"The hospital's mission and concern extends to married couples who desire to have a child but who are unable to do so without the aid of medical intervention. The hospital endorses the right and proper use of available technology to help married couples achieve one of the natural goals of marriage, the begetting and raising of children. To that end, technological assistance to married couples can embody Christian values and the Christian meaning of human life, the presence of care with integrity, and offer concerned witness to the community the hospital serves.

"Children are a gift of God gratefully to be received. They are not to be made or exchanged as property; they are persons whose rights and needs must be respected—and among those rights and needs is the possession of an identity as specific as possible. In order fully to be themselves, persons have the right to know their lineage and the biological—as well as the spiritual—heritage which is theirs. The family is the basic unit of human society and should be respected and upheld. Parents have responsibilities to their children, and the hospital seeks to encourage familial mutual responsibility as an important dimension of health in human beings."

The statement introduced a program at Saint Luke's of in-vitro fertilization and cryopreservation (preservation by freezing) of the resulting embryos, subject to certain stated principles compatible with the foregoing credo.

The Center for Health Enhancement opened in February, in a Butler building in the Westport area a block north of the hospital. The facility houses Lifewise activities including a track, gymnasium, lap pool, and a myriad of exercise equipment. It is also an important rehabilitation resource, used by cardiac and orthopaedic patients, the Sports Medicine Department, and others.

The Missouri Health Facilities Review Committee unanimously approved a five-story addition to the Robert Wilson Wagstaff Building housing the Mid America Heart Institute at Saint Luke's. Local planning agency approval no longer was required. The building would now reach the size sought in the original application denied by MAHSA, but at a total cost of many million dollars more than the rejected proposal.

The following month the hospital completed its twenty-fifth heart transplant, with all recipients doing well.

In March, 1988, Wiese Research Associates completed a consumer study for Saint Luke's. The study confirmed that the hospital's "presence" in its primary service area was stronger than any competitor and that overall as well as for specific performance attributes, Saint Luke's enjoyed an extremely strong image. This was especially true with respect to its quality medical staff, special skills available, complete range of services offered, quality nursing, and up-to-date equipment and technology. The Mid America Heart Institute was the most dominant of any medical-specialty category in the Kansas City area. A slow but constant growth of HMOs and PPOs would occur in the next several years, and it was advantageous to managed-care organizations to include Saint Luke's in their plans. As a special report in *The New England Journal of Medicine* would later note (August 8, 1996):

> "Large teaching institutions are also sheltered in part by the fact that insurers have trouble telling subscribers and physicians that distinguished local hospitals are off limits."

The Wiese survey also noted that location was not nearly as often a reason for utilization of Saint Luke's as for many other hospitals; the hospital should make access more convenient. Careful consideration of the southwest sector of the metropolitan area for a primary-care clinic was recommended.

The reigning Miss America, Kaye Lani Rae Rafko, was a nurse; in April she visited Saint Luke's and encouraged the nursing students in their choice of careers.

The Heart Institute received a grant for clinical-trial use of a laser catheter to dissolve plaque in coronary arteries. In May, the Saint Luke's directors viewed a nationally televised demonstration of the new procedure originating from the Heart Institute.

The Heart Institute partnership with Marion Laboratories for clinical research produced a study of coronary angioplasty in diabetic patients, based on the largest group of such patients anywhere to have undergone review. There were also studies of the effects of the drug Cardizem on restenosis (return of blood vessel constriction) and on acute irregular heartbeats in postoperative patients.

Also in May, the board approved a partnership by Saint Luke's for-profit subsidiary with Saint Luke's physicians in a free-standing dialysis unit in Harrisonville, Missouri.

• • • • •

An article in *The Kansas City Business Journal* for the week of May 23, 1988, noted that area hospitals had seen sharp declines in profits in 1987.

Saint Luke's continued to generate the city's highest total profit—$16.8 million—but it also had suffered the largest decrease from 1986 profit totals. And only $3.5 million of Saint Luke's 1987 profit came from patient care. Gone were the prosperous years—Medicare no longer provided money for reserves but was once again a drag on the bottom line.

However, the hospital board did not measure success by financial results.

Endorsement of Medicare by the hospital community was predicated on predictability. Hospitals believed that the time had come for an incentive-based system with rules that rewarded the efficient. For a while the new system worked well for hospitals. But not for long. Medicare DRGs were supposed to be adjusted from time to time, but in 1987 only ten were increased and none with any significant relief. For example, one of the ten dealt with postchildbirth and postabortion problems, which in Medicare-age patients seemed unlikely to occur.

The Missouri Hospital Association mailed letters to community business leaders pointing out that, due to discounts and other factors, Missouri hospitals were paid only seventy-four cents of each dollar they charged for health care. The largest disparity came from Medicare shortfall and from the growing burden of charity care. The hospitals' recourse was cost-shifting to other patients. The MHA communication went to health care purchasers throughout the state in an effort to acquaint them with the consequences of Medicare and Medicaid contractual adjustments.

Locally, the managed-care systems took their toll in discounted services, with hospitals in a bidding war to secure additional patients from Blue Cross/Blue Shield, HealthNet, Preferred Health Providers, Prime Health, and others.

An exception to the decline was the for-profit Humana hospital, which enjoyed a 1987 profit of $7,119,000 (up from $6,353,000 in 1986) despite an occupancy rate of just 29.2 percent. Humana attributed its success to a low-overhead operation, the buying power of a national hospital chain, and contracting out for many professional services. However, the national debate continued over the real reasons for profitability of the proprietary hospitals; some studies attributed their financial success to higher prices.

One such study was conducted by the Federal Trade Commission's Bureau of Economics. The conclusion of another study, generated by the Institute of Medicine of the National Academy of Science, was described by Princeton Professor Uwe Reinhardt in a March 25, 1987, letter to *The Wall Street Journal:*

> "After surveying the published literature on the issue, and on the strength of commissioned additional research, the panel concluded in its final report, published in June of 1986, that for-profit hospitals were typically not more efficient than their nonprofit counterparts but simply charged somewhat more than nonprofit hospitals for their services."

Another factor was the community-service mission of the nonprofit hospitals such as Saint Luke's, with millions spent on charity care, and the provision of unprofitable services such as Level One trauma care, pediatric and neonatal intensive care, medical education, and a range of social services.

· · · · ·

Responding to pressures by national nursing professional organizations, the board initiated a feasibility study of converting the School of Nursing to an accredited, degree-granting college.

On June 17, some 500 people attended the William Coleman Branton Memorial Forum featuring Dr. William Castelli, medical director of the Framingham Heart Study that had first demonstrated the connection between high levels of cholesterol in the bloodstream and heart disease.

The outpatient center was named The Peet Center in recognition of the historic generosity and service to the hospital of the Peet family. The latest philanthropy was a $500,000 gift to the capital fund campaign arranged by Marguerite Peet, widow of Herbert O. Peet. A portrait of Herbert O. Peet, painted by Mrs. Peet, joined her earlier portrait of A.W. Peet in the Peet Center lobby. The Center was awarded a design citation by *Modern Healthcare Magazine.*

The ER's trauma center was busy. Accidental injuries were the fourth-leading cause of death in the nation and the third-leading cause locally—trailing only heart disease and cancer.

A *Time Magazine* article on July 4, 1988, discussed the plight of hospital trauma centers:

> "Beset by high costs and poor patients, often ignored by paramedics and abandoned by doctors who fear malpractice suits, the nation's trauma centers—specialized 24-hour emergency rooms—have been especially hard hit."

Dr. Howard Champion, chief of trauma services at the Washington D.C. Hospital Center, said:

> "Why the hell should the hospital dish out $50,000 for the care of a patient if there's no way of getting it back?"

The answer, so far as Saint Luke's was concerned, lay in the hospital's mission. And so it continued to function as a Level One trauma center.

In response to the Wiese recommendations, a Saint Luke's primary-care clinic opened in Lenexa, Kansas, on September 12. This was the first such primary-care outreach effort by the hospital.

In September, the board approved a proposal for development by the Medical Plaza Partnership of a third medical office building on the campus, Medical Plaza III. A new multi-story parking garage would complete the office-building enclave, with an entrance off Broadway.

Heart Institute programs continued to grow. Four new cardiologists joined the medical staff. Bids for the Robert Wilson Wagstaff Building expansion were invited for submission on or before February 1, 1989, with completion of the project expected by October 1991. Mrs. Lelia Normandie, a cardiac patient of Dr. James Crockett, funded a Heart Institute mini-auditorium conference room in Crockett's honor and bearing his name.

For eighteen years, Saint Luke's had conducted animal research, including hundreds of surgeries. Animal-rights activists discovered that the program was not registered with or regulated by the United States Department of Agriculture despite receipt of research grants from the National Institutes of Health amounting to $225,000 per year. The USDA was contacted, an inspection ensued, and changes were introduced.

The nursing-baccalaureate feasibility study produced encouraging results, and a college of nursing was authorized at Saint Luke's that would grant a baccalaureate degree. Board member Marshall H. Dean, chairman of the Saint Luke's College Committee, directed the development of the college.

THIRTY-FOUR
1989

John Clark Buchanan ... UMKC major
teaching hospital ... cardiovascular clinical research ...
Dr. Arthur W. Robinson ... Saint Luke's College

Since 1975 the president of the auxiliary had been an ex-officio member of the board of directors. In January, 1989, Marilyn McMullen, a past president of the auxiliary, was elected to the board in her own right. She was joined by civic leader Ellen Hockaday. Both women would serve as board committee chairs as well as members of the Executive Committee.

John Clark Buchanan, a native of South Carolina and doctor of jurisprudence, was elected Bishop Coadjutor of the Diocese of West Missouri and would succeed Bishop Vogel as diocesan bishop and hospital board chairman upon the latter's retirement. The new bishop attended the February board meeting.

•••••

Spelman/Saint Luke's Hospital opened in February. The J.E. Dunn Construction Co. brought the project in ahead of schedule and below budget. A dedication ceremony was held in April.

It did not take long for the new hospital to prove its worth. In April the administrator received a letter from Dr. Leonard Nadler of College Park, Maryland, which read as follows:

> "On Saturday, April 15, I had to be evacuated from a Piedmont flight for medical reasons. I was taken to your facility.
>
> "I just wanted to take this opportunity to express my thanks, and my compliments, for a job well done. All your staff that handled my situation were outstanding and provided service that I consider well above-average.

In addition to their medical competency, they also showed a warm understanding of the human side."

For the ten-year period 1979-1988, patient revenues at Saint Luke's Hospital totaled $1.33 billion. However, a predicted downturn in operating revenues had come to pass, underscoring the importance of other financial resources such as the Saint Luke's Hospital Foundation, the current capital campaign, and investment income. Also, auxiliary support continued to be significant: the 1988 Holly Ball generated almost $36,000, turned over to the foundation's "Presence of Care Fund." Seven hundred dollars were donated for support of the Richard Cabot Clinic.

The capital campaign produced generous responses from people in all walks of life and all circumstances. An example was a poignant letter which read:

4/25/89

"Dear Sirs:

"I am writing for the First Presbyterian Church Women of Frankfort, Kansas. We are small in number—average attendance at our monthly meeting is eight. When we heard of your worthy endeavors to help ease the pain and suffering, we wanted to help in our small way.

"Sincerely,

Lela L. Padden"

A check was enclosed. There was a postscript:

"P.S. We are purely agricultural. Our wheat is dying; no pasture for the animals, and the ponds contain small amounts of muddy water. Unless the Dear God sends rain, it will grow worse. But we feel ourselves much more fortunate than others."

Advances in medical science were accompanied by ethical and financial dilemmas. The previous year, blood for a single hemophilia patient cost more than $400,000. In April, the Ethical Concerns Committee, chaired by Fred H. Olander Jr., advised the board of a meeting with representatives of Jehovah's Witnesses regarding hospital blood transfusions, forbidden by their religion, and a special consultation with family, physician, and nurses about withholding treatment from a dying patient.

The committee also addressed the subject of "living wills." Later in the month the committee heard a presentation on donations of fetal tissue, and in May information was presented on the Uniform Anatomical Gift Act and the procedure for and importance of donating body organs. The hospital was asked to participate in an appellate brief to be filed in the U.S. Supreme Court in connection with the Cruzan "right-to-die" case.

Bishop Vogel retired July 1, 1989. A board resolution recognized his "superlative" performance of the duties of chairman ... "presiding over the meetings of the board of directors with wisdom and wit, and providing guidance and counsel to the hospital in the accomplishment of its healing mission all in accord with the doctrines of the Episcopal Church." The resolution also noted that he "provided the hospital with its motto, 'The Presence of Care.' " The bishop was presented with a captain's chair inscribed with the hospital's logo.

· · · · ·

It was becoming increasingly evident that without formal university affiliation, including merger of residencies, the hospital's graduate medical-education program would ultimately lose accreditation and be doomed. Consequently, there was keen interest on the part of the medical staff in discussions with both the KU Medical Center and UMKC concerning affiliation. The physicians' Education and Research Committee was involved in the process. The Executive Committee of the medical staff recommended a UMKC alliance, perceived to be more advantageous than the limited KU proposal.

At a special board meeting on August 17, 1989, attended by Bishop Buchanan in his first appearance as chairman, a landmark resolution was adopted:

> "RESOLVED, that the board of directors authorize administration of the hospital to negotiate an affiliation agreement for medical education with the University of Missouri at Kansas City School of Medicine, such agreement to be for a term of two (2) years, provide for payments of $500,000 to the University of Missouri at Kansas City during 1989, $1,800,000 during 1990, and $3,000,000 annually thereafter if the agreement is continued beyond its initial two-year term, and contain such other terms and provisions as may be negotiated by administration. The final contract shall be subject to the approval of the board of directors."

An affiliation agreement was signed September 7, 1989, in a ceremony attended by the president of the University of Missouri System and members of the University of Missouri Board of Curators. The new partnership brought together Kansas City's two largest medical residency programs and designated Saint Luke's a primary teaching hospital for UMKC.

A laudatory *Kansas City Star* editorial entitled "Building At Last On Hospital Strengths" observed that the affiliation promised a long-range bonus to patients and would "boost both a good medical school and a good private hospital."

Dr. James J. Mongan, dean of the UMKC medical school, was an important asset. While serving on the staff of the Senate Finance Committee during the Carter administration, Mongan was recruited by an admiring HEW Secretary, Joseph A. Califano, Jr., to help shape a national health proposal. The proposal never was adopted, but Mongan demonstrated organizational skills and a grasp of health care issues that now served him well.

Dr. John L. Barnard, Saint Luke's Director of Medical Education, became associate dean for Saint Luke's Affairs, to direct Saint Luke's medical-education department and work closely with the leadership of both institutions in merging their undergraduate, graduate, and medical-education activities. Robert H. West and publisher/philanthropist Morton I. Sosland were appointed the hospital's representatives on the Oversight Committee, to monitor performance under the affiliation agreement. The committee was chaired jointly by hospital president Edward T. Matheny, Jr., and UMKC Chancellor Dr. George A. Russell.

Later in the year, a staff report prepared for the Association of American Medical Colleges (of which Saint Luke's was a member) stated:

> "The reputation of the teaching hospital for providing high-quality care at the cutting edge of medical knowledge and skill is its primary asset in the competitive health care environment." (American Medical Education: Institutions, Programs and Issues, October 1989, page 31)

The same authority noted that the core mission of teaching hospitals is the delivery of high-quality patient care. They were said to contribute uniquely to the nation's health care delivery system by the patient populations they serve and the types of service they offer. The latter include a disproportionately large share of the most sophisticated and intensive hospital services. These are attributes of Saint Luke's Hospital.

• • • • •

On August 22, Drs. McCallister and Hartzler were advised of two $50,000 grants from the Saint Luke's Hospital Foundation for their clinical-research unit at the Heart Institute. One grant was received in 1989 and one in 1990. In addition, the unit received another $50,000 generated by the PTCA courses presented by the Cardiovascular Consultants group. Foundation director Charles Duboc and his wife Barbara contributed funds well in excess of $400,000 for the support of this research effort. The unit underscored the stature of Saint Luke's in national and international cardiology and was deemed essential to the continued development of the Mid America Heart Institute as a major cardiac diagnostic and treatment center.

When North Kansas City Hospital became the eighth Kansas City hospital to offer heart-bypass surgery for adults, an article in *The St. Louis Post-Dispatch* noted that only one hospital in the city met state guidelines for a minimum number of procedures a year:

> "Only Saint Luke's Hospital of Kansas City, whose surgeons performed 852 bypasses and other heart operations last year, exceeded state guidelines. No other Kansas City hospital performed more than 229 open-heart surgeries during their 1988 fiscal years."

Implementation of the affiliation agreement with UMKC proceeded. Several members of the Saint Luke's medical staff were appointed to serve on committees and councils at the School of Medicine, and the mergers of various residency programs were underway.

Dean Mongan attended the October board meeting and, in behalf of the UMKC School of Medicine, accepted the hospital's initial financial contribution to the affiliated program. Dr. Don Blim—now a thirty-three-year veteran of the Saint Luke's medical staff—was welcomed to the meeting in his new role as Director of Medical Affairs, succeeding Associate Dean John Barnard.

The 1990 budget projected a contribution to the reserve for growth and development of $10,259,000. However, the lion's share of this—$8,186,100—would come from nonoperating revenue.

Dr. Arthur W. Robinson, a gifted Mayo-trained internist and medical-staff leader, did yeoman duty in support of the Medical Education Endowment Society. He encouraged board members to join with the medical staff in society membership.

In December, it was proposed that the School of Nursing be renamed "Saint Luke's College" once the baccalaureate program was in place. Meanwhile the transition toward college status continued, there was an upward trend in the school's enrollment, and nursing graduates were heavily recruited for employment at Saint Luke's Hospital.

THIRTY-FIVE
1990-1991

belt-tightening ... Saint Luke's Health System ...
William L. Atwood ... Medicare heart-transplant center ...
reproductive technology ... shared governance ...
imaging center ... Wagstaff Building addition

*T*he AIDS epidemic continued to grow. The State of Missouri enacted legislation requiring all physicians and hospitals conducting HIV tests to consult with the patients prior to taking samples and when reporting the results. The board adopted a resolution directing Saint Luke's administrators to insure compliance.

Meanwhile, doctors and nurses at Saint Luke's received letters praising the care of AIDS patients at the hospital. Dr. Joseph H. Brewer forwarded one such letter, expressing thanks to Saint Luke's personnel for the care and treatment of his patient. The letter commented that, "Each and every one of you responded to Shannon's needs with warmth and compassion such as I have never seen under similar circumstances," and concluded:

> "There are too many of you to mention individually. Shannon was hospitalized four times at Saint Luke's. We came in contact with many of you; you left a lasting impression on us. We're grateful you were there for him. We hope and pray you continue to provide your exemplary support and care.
> "You have our deepest and most sincere respect and admiration."

Dr. Brewer's transmittal letter was as follows:

> "Please find enclosed a copy of a heartwarming letter that I received regarding the care of one of our AIDS patients who recently died at Saint Luke's.

I think the content of the letter is rather self-explanatory. Certainly, it is reassuring to know that our hospital, our nurses, and ancillary staff stand behind us in our fight against this tragic epidemic. We not infrequently receive letters like this these days; however, I thought this one was particularly to the point. I wanted to share it with you, and feel free to share it with any other individuals in the Saint Luke's hierarchy. Many thanks personally for your support in the battle against this disease."

The anesthesiology residency added two positions, enabling Truman Medical Center to participate in the program. Saint Luke's would fund one of the additions. Under the leadership of Dr. Gerald F. Touhy, the Saint Luke's Department of Anesthesiology was restructured; Saint Luke's now would provide anesthesiology service to Truman Medical Center, supply two professors for the medical school, and coordinate the anesthesiology departments at the medical school and Saint Luke's.

• • • • •

Robert West reported the successful completion of the capital campaign, with a total of $12,880,500 raised. Thirty percent came from the Saint Luke's "family" … hospital and foundation boards and personnel, and medical staff. Philanthropy in other forms continued to make an important contribution to hospital programs, enabling Saint Luke's to do many things that would otherwise be precluded by financial constraints. In particular, the McWilliams Trust periodically forwarded large sums for indigent neonatal care; and at the January board meeting two grants were announced: a Speas Foundation grant of $350,000 to fund a geriatric assessment program, and a bequest of approximately $463,000 from the estate of Pansy Pratt.

The final numbers for the previous year were reported in March by the chairman of the Budget Committee. From an operating-revenue standpoint, 1989 was dismal, with expenses exceeding revenue by $1,393,800. Contributing to the operating loss were: continuing decline in patient days, shorter lengths of stay, rapid growth of managed care and accompanying discounts, and medical-supply cost increases. Another major factor was the increasing shortfall in Medicare reimbursement. Independent auditors advised that while the hospital's expenses per discharged patient had increased since 1985, Medicare payments to the hospital were actually lower than their 1985 level.

To some extent, the decline in patient days and lengths of stay was off-set by a significant increase in outpatient care. UMKC's Dean Mongan, noting this to be a trend nationally, attributed the shift to a combination of clinical advances and economy measures.

Fortunately, nonoperating revenue (largely investment income) again provided a safety net—$7,049,800 in 1989—resulting in positive bottom-line results.

The board approved an additional allocation to increase the working capital of Saint Luke's Health Ventures, the hospital's for-profit subsidiary, primarily to support the Lenexa Clinic. That primary-care outpost in Johnson County was a financial drain.

An April 23, 1990, article in *The Kansas City Star* reported that the median profit margin for Kansas City's twenty-four general acute-care hospitals had fallen to a scant 1 percent in 1989. Such a meager return would reflect failure in the business world, but it indicated that the city's nonprofit hospitals continued to do their job despite financial pressures. The drop resulted primarily from increasing patient-care costs, including expensive new federal guidelines prompted by concerns over AIDS.

· · · · ·

An article in the perceptive but short-lived *Kansas City Health Care Times* was based on an interview with hospital president Edward Matheny, CEO Charles Lindstrom, and chief operating officer G. Richard Hastings. It noted Saint Luke's deliberate approach to growth:

> "Saint Luke's, when system-building is involved, is more a builder than a buyer."

Describing the board, the writer stated:

> "That board is easily one of the most powerful groups of business, political and society leaders assembled by any organization in town in the same room."

And, after describing Saint Luke's plans for future development, the article concluded:

> "As changes do occur at Saint Luke's, Matheny believes the hospital will remain true to its mission of educating doctors and offering high-quality care accessible to all.
>
> "'We're not going to achieve our goals by reducing our commitment to what makes Saint Luke's what it is,' he said."

In May, Saint Luke's lost the Kaiser Permanente managed-care contract, awarded to a lower bidder. This would have a limited impact upon the hospital in view of the heavy discounting of Kaiser billings, but a number of the Saint Luke's physicians would experience reduced patient volume.

Despite continuing diminution in admissions and patient days, the hospital's bottom line remained ahead of budgetary projections. Investment income helped, and the "patient mix" included fewer discounted and more full-pay inpatients. No longer could financial results be predicted from inpatient volume alone.

At the annual board/medical staff dinner on June 11, 1990, Edward Matheny noted that the Saint Luke's organization encompassed much more than a single hospital on Wornall Road. He urged that the evolution of the "Saint Luke's Health System" be recognized and emphasized in the future.

• • • • •

William L. Atwood, longtime Saint Luke's officer and director, and prominent civic leader and investment advisor, was elected to succeed David H. Hughes as Foundation president. The hospital board adopted a resolution expressing appreciation to Mr. Hughes for his five years of leadership and distinguished service.

Union efforts to organize nurses at nearby KU Medical Center were successful. This was expected to stimulate renewed union activity among Saint Luke's nurses. New National Labor Relations Board rules permitting organization by hospital departments also could facilitate union efforts. On the other hand, the introduction of shared-governance concepts in the nursing department, while not adopted as a strategy to counteract unionization, were in fact a deterrent. There were no union successes among Saint Luke's nurses.

The Division of Experimental Medicine was shut down June 30, 1990, as an economy measure. There would be no more animal surgeries.

This enterprise was unique among area private hospitals and one of the few in the nation. It had, through the leadership of its director, Dr. Kenneth Goetz, produced valuable basic research results that commanded worldwide attention. The closure marked the end of a time when laboratory experiments were affordable at Saint Luke's. There continued to be a great variety and volume of clinical research at the hospital, however.

As a trade-off in the application of hospital resources, the board approved renewal of the liver-transplant program to begin no later than July 1, 1990.

Effective July 1, 1990, smoking was banned entirely within hospital buildings. Henceforth dedicated smokers, including patients and hospital personnel, would be seen forlornly puffing away outside the hospital entrances … rain or shine. Not surprisingly, their dismal circumstances did not seem to be a deterrent; published statistics indicated that 70 percent of all smokers wanted to quit but only 8 percent succeeded.

Dr. Jon Browne, sports-medicine specialist and newly appointed team physician for the Kansas City Chiefs, brought the football team to Saint Luke's in 1990. The arrival of Coach Marty Schottenheimer the previous year improved the Chiefs' fortunes enormously, and the move to Saint Luke's coincided with a resurgence of community interest bordering on mania among sports fans.

The Mid America Heart Institute qualified as Kansas City's only Medicare heart-transplant center. Despite a tardy start, Saint Luke's transplant program had outstripped any others in the area—fifty-four transplants accomplished since the program's initiation in 1985. Pre-eminence was reaffirmed when the Heart Institute was approved as a heart-transplant center for CHAMPUS (Civilian Health and Medical Program of the Uniformed Services).

The reinstated liver-transplant program was on the verge of implementation; a Mayo liver-transplant surgeon would join the Saint Luke's staff in July, 1991. Meanwhile, in December 1990, the board approved hospital payment of the surgeon's $175,000 salary for one year, to be offset by billings for professional services, and also authorized hospital support services in the amount of $107,373.

On December 11, 1990, the Medical Staff Development Committee met to consider the admission of nonphysician health care practitioners to the medical staff, an issue confronting hospitals across the country. As a result of their deliberations, a policy statement was adopted by the board limiting medical-staff appointments to properly qualified physicians and dentists.

• • • • •

The hospital revised its statement of philosophy with respect to reproductive technology, at the recommendation of the Ethical Concerns

Committee. The operative portion of the new edict was extensive, demonstrating the complexity of the new program and its consequences:

"Oocytes from a prospective mother will be fertilized by sperm from her husband, or by sperm from an agreeable donor only if the husband is unable/incapable of impregnation of his wife. The pre-embryos will be frozen for future implantation in the prospective mother. If the prospective mother is incapable of producing healthy retrievable oocytes, oocytes from an agreeable donor may be utilized and fertilized by sperm from the husband of the prospective mother and the pre-embryos frozen for future implantation in the prospective mother. Exceptions to the above conditions will be considered case by case by the Ethical Concerns Committee of Saint Luke's Hospital.

"The knowledge of reproductive technology, freely given by God, accompanies a demand by mankind to develop concurrently healthy moral and sociological insights that will:

"(1) fully protect those who cannot protect themselves, the offspring of the technology;

"(2) assure that the long-range effects of use of these technologies are fully explained to the prospective parents;

"(3) neither offend nor destroy individual dignity and values of the prospective child or either prospective parent.

"This can best be done when:

"A) The practicing physicians, in conjunction with Saint Luke's Hospital, establish and adhere to a required genetic and psychological counseling for the infertile couple during a mandatory waiting period.

"B) The practicing physicians and the hospital jointly develop uniform guidelines for donor selection and screening. This will include procedures required for the obtaining and maintaining of confidential information as to:

"(a) Complete medical and genetic history,

"(b) Profile of donor's family members' ages, interests, occupations, levels of schooling, etc.

"(c) Donor acknowledgment of awareness that the resulting child might have access to these records.

"C) The practicing physicians and the hospital will determine the maximum number of pregnancies per donor that can be allowed and will establish controls to not allow the mixing of sperm from two donors or the father and donor.

"D) The practicing physicians and the hospital will develop legal papers that will uniformly and adequately be protective of all members of the infertile family, of the donor, and establish the legal rights of the parents with respect to the pre-embryo(s) in case of death of either parent or the separation or divorce of the parents.

"E) Saint Luke's Hospital and its constituents recognize 'honesty' as the fundamental ethic. We will conscientiously attempt to open the subject of alternative methods of conception to the general public so that these may be understood techniques, recognized as ones that offer great rewards to loving families while carrying with them great responsibilities.

"F) Saint Luke's Hospital and its practicing physicians must establish a record-keeping program of these families and their children as a basis for research and possible eventual future guidelines.

"G) Saint Luke's Hospital and its practicing physicians will utilize The Guidelines for Donor Insemination as established by The American Fertility Society, March 1990 and future updates. Consent forms along the lines of their examples will be prepared to cover Saint Luke's requirements as well as local requirements and conformity with state laws. Instructions for the use of consent forms will include an allowance of ample time for thoughtful consideration of the forms' contents.

"H) The cryopreservation of pre-embryos will involve fertilized ovas only through the fourteenth day of development, while twinning is still possible.

"I) Pre-embryos will be stored only for a maximum of three years. Upon the earliest successful delivery of a child (unless within thirty days of such delivery both husband and wife request continued maintenance of the remaining pre-embryos for the remainder of the three years) or upon the death of either spouse, or upon the dissolution of the marriage, all remaining pre-embryos will be allowed to thaw and deteriorate. Under no circumstances will pre-embryos be sold.

"J) Surrogate motherhood, defined as use of volunteer female to carry a child for a couple, will not be considered for the program at Saint Luke's Hospital.

"K) There will be no sale or purchase of human gametes where monetary incentive is the primary factor in the exchange.

"L) An annual review of the policy and of compliance with it will be made by the Ethical Concerns Committee of the Hospital and those medical groups involved in the programs."

Application of the foregoing principles avoided legal entanglements that afflicted reproductive programs at other institutions.

· · · · ·

The Mid America Dialysis Center in Harrisonville, a partnership between the for-profit Saint Luke's Health Ventures and certain hospital physicians, was unprofitable per se. However, it was a patient-referral source for Saint Luke's. In January, 1991, the hospital board authorized termination of the enterprise, which was then assigned to the hospital. Saint Luke's paid no additional consideration or compensation but assumed the existing lease and provided operating funds and management.

Ambassador Charles H. Price II chose not to stand for re-election to the hospital board upon the expiration of his term, and at the annual meeting on January 18, 1991, he was elected an honorary director.

Dr. Thomas M. Holder, Associate Dean at Children's Mercy Hospital, attended meetings of the Saint Luke's/UMKC Oversight Committee. Part of the Saint Luke's financial support for the medical-education affiliation benefited the residency programs at the children's hospital.

Once again, war disrupted the delivery of medical services at Saint Luke's Hospital. Six registered nurses and three physicians were called to active duty in Operation Desert Storm in the Persian Gulf, including Dr. Charles VanWay, the program director of surgery. However, the war and the disruption were of short duration.

Nurses were enthusiastic over the prospect of shared governance, increasing their participation in management. A steering committee was appointed to give direction to the endeavor; practice and management councils were formed, and others would follow. Meanwhile, nurse recruitment was successful to the point that agency nurses no longer were needed to supplement the hospital RNs. The Holly Ball proceeds from the event of the previous December—$35,000—were used to initiate an endowment fund for the fledgling college of nursing.

A Joint Planning Committee, with board, medical-staff, and administration representation, determined that the ultimate strategic aim should be an integrated physician/hospital system. Several interim strategies were pursued, including affiliation with other hospitals and doctors and development of clinics at various locations in the area.

At the March, 1991, board meeting, CEO Charles Lindstrom discussed the new "Heritage Health" organization, a collaborative concept pursued with Independence Regional Hospital, St. Joseph Health Center, and Shawnee Mission Medical Center. One of the first goals of this entity was the development of a managed-care company. It also was hoped that the four institutions would be able to cooperate in providing cost-efficient, quality health care to the community. All were strong, successful competitors, and the cooperative concept was challenging.

Medical-staff integration required the development of a Physician's Organization (PO) and formation of a joint Physician Hospital Organization (PHO). Physician initiatives also included coordinating the Northland hospitals' medical-staff procedures and activities with those at Saint Luke's and developing a Department of Family Practice at Saint Luke's. The latter was significant because of the historic role of Saint Luke's as a tertiary-care center made up almost exclusively of specialists and subspecialists.

Interest rates fell to a level at which refinancing part of the hospital's debt was advantageous, and the board adopted a Finance Committee recommendation providing for this in April. Meanwhile, an increase in the volume of monitored outpatients, while offsetting declining inpatient admissions to some extent, necessitated a reallocation of personnel and facility resources.

In April, 1991, Saint Luke's submitted a certificate-of-need application for an imaging center to be housed in the Medical Plaza III building. A rival effort was mounted by physicians who staffed an imaging center in Medical Plaza I. The competing doctors proved to be more adroit than the hospital in threading through the bureaucratic and political maze in Jefferson City, and, rather than face rejection, the hospital withdrew its application and sat down to negotiate a compromise joint-venture arrangement with the physicians. A lesson was learned—no longer could Saint Luke's rely entirely upon its considerable prestige to insure success in dealing with the Missouri Health Facilities Review Committee.

• • • • •

On April 21, a five-story addition to the Robert Wilson Wagstaff Building housing the Mid America Heart Institute was dedicated. *The Kansas City Business Journal* published a letter from the Executive Director of the Mid-America Coalition on Health Care, noting the expansion underway and the "positive impact" that it might have in the Kansas City area. He commented:

> "In my view, there is a direct correlation between the volume of service and the quality of care with respect to open-heart surgery. The mortality and morbidity rates from open-heart surgery decline when an increasing number of operations are performed by the same surgical team. The improvement of survival rates can be attributed to the increased skill level and efficiency of the operating and recovery-room staff.
>
> "Thus, as Saint Luke's Mid America Heart Institute continues to increase the number of open-heart surgeries it performs, the quality of its services should also increase."

These comments were right on target. An earlier article in *Hospitals* magazine by William Jessee, M.D., vice president of the Joint Commission on the Accreditation of Hospitals, noted:

> "There is a tremendous amount of research that shows mortality and mor-

bidity are inversely proportional to the volume of procedures performed ... The frequency of performance of procedures, particularly surgical procedures, has to be examined as part of the privileges-renewal process, because it is necessary to demonstrate current competence. A hospital should decide to limit its practice and the practice of its physicians to procedures that can be performed with a sufficient frequency to maintain that competence."

In the course of the dedication ceremony a number of facts were noted about the high volume of Heart Institute procedures:

In 1989, Saint Luke's performed 2,212 balloon angioplasties (63 percent of those done in the Kansas City area); in 1990 the number was 2,235.

In 1989 Saint Luke's surgeons performed 866 open heart surgeries; the closest pursuers performed 210, 205 and 201, respectively, and no other local programs performed as many as 200—the minimum annual number recommended by the American Heart Association and the American College of Cardiology for maintaining proficiency. In 1990, there were 951 such procedures at the Heart Institute.

The Heart Institute was the site of 3,340 echocardiograms in 1990 and 182 pacemaker implantations.

There were other notable cardiac accomplishments as well:

Saint Luke's had the only dedicated electrophysiology lab in the Kansas City area, where it was one of only twelve hospitals in the country performing radio-frequency ablations.

At the Heart Institute several recently developed procedures were also underway: implantation of automatic internal cardiac defibrillators to correct life-threatening irregular heartbeats; implantation of stents in coronary arteries to prevent the buildup of clogging plaque; use of lasers to burn out plaque in blood vessels; and removal of plaque by athrectomies, where a tiny "roto rooter" cut out plaque.

And, of course, Saint Luke's doctors were the principal heart-transplant surgeons in the Kansas City area.

A review of patient origin data for the year 1989 disclosed that there were 5,919 Heart Institute admissions with primary cardiac diagnosis. Forty-nine percent of these were from outside Saint Luke's primary service area. Patients came from thirty-eight states. There were also government officials from other countries, including Thailand, Malaysia, Nigeria and India, and ambassadors, businessmen, physicians, and surgeons from all over the world. One inpatient summary accurately listed the patient's occupation as "Royal Highness"; another royal heart patient caused a stir when he appeared accompanied by three attractive wives.

Angioplasty programs educated heart specialists from all fifty states, the District of Columbia, the Virgin Islands, and thirty foreign countries ... all in all, 15,000 physicians and nurses.

• • • • •

Dr. Don Blim, Director of Medical Affairs, advised the board in June that several internists were interested in forming a primary-care group on the Saint Luke's campus. This resulted in Saint Luke's Medical Associates, Inc., a nonprofit subsidiary of the hospital.

Dealing with the Medicare bureaucracy was one of the biggest challenges for Saint Luke's doctors and administration. The inadequate payment level was only part of the problem; there was also the torture of dealing with Medicare audits.

The auditors were never finished—they came back again and again, reopening matters that had passed muster previously. Medicare revisited Saint Luke's 1984 cost report five times—somehow the auditors had gotten the idea that the medical residents' teaching clinic, located in the Medical Plaza office complex across from Saint Luke's, in fact occupied space in a shopping center. This led to disallowance of reimbursement for all education costs associated with the clinic, on the premise that the facility catered to the general public. The hospital contested the ruling; the amount at stake was significant—$250,000 to $300,000 per year, for several years.

The Medicare intermediary also disallowed some 300 claims for patients who had attained age 65, on the unsubstantiated theory that they were still gainfully employed and ineligible for Medicare benefits. This required Saint Luke's to obtain retirement dates from all of these patients before Medicare would pay the account.

If the hospital appealed an adverse decision, there was a protracted delay before the matter was considered. In the spring of 1991, the hospital filed applications for formal appeals of Medicare audit adjustments relating to 1988; the first hearing date would be June, 1995.

The board also adopted a resolution mourning the sudden and unexpected death of Robert M. Patterson, a wise and conscientious director and a generous philanthropist.

Hospital visitors heard the introductory strains of *Brahm's Lullaby* as they walked Saint Luke's corridors, announcing the arrival of a baby in one of the second-floor birthing rooms. This innovation resulted from a nurse's suggestion; she had heard the lullaby in the obstetrical department of a Nebraska hospital.

An August 8, 1991, *Kansas City Star* article noted that, although area hospitals had seen a slight improvement in overall profitability in 1990, they continued to suffer losses on patient-care services.

In September, two new treatment modalities were available at Saint Luke's: stereotactic radiography to treat growths within the brain, and a mammotest precision mammographic needle biopsy system.

The 1992 budget was presented for board approval in October, 1991. The projected return on patient revenue was a mere 1 percent, due primarily to insufficient reimbursement for Medicaid and Medicare, the hospital's major commitment to community service, and the types of programs offered by the hospital. Particular attention was called to the $33.8-million community services budget (primarily free care, and medical and nursing education), and to the $89 million in Medicare contractual allowances.

At a special board meeting on October 30, 1991, Saint Luke's participation in the Heritage Health project was approved, with funding from the hospital authorized in the amount of $3.4 million. The vote was preceded by presentations on the evolution of managed care in the Kansas City-area marketplace and certain characteristics common to all four Heritage partners—shared values and traditions, excellent medical staffs, and the practice of high-quality medicine. Although Heritage might engage in other activities, initial efforts would concentrate on the formation and operation of a managed-care company.

Heritage Health was incorporated in Missouri and qualified also to do business in Kansas.

The board was advised in November of the status of PHO efforts, including the appointment of a nominating committee to propose PHO officers, and a scheduled presentation to the medical staff on November 25, 1991. Kenneth Fligg and Daniel Dibble were chosen as the hospital board's representatives on the PHO board. A PO also was formed with a board of fourteen physicians. Dr. Thomas T. Crouch played a pivotal role in these efforts.

The first televised informational broadcast between Saint Luke's and the UMKC School of Medicine—a cardiology presentation—occurred on November 21. Meanwhile, revenues from coffee-shop operations enabled the auxiliary to contribute $30,000 to hospital programs and services of particular interest to that organization.

$$\bullet \ \bullet \ \bullet \ \bullet \ \bullet$$

Robert Wilson Wagstaff died on November 29, 1991, after a long illness. He was a kind, caring man, a civic leader, and a philanthropist who by his own life and example set a high standard of excellence. He served on the Saint Luke's board for more than forty years and was a major donor to the hospital. As a gesture of respect, the board attended his funeral as a body and later adopted an appropriate commemorative resolution. The Heart Institute building bearing his name is a lasting memorial.

Efforts to obtain approval for the proposed imaging center in Medical Plaza III continued. A partnership agreement was negotiated among Saint Luke's Hospital, its radiologists, and the Western Missouri Radiological Group, currently operating the imaging center in Medical Plaza I. This shotgun marriage had the blessing of the Missouri regulatory agency, insuring the issuance of a certificate of need authorizing the new center.

The hospital's Christmas activities for 1991 included the Cathedral Project sponsored by Grace & Holy Trinity Cathedral. Saint Luke's personnel provided, cooked, and helped serve meals to the homeless on Christmas Day. Later, eighty-four hospital volunteers delivered socks, underwear and clothing donated by hundreds of Saint Luke's personnel.

A survey of some 800 residents in the metropolitan area confirmed the hospital's preferred status among area consumers.

The board sustained another loss with the unexpected death of director Stan Ladley. In recognition of his interest in and valuable contributions to nursing at Saint Luke's, a "Stan Ladley Memorial Scholarship in Nursing" was established.

The hospital's Articles of Incorporation were amended to reduce to thirty-nine the number of diocesan communicants required out of the board's total membership of fifty-one. The additional flexibility, which had the blessing of Bishop Buchanan, would permit election to the board of two representatives of Spelman Memorial Hospital. Saint Luke's corporate officers would continue to be Episcopalians.

THIRTY-SIX
1992-1993

PO-PHO ... primary care group ... charity care ...
Crittenton ... Atchison Hospital ... Senior Tour ...
helicopter crash ... Dr. Robert J. Belt

*T*he board's annual meeting in January, 1992, was attended by Dr. Charles Rosen, director of the resurrected liver-transplant program. He had performed just three liver transplants at Saint Luke's. Late re-entry into the field handicapped attempts to establish an adequate referral base. To increase volume, application was made for Medicaid certification of the transplant program for the 1992 calendar year, even though Medicaid reimbursement was not likely to cover all charges. However, despite these efforts and despite the excellence of the program, there was never sufficient volume to justify its continuation, and it was abandoned.

A neonatal-transport system was initiated, to serve Saint Luke's ten-year-old, 200-mile-wide perinatal-referral organization. Saint Luke's was the only hospital in the Kansas city area providing twenty-four-hour in-house coverage with board-certified neonatologists in addition to its neonatal ICU.

Children's Mercy Hospital was invited to join Saint Luke's as a partici-pant in the transport system. Relations between the two hospitals were strained after neonatologists formerly based at Children's Mercy but working primarily at Saint Luke's severed connections with Children's Mercy and established full-time practices at Saint Luke's. Saint Luke's tried to dissuade them from decamping but to no avail. And so Saint

Luke's reluctantly accepted the change, needing continued neonatal coverage for its center. But there was resentment at Children's Mercy, where some believed that Saint Luke's had "stolen" their neonatologists.

The board's committee on medical-staff credentialing and development attended meetings of the medical staff's Credentials Committee in order to be more familiar with the credentialing process and to make independent recommendations to the board concerning new applications, status changes, and additional privileges. This was a burdensome responsibility for committee members under Chairman (and hospital Vice President) Graham T. Hunt, but necessary in order to avoid criticism and legal problems based on conflicts of interest and antitrust charges. The board committee convened its sessions immediately following the meetings of the medical staff committee on the first Monday of each month.

Despite favorable physical facilities, location, and demographics, the Lenexa Clinic's operation was disappointing, and it was closed. However, on-campus development of the primary-care group—Saint Luke's Medical Associates—proceeded, with 15 physicians under contract. They opened offices in Medical Plaza III.

The PHO and PO were incorporated in April, 1992. The PO unified the medical staff, and the PHO joined the physicians with the hospital in a mechanism for dealing with managed-care contracts.

· · · · ·

Final steps in the acquisition of Spelman Memorial Hospital and Spelman/Saint Luke's Hospital were taken in April, with Saint Luke's becoming the sole member (owner) of both Northland hospitals. Mack A. Porter and H. Frank Halferty from Spelman Memorial were elected to the Saint Luke's board. The two Spelman hospital corporations did not initially merge but remained separate entities. A series of meetings and other measures bonded the cultures, medical staffs, and boards of all three hospitals. An April 27 open house at Spelman Memorial celebrated the affiliation.

There were significantly fewer physicians in burgeoning Platte and Clay counties than elsewhere in the state, forcing residents to travel to Kansas City for medical services. This would be remedied by the Northland hospitals.

Saint Luke's took a step forward in managed care with the acquisition of Lincoln Health Plan of Kansas City, a health maintenance organization (HMO). Heritage Health ultimately would accept transfer of Lincoln, reimbursing Saint Luke's for the acquisition costs. However, Heritage would not be operational for six months, and meanwhile the opportunity to acquire Lincoln would expire. The purchase carried with it certificates of authority for HMO licenses in Missouri and Kansas, saving time and start-up costs and positioning the purchaser to renew managed-care contracts in January, 1993.

The April, 1992, issue of *Prevention* magazine contained an article entitled "Doctor Shopping '92," which advised:

> "Check out the hospitals. Good doctors are more likely to be affiliated with good hospitals ... The teaching hospitals of major medical schools are considered the cream of the health-care-institution crop ... Most people have a choice of hospitals but no way of distinguishing between them. For the purpose of picking a doctor, you want to find out which hospital has the best overall reputation. Ask your medical center contacts about the 'centers of excellence' at hospitals in the area. Where's the best place to go for heart surgery? Who has the best trauma center?"

Saint Luke's, a major teaching hospital, checked out very well with its Mid America Heart Institute and Level One trauma center.

The cover story in the June 15, 1992, issue of *Modern Healthcare* discussed charity care by American hospitals. The story reflected favorably upon Kansas City's acute-care hospitals:

> "Statistics from the Kansas City Area Hospital Association show that the thirty-two acute-care hospitals in the Kansas City area, excluding 308-bed Veterans Affairs Medical Center, spend a substantially larger share of their money on charity care than hospitals nationally."

The magazine devoted one section of the article to a comparison between Saint Luke's and for-profit Humana Hospital:

> "Two hospitals in the Kansas City area provided an interesting lesson on how individual hospitals handle the dissemination of charity-care information.
> "The hospitals are 560-bed Saint Luke's Hospital of Kansas City (Mo.) and 400-bed Humana Hospital of Overland Park (Kan.).
> "Saint Luke's is an inner-city facility in Jackson County, which has a population of about 636,000. Humana Hospital is in nearby Johnson County (Kan.), a decidedly affluent suburban county of about 355,000."

The article disclosed that for calendar 1992, Saint Luke's had budgeted $27.9 million for bad debt and charity care, of which $21.2 million was spent on charity care alone.

" 'In the interest of clarity, I've always felt that charity care should be broken out from bad debt,' said Edward Matheny, Saint Luke's president. 'Of course, there's an element of charity in bad debt, but you have to distinguish that from real charity.'

"Meanwhile, Jay Williams, executive director of Humana Hospital-Overland Park said his facility spends 6 percent of total net revenues on bad debt and charity care. He declined to disclose any specific dollar figures or a breakdown of bad debt and charity-care expenditures."

The president of the medical staff, Dr. Joseph A. Pinkerton, announced in September, 1992, that physician enrollment in the PO was nearly complete. The PHO turned its attention to soliciting managed-care contracts with business enterprises. The employment of Pamela Cole as PHO Executive Director facilitated this effort. In the development of the PHO, utilization review and quality assessment received high priority.

There was urgent need to develop Saint Luke's clinics and primary-care practices throughout the area. A medical practice a few miles from the hospital was acquired, and recruitment of a chairman for the Department of Family Practice began.

The hospital's on-campus primary-care organization, now called Saint Luke's Internal Medicine Group, experienced growing pains. These included snarls with billings, scheduling, telephone calls, and reception-desk staffing. The result of the coalescence would be worth the effort, but meanwhile, the learning process was painful for physicians and administration, and unsatisfactory for some patients.

• • • • •

Crittenton was in financial distress. The largest private mental health organization in the metropolitan area, it served the emotional needs of children and their families in six counties. Services ranged from outpatient treatment to acute hospital care. Located for many years on the Saint Luke's campus, Crittenton moved in 1979 to an attractive 156-acre site on the southern edge of Kansas City. As the only free-standing non-profit mental health resource in the area, it attracted donors including the Hall Family Foundation, Boatmen's Foundation, national foundations such as Kresge and Ford, and the local United Way organization. After reviewing somber financial projections but mindful of Crittenton's importance in the community, the board approved acquisition of the center.

Assimilation of the Spelman hospitals continued in October, with a retreat for the boards, medical staffs, and administrators of all hospitals. The decision was made to merge the corporate structures of the two Northland hospitals while retaining both campuses.

The residents' clinic in the Medical Plaza III building, which furnished so much charity care, changed its name to the more descriptive "Medical Education Clinic of Saint Luke's Hospital."

The 1993 budget was adopted in October, 1992; it anticipated system-wide patient revenues in excess of $400 million and a contribution of $38 million in free care and other services to the metropolitan area.

Changes in guidelines promulgated by the Center for Disease Control in Atlanta, governing hospital employees infected with HIV and AIDS, necessitated revisions in Saint Luke's personnel policies. Involuntary reassignment would provoke resentment, and the matter was approached with sensitivity. The board instituted changes protecting employee rights without jeopardizing patient health ... infected employees would not be assigned to positions that endangered patients.

The Ethical Concerns Committee continued to labor on the frontiers of medicine, not making medical decisions but exploring reasonable ethical options where appropriate. DNA, the molecular basis of heredity, would be the mystical subject of a committee-sponsored seminar in the spring of 1993.

The Joint Education Committee of the hospital board and medical staff approved the expansion of the UMKC School of Medicine ophthalmology residency to include Saint Luke's. This entailed a closer relationship between Saint Luke's Hospital and Dr. Felix N. Sabates' nonprofit Eye Foundation on Kansas City's Hospital Hill. John D. Hunkeler's Hunkeler Eye Clinic, relocated on the Saint Luke's campus, also offered excellent ophthalmology care and additional educational experience for the medical residents.

Managed-care plans were in the ascendancy. They offered profuse incentives to shortchange patients, with a contracting hospital's profitability dependent upon minimizing the use of its resources. There was temptation to utilize second-rate providers and to subtly underserve patients. Nevertheless, attention to quality was constant at Saint Luke's.

The board's Quality Assessment Committee, aided by the dedicated Dr. Eugene E. Fibuch, scrutinized activities such as Code Blue procedures, infection control, and quality statistics relating to ambulatory surgery, outpatient care, and respiratory therapy. In nursing, a strong connection was noted between shared governance and quality improvement.

• • • • •

An October 12, 1992, article in *Modern Healthcare* reported the results of a study by the Rand corporation published earlier in *The Journal of the American Medical Association.* The study used three types of quality-measurement criteria and concluded:

> "All three measurement techniques yielded 'strikingly' consistent findings … 'Quality improved steadily with the size of the hospital and the population of the community in which it was located,' and the best care was delivered at the urban teaching hospitals."

One reason for the high-quality patient care at Saint Luke's was the advanced technology employed. However, this could bewilder the uninitiated. An October, 1992, story in the *Benton County Enterprise,* published in Warsaw, Missouri, told of two Ozark area ladies who boarded an elevator at Saint Luke's and were joined by a man pushing a complex piece of equipment with a multitude of spouts, hoses, and lights:

> "One lady turned to the other and exclaimed, 'Lord, I'd hate to be hooked up to that thing!'"
> "'So would I, lady,' the hospital worker said. 'It's a carpet cleaning machine.'"

Saint Luke's lobby carpets require a great deal of cleaning. Several million pedestrians walk over them in the course of a year.

• • • • •

A 1992 Medicare Hospital Information Report on the Heart Institute confirmed the excellent mortality results experienced by the Saint Luke's heart program. Deaths from myocardial infarction at Saint Luke's are far fewer than the national average. Emergency treatment has become much more sophisticated during the years since the introduction of the original, jury-rigged Code Blue cart.

A Kansas Citian attending a medical meeting in San Francisco heard an expert declare that "the best place in the country" for someone suffering a heart attack is Saint Luke's Hospital in Kansas City, Missouri.

A special meeting of the board was held in December, 1992, to consider information on financing the emergency room, surgery, and parking projects approved earlier subject to a determination of feasibility by the Finance Committee. Robert H. West, hospital Treasurer and Finance Committee chairman, reported that the projects were financially feasible. He also advised that it might be advantageous to borrow part of the funding for the projects through a tax-exempt bond issue. However, the Missouri Health Planning Agency recently had pressured hospitals to use their cash reserves for such purposes. Since the ER project would provide better facilities for the state-designated Level One trauma services, it appeared unlikely that the CON application would be rejected in any event. The matter would receive further consideration.

The Crittenton acquisition was completed December 17, 1992.

A December article in *The Kansas City Health Care Times* announced an affiliation agreement between Saint Luke's and the 85-bed Atchison Hospital, noting that the arrangement would aid both institutions. Saint Luke's would provide medical education, help in establishing physician specialty clinics, and offer support in dealing with managed-care programs. In return, Atchison would continue its long-standing practice of sending patients needing tertiary care on the fifty-five-mile trip to Saint Luke's. The Atchison Hospital's physicians were well-acquainted with Dr. Hugh Bell, a prominent Saint Luke's cardiologist who grew up in Atchison.

In January, 1993, the W.T. Kemper Foundation announced two significant research grants, one to Dr. Paul Koontz for breast-cancer prevention and the other for clinical investigation of heart arrythmia. The research would be conducted at Saint Luke's.

Cardiologist David M. Steinhaus, who would conduct the arrythmia research, implanted the first investigative device in the world for monitoring heart function in patients with congestive heart failure.

The Dickson-Diveley Clinic and the Midwest Orthopaedic Clinic, the two major orthopaedic groups at Saint Luke's, merged to form the Dickson-Diveley Midwest Orthopaedic Clinic.

There was concern at the hospital when Dean James J. Mongan of the UMKC School of Medicine was offered the position of assistant secretary for the Department of Health and Human Services, and relief when Dr.

Mongan declined the invitation. His presence at the medical school during the formative years of affiliation was important to the medical-education programs at both institutions and also to a congenial relationship between the hospital and UMKC.

The board approved a policy for dealing with physicians infected with blood-borne pathogens, including HIV and AIDS. There was no known problem, but it was prudent to have a policy in place for patients' protection.

Robert West presented the Hospital with a portrait of Edward T. Matheny, Jr., in recognition of the latter's service as hospital president and Foundation chairman since January, 1980, and service on the board commencing in 1961. The portrait was hung in the hospital's main lobby.

An ad hoc committee reviewed the cost of medical education to determine whether, without significantly weakening the program, cost savings and income generation were possible. Committee chairman Daniel M. Dibble reported that extensive study by the committee disclosed no areas in which current funding could be reduced without harm to the program and pointed up the need for exploring other sources of income.

• • • • •

UMKC's Dean Mongan acted as facilitator for a retreat of the U.S. Senate Finance Committee to consider financial aspects of the health care "reform" legislation under discussion in Washington. And Dr. Blim was part of a small group receiving a White House briefing on the same subject. In April, both expressed to the board skepticism over prospects for passage.

The publisher of *Modern Healthcare* defended the existing system:

> "The healthcare industry has nothing to feel ashamed about. It has done an incredible job of bringing first-class healthcare to the majority of Americans in an efficient and heroic manner. We have the finest physicians in the world; we have the finest hospitals in the world; we have the finest pharmaceutical industry in the world. Everything is first class because Americans demanded these things, but now we're mad because the cost is too high. Just remember that to increase longevity as we have, to save premature babies from certain death, and to make liver, heart, lung and pancreas transplants an almost common occurrence takes a lot of money and dedication. Let's not turn back the clock and let the bureaucrats control the system. They'll eventually destroy it in the name of reform." (October 11, 1993)

Saint Luke's anticipated special problems with the "reform" proposals because of their impact on medical education and on tertiary-care hospitals staffed largely with specialists. Cost-containment provisions in the bill cut the number of doctors in the country by a quarter and halved the number of specialists. Control was exercised by capping the number of residents in training. Critics complained that "controlling demand by limiting supply is perverse."

Walter Reich, M.D., director of the Program on Health, Value and Public Policy at the Woodrow Wilson International Center for Scholars, wrote to Senator Daniel Patrick Moynihan:

> "The idea that one should avert the expense of medical procedures by getting rid of the specialists who understand or carry them out, or by making sure that new specialists aren't trained, makes as much medical sense as getting rid of the possibility that a person will experience future illnesses by prophylactically removing all his healthy organs at an early age."

He characterized an "attempt to dismantle the edifice of specialization" as "akin, somehow, to the torching of the great library in Alexandria."

• • • • •

The hospital's operating margin for the first quarter of 1993 was less than anticipated, primarily because of increased length of stay by underfunded Medicare patients.

Crittenton losses were greater than budgeted, necessitating an infusion of $500,000 in operating funds and an additional $100,000 for critical capital needs. However, Crittenton was the charity beneficiary of the Southwestern Bell Classic, a golf tournament on the popular PGA Senior Tour, and in June that event produced badly needed financial support for the center. It also generated favorable publicity for Crittenton and for the parent Saint Luke's Health System.

Following the failure of the Lenexa clinic, the hospital looked for a primary care site in Johnson County, Kansas. A twenty-seven-acre tract in southern Johnson County—sufficient land to permit future expansion, including ancillary and diagnostic clinics—was purchased for approximately $3.8 million.

The long-standing dream of an Episcopal retirement facility—Bishop Spencer Place—was closer to reality thanks to the support of Bishop Buchanan, who had seen such a project brought to successful completion in South Carolina. A tract of land near Saint Luke's, at 43rd and Madison, was identified as the site.

Hospital Corporation of America had purchased Humana Hospital in Johnson County. Now for-profit Columbia Hospital Corporation, through merger with HCA, acquired the hospital—renamed Overland Park Regional Medical Center. Increased for-profit competition in the community was anticipated as Columbia/HCA showed an interest in expanding its presence and its operations in the metropolitan area. In a disappointing sequel, the RLDS Church in Independence elected to sell its 80-year-old Independence Regional Health Center (formerly Independence Sanitarium) to Columbia/HCA. This ended discussions between Saint Luke's and RLDS representatives of merging in a single nonprofit health care system.

The Saint Luke's Life Flight helicopter crashed after picking up an accident victim in rural Missouri. The patient and pilot were killed, and the flight nurse and a paramedic were critically injured. This was the first helicopter tragedy for Saint Luke's, and the friends and colleagues of the crew among hospital personnel were devastated. However, Life Flight operations continued unabated.

The board approved purchase of the Clinton Medical Doctors Clinic, a successful primary-care group practice in Clinton, Missouri. This brought to fourteen the number of medical clinics in the Saint Luke's system, located throughout the area at sites providing high-quality care and access to the clinical resources of Saint Luke's Hospital.

• • • • •

For years there were unsuccessful efforts to identify and employ a medical director for the oncology program at Saint Luke's. "Turf" problems and other concerns of medical-staff members thwarted committees charged with the search effort. However, with the outspoken support of Dr. Pinkerton, an ad hoc committee was appointed to develop a job description and find a medical director.

The work of the ad hoc committee culminated in September, 1993, with the employment of a director of oncology, Dr. Robert J. Belt. Dr. Belt had two areas of special interest: clinical research into new cancer treatments and strategies, and establishment of a high-dose therapy clinic, including bone-marrow transplant capabilities.

With continued favorable interest rates, the advantages of tax-exempt financing for the emergency and surgery renovations and new parking facility were too great to forgo. The board authorized the issuance and sale of bonds in an amount not to exceed $140 million, again using the Health and Educational Facilities Authority of the State of Missouri as the vehicle.

Also included in the package were funds for future capital improvements and the refinancing of all existing debt.

The system budget for 1994, adopted in October, 1993, provided in excess of $23 million for community services, including charity care—several million dollars less than the previous year but nevertheless a very significant commitment to Kansas City.

One announced area of retrenchment was the Developmental Preschool sponsored by the hospital. However, community and parental pressure led to reconsideration and preservation of the preschool, upon assurance of broader philanthropic support and reduced hospital financial commitment. A looseleaf notebook compiled by parents and filled with case histories and pictures was poignant and persuasive. The program was unique in Kansas City and a resource well worth preserving. Parental involvement and support from the Greater Kansas City Community Foundation, the Bacchus Ball Foundation, and the Jacob and Ella Loose Trust promised future financial stability for the program—renamed The Children's SPOT.

UNICEF (United Nations Children's Fund) awarded Saint Luke's Hospital a certificate for its breast-feeding education efforts—one of eighty-two U.S. hospitals to be so recognized.

The merger of Spelman Memorial Hospital and the Spelman/Saint Luke's Hospital was accomplished, forming Saint Luke's Northland Hospital. The merged entity retained both its Smithville campus, the former Spelman Memorial Hospital, and its Barry Road campus, the former Spelman/Saint Luke's Hospital. The Northland board of directors perpetuated the "Spelman" heritage by voting to name the three-story patient tower on the Smithville campus after Arch Spelman, M.D., in recognition of his outstanding contributions to medicine in the Northland area.

Judge Frank W. Koger, chairman of the Insurance Committee, recommended a new excess general liability insurance policy of $30 million above the amount provided by the hospital's self-insurance trust, and additional $25 million claims-made coverage beyond that. The recommendation was approved. Judge Koger reported that no additional funding would be required for the self-insurance trust and noted that no hospital contributions had been required for the past five years. The emphasis on quality was financially rewarding.

• • • • •

A major stroke program was established December 11, 1993, when a twelve-bed Stroke Center was opened at the hospital. Neurologist Marilyn Rymer, M.D., who in two years would become the first woman to head the medical staff, was a visionary leader of the enterprise. A core curriculum in cerebral vascular disease was installed, and each bed was equipped with monitoring equipment. The program complemented Saint Luke's outstanding cardiovascular program and the surgery of Dr. Joseph Pinkerton, who had amassed one of the largest series of carotid endarterectomies in the country.

THIRTY-SEVEN
1994

family practice ... midwifery ... proliferation ...
Wright Memorial Hospital ... Columbia/HCA ...
Bishop Spencer Place ... G. Richard Hastings ...
Anderson County Hospital

*D*r. John M. Miles, Mayo endocrinologist, joined the Saint Luke's Internal Medicine group the first of January, 1994. A significant part of his time was devoted to research.

The parent company for the Saint Luke's Health System was Saint Luke's Hospital itself, serving as a holding company with a number of subsidiaries. On January 7, 1994, a special meeting of the Saint Luke's Hospital board discussed the formation a new "umbrella corporation" under which the parent hospital and all other parts of the system would be placed. Some of the components, such as Saint Luke's Northland Hospital and Crittenton, would remain subsidiaries of Saint Luke's Hospital.

The holding company would facilitate integration of Saint Luke's physicians with the hospital ... they would be represented on the holding-company board. It also would allow other hospitals to join the Saint Luke's system without becoming subsidiaries of Saint Luke's Hospital. The ensuing discussion was spirited ... it was clear that many board members were not persuaded of a need to change the structure. The concept was shelved.

Also on January 7, the hospital and the community lost a stalwart with the death of Dr. Charles N. Kimball.

At their annual meeting on January 21, the board allocated $3.3 million to Bishop Spencer Place, for site acquisition. This anchor grant was the catalyst in making the retirement home a reality.

Networking among hospitals was in vogue, and relationships with other health care institutions constantly were explored. Formal affiliation with the prestigious Mayo Clinic was perceived as advantageous from the standpoint of image and improved quality of care in some specialties; representatives of the hospital spent a wintry day at the Mayo Clinic in Rochester, Minnesota without tangible results.

The advantages and disadvantages of participation in a Blue Cross plan called "HealthSource" also were carefully considered. The plan was attractive from a marketing perspective, joining together twenty hospitals from a wide geographic area under a master partnership agreement that provided for 52-percent ownership by Blue Cross and 48 percent divided equally among the hospital participants. Blue Cross enrollees in HealthSource numbered 70,000 HMO patients and 370,000 PPO patients in the Kansas City area. Blue Cross urged the hospital to join. However, there were problems associated with Saint Luke's participation, including an offensive two-year "probationary" membership, exclusion of the Northland Hospitals, loss of a significant hospital investment in HealthNet, uncertainty as to the degree of physician participation, and realignment of the hospital's alliances both statewide and locally.

An alternative to the BlueSource opportunity was membership in a new alliance being formed primarily by old friends from HealthNet, replacing the more limited Heritage Health: Bethany Medical Center, Children's Mercy Hospital, Liberty Hospital, Saint Joseph Health Center, Saint Mary's Hospital of Blue Springs, and Shawnee Mission Medical Center. The goal was creation of an integrated health system that would establish an accountable health plan. Two consulting firms were engaged to work with the alliance, tentatively named Community Health Partners, in devising the accountable health plan and focusing on physician integration with the system.

The members of Community Health Partners signed a statement of intent to engage in a long-range strategic planning process over a period of several months.

Dr. Greg Chambon, a UMKC medical-school alumnus, was employed as chairman of the new Family Practice Department of the hospital.

The first set of triplets delivered at the Barry Road campus of Saint Luke's Northland Hospital were born on March 1.

The Saint Luke's Hospital Foundation retained Robert F. Hartsook and

Associates to study the feasibility of an endowment campaign for medical education at Saint Luke's. Hartsook concluded that the proposed campaign would require much effort but would affirm the hospital's premier position in the community.

An additional facility in Johnson County—the Southcreek Office Park ambulatory care site—was approved for development at 129th and Old Metcalf, with a fall opening scheduled.

Dr. John L. Barnard announced his retirement as associate dean for the affiliated medical-education program with UMKC, and Dr. Ralph R. Hall was employed as his replacement. This marked the return to the campus of a long-time supporter of Saint Luke's and its medical education program. Dr. Hall was first employed in 1961 as director of medical education and research at Saint Luke's and served for many years in that capacity.

The Barry Road campus of the Saint Luke's Northland Hospital enjoyed marked success. Primary-care physicians at the Gashland Clinic contributed substantially to this. The latter determined to sponsor a medical office building, North Oak Medical Park, and the board approved an expenditure by the Northland Hospital of $600,000 for an ownership position in the project. This not only was a promising investment but also would solidify relations with important members of the Northland medical staff.

· · · · ·

Saint Luke's College, successor to the hospital's diploma School of Nursing, graduated its first class on May 13. Edward Matheny presented the inaugural commencement address. Forty-five students received nursing degrees. The college was accredited by the North Central Association of Colleges and Schools for the maximum five-year period. Patricia Teager, R.N., M.S., director of nursing education, was the Provost of Saint Luke's College. The new graduates were heavily recruited for employment at Saint Luke's Hospital.

Over the years, the nursing supply available to the hospital fluctuated, with shortage followed by surplus. But for quite some time stability had reigned, with an upward trend in the School of Nursing enrollment during the transition toward college status. However, college applications for the fall of 1995 were significantly fewer, despite recruitment efforts at thirty-four college/career fairs attended by students from 247 high schools. The diminution was not limited to Saint Luke's College and was attributed to decreased nursing opportunities for graduates. As health care providers tightened their belts, counselors referred high school students to other academic majors.

The medical staff supported the establishment of a certified midwifery program at Saint Luke's, and the Speas Trust provided a $300,000 grant for this purpose. The program, the first of its kind in the area, received board approval on May 20. Midwives would be employed by the hospital and supervised by the program director, with back-up coverage provided by obstetricians who furnished coverage for the OB residents. The cost-effective program was designed to provide prenatal care for women unable to participate in the resident clinic's OB program due to shortage of physicians as well as for women desiring this alternative delivery procedure. Only women with low-risk, uncomplicated pregnancies would be accepted. The midwives would be certified and credentialed by the hospital.

Meanwhile, the high-tech neonatal intensive-care unit continued to save many struggling newborns, earning the undying gratitude of anxious parents:

> "Allison came into this world fighting for her life. Fortunately, she came into this world at Saint Luke's Hospital. Immediately after she was removed from the womb, she was given to the care of Dr. John Callenbach. For the next five-and-one-half weeks, he, his colleagues and the wonderful staff took care of Allison ... not to mention her parents and extended family. I am truly convinced that they saved her life and somehow assisted in preserving our sanity during that time. (Not incidentally, and to our vast relief, her subsequent check-up with physicians and the Saint Luke's Developmental Clinic have been extremely reassuring.) The depth of our gratitude to Dr. Callenbach, his associates, the staff of Saint Luke's and the hospital itself is immeasurable."

HealthNet, originally a Saint Luke's preferred-provider organization, expanded to include several other hospitals. The largest PPO in the area, it was the source of one-third of Saint Luke's managed-care business. However, to maintain its market share and remain competitive, the PPO needed an HMO component. This was provided when HealthNet merged with Healthmark, an HMO owned by several HealthNet participants, including Saint Luke's and its Heritage partners. For several months a merger committee worked out the terms ... it was difficult to satisfy the varying needs of the participants, including Saint Luke's.

The Saint Luke's board authorized execution of the merger documents and investment in the new company. Saint Luke's Northland Hospital also participated; Saint Luke's Hospital advanced the funds to permit this. Dr. Andrew Dahl was employed as HealthNet's CEO, and Saint Luke's Lincoln Health Plan was transferred to the merged entity.

The medical-education oversight committee conducted its periodic review of the financial aspects of the UMKC-Saint Luke's affiliation, including distribution of the annual funding supplied by Saint Luke's under the affiliation agreement. For 1993, after crediting the hospital for certain expenses, the remaining $2,778,118 was allocated as follows: $1,852,078 to Hospital Hill Health Corporation Services to continue support of faculty, research, and other education efforts based at UMKC/Truman Medical Center; $694,530 to Truman Medical Center to fund insurance protection against malpractice exposure related to medical residents and other costs of residents' involvement in medical education; and $231,510 to Children's Mercy Hospital to continue support of costs of residents' participation in medical education at CMH.

• • • • •

Graham Hunt's Committee on Medical Staffing recommended elimination of the policy requiring Saint Luke's cardiologists to practice exclusively at Saint Luke's subject to minor exceptions involving noninvasive procedures. Some Saint Luke's cardiologists were performing complex cardiology procedures at other institutions, and the recommended policy shift recognized the change in their practice. The board approved the modification.

For many years there had been a problem with integrating Heart Institute physicians into the mainstream of Saint Luke's Hospital and its medical staff. Cardiologists in particular tended to regard the Heart Institute as a separate institution and occasionally argued that it should be an independent corporate entity with a separate board of directors and officers.

Many of the younger cardiologists practicing in the Heart Institute, while extremely able physicians, were not conversant with all of the hospital effort and support that had gone into the development of that remarkable facility and its exemplary programs. They did not entertain the same loyalties to the Saint Luke's facility as Jim Crockett, Ben McCallister, Geoff Hartzler, Hugh Bell, Lynn Kindred, and other older cardiology colleagues. There was no longer the attitude of "sink or swim" with the hospital that had prevailed with another generation of physicians. Nor did they appear to have the concern that itinerant physicians might adversely affect quality and cost-effectiveness at the Heart Institute that led to the adoption of the now-abrogated policy. In an environment where high-volume "centers of excellence" were recognized as desirable, if not necessary, they proceeded in the opposite direction. Heart programs proliferated further.

One factor contributing to the escalating cost of health care was medical-malpractice litigation. It was necessary to increase the minimum malpractice insurance coverage required of Saint Luke's physicians as a condition of their membership on the hospital's medical staff. The board approved the recommendation of the Insurance Committee that policy limits be raised to $1 million per occurrence, $3 million in the aggregate. This led to the resignation of a handful of physicians, but most doctors complied.

Community Health Partners was renamed Mid-America Health First—Health First for short. Efforts to launch Health First successfully were constant, consuming a great amount of administrative time. In addition, Edward Matheny attended meetings with lay leaders of the other participating hospitals. Physician integration was an essential and challenging element in the Health First effort, and medical staff president Dr. Warren Johnson exercised an important leadership role among his peers at the various member hospitals.

The Health First hospitals were the most financially stable in the Kansas City area, and each enjoyed considerable success in terms of patient volume and image, but the winds of change were blowing: competitive pressures and managed-care demands threatened hospital futures. There was considerable incentive to address and solve the complex problems of integrating several strong, fiercely independent institutions ... to "hang together, lest they hang separately."

Meanwhile, some notable events occurred at Saint Luke's. On Valentine's Day, surgeons at the Mid America Heart Institute successfully completed their 100th heart transplant. The hospital's kidney-transplantation program celebrated its twenty-fifth anniversary ... 650 people had received new kidneys over that span. Quadruplets, conceived without fertility therapy, were born in the hospital's intensive-care nursery—babies ranging in weight from two pounds eight ounces to three pounds seven ounces, all in good health. The Saint Luke's gynecologic oncology physician group was accepted as an affiliate member of the national Gynecologic Oncologic Group (GOG)—the only practice in Kansas City with such affiliation. The Women's Cardiac Center, one of the first in the nation to provide cardiac-risk assessment and research specifically for women, provided risk-profile assessments for 2,400 women and scheduled 275 appointments in the first three months of the program's existence.

Helen Anna Jepson, Ed.D., R.N., was named chief education officer and Dean of Saint Luke's College.

Saint Luke's Health System entered into a lease agreement with fifty-three-bed Wright Memorial Hospital of Trenton, Missouri. The Trenton hospital now is operated as part of the system. A long-standing referral relationship exists among physicians of the two institutions, and the lease supports Saint Luke's network strategy in the State of Missouri in general and enhances the competitive position of the system in the Northland area in particular.

Saint Luke's affiliated hospital in Atchison, Kansas, opened a family medical center in Weston, Missouri. Warrensburg Family Care, with three family practitioners in Warrensburg, Missouri, was purchased. And two nurse practitioners were added in the Northland communities of Kearney and Plattsburg.

For financial reasons, Southwestern Bell Telephone Company withdrew as the sponsor of the Kansas City stop on the Senior PGA Tour. This was a serious blow to Crittenton, which, as the charity beneficiary of the Southwestern Bell Classic, had enjoyed several hundred thousand dollars per year in much-needed income. (The 1994 tournament had netted $441,667.) It was also a loss for Kansas City. So there was jubilation when Mayor Emanuel Cleaver announced that the Kansas City-based Veterans of Foreign Wars of America had agreed to assume the tournament sponsorship for the ensuing two years. It would be called the "VFW Senior Championship."

• • • • •

Despite participation in Health First, the board attempted to keep open other options, including a relationship proposed by Columbia/HCA. However, disturbing rumors circulated of pending sale of Saint Luke's, or other ventures involving transfer of control or ownership of the hospital, to for-profit Columbia. All of this was unsettling—to Health First partners, to hospital patrons and potential donors, to Foundation trustees and officials preparing for a fund-raising effort, and to the community at large. It was no longer possible to maintain the status quo. Accordingly, at the September board meeting there was comprehensive discussion of the advantages and disadvantages and the implications for Saint Luke's as a nonprofit, major teaching institution of a relationship with Columbia. The board voted unanimously to decline Columbia's overtures and directed Mr. Matheny to write a letter to that effect. The letter ended:

> "We are gratified by your interest in Saint Luke's but have concluded that our mission and our community will be better served by our participation in the development of Mid-America Health First."

A press release was issued in a further effort to dispel rumors.

There were numerous problems with the Columbia proposal from a business standpoint as well as the conundrum of putting a price tag on an institution whose present worth represented well over a hundred years of philanthropy, forgone taxes, other public outlays, and the contributions of thousands of volunteers and professionals. But the board's action was predicated less on those problems than on a reluctance to convey or share control or ownership of the hospital with a gigantic for-profit corporation headquartered in a distant city.

An article in the *Wall Street Journal* reported the decision as follows:

> "Saint Luke's Hospital, Kansas City, Mo., declined Columbia/HCA's advances last month after several months of exploratory talks over being acquired. Saint Luke's heart program, the Mid America Heart Institute, is a major provider of cardiac services in the Midwest and would have been a plum for Columbia.
>
> " 'It was impossible for us to reconcile their bottom-line motivation,' says Edward Matheny, president of Saint Luke's. 'They're answerable to their stockholders, and what we're trying to do is to take care of the community.' "

The Mid America Heart Institute would indeed have been a "plum" for Columbia. Its 2,000 angioplasties performed in 1993 once again placed it among the world's leading heart centers.

Columbia/HCA was a relatively new phenomenon, and it remained to be seen what its ultimate success would be. A few years earlier a skeptical article in *The Harvard Business Review* (May-June 1989, p. 105) observed:

> "Those who have predicted that American health care would be dominat-

ed by a handful of large, vertically integrated organizations have come to realize that there is little that is meaningful about health care which is national. Health services are a neighborhood business, beginning and ending with a doctor and a patient."

Similarly *Best's Review,* an insurance-industry publication, in April, 1987, predicted "the demise of the supermeds," mainly because health care is a "local business." The glaring failure of the supermeds was said to be inability to lower health care costs; their higher profits resulted from higher prices, not efficiency.

Now it was clear that the obituaries of such organizations had been premature. The for-profits were very much alive in 1994, having continued to evolve over a period of years. The majority of the American public did not recognize the size and scope of the proprietary advances or their implications. Man's nervous system developed to respond to immediate danger at his cave's mouth, and he finds it difficult to react to anything that takes years to transpire. If the arrival of for-profit medicine is a mammoth tiger on the doorstep, it has not yet been identified as such.

Meanwhile, Columbia would not go quietly from the local scene. It would compete intensively, using its considerable financial resources and its leverage based on size and national managed-care contracts.

To allay concerns of potential donors to the Saint Luke's Foundation aroused by the Columbia experience, this response was suggested by Foundation legal counsel:

> "I think you can find reassurance in the fact that the foundation Articles and By-Laws identify Saint Luke's Hospital by name as the beneficiary of the Foundation's philanthropy and go on to identify the hospital as a public charity of the type benefited by Sec. 501(c)(3) of the Internal Revenue Code. The Foundation trustees have a fiduciary obligation to carry out the purposes of the Foundation. Any substantial change in the operation of the hospital would leave the Trustees with an obligation to find a way to follow the intentions of the donors. Their actions in so doing are subject to review by the Internal Revenue Service and the State of Missouri Attorney General. In addition, through the Missouri Court system, any individual donor can challenge the Trustees' actions.
>
> "We hope you will also have confidence that your intentions will be followed because of your regard for the individuals who serve as trustees and employees of the Foundation. Because of the commitment of these individuals to keep faith with the donors and the fact that the stated purposes of the Foundation are tied to the hospital as a charity, we are comfortable in recommending to donors that they make unrestricted gifts to the foundation."

Such assurances and the actions and comments of Saint Luke's directors and officers laid to rest concerns of the public in general and of the hospital's patrons and allies in particular.

• • • • •

The prognosis was promising for the Southcreek Clinic (Saint Luke's Outpatient Care-Johnson County), projected to open October 3. Eight primary-care physicians and several specialists were scheduled to practice there.

Saint Luke's acquisition of physician practices continued, with three more approved and six additional acquisitions under consideration.

Friday, September 30, was a significant date for the supporters of Bishop Spencer Place. Financing was finally in place, and there was a groundbreaking ceremony at the construction site. After remarks by Kansas City Mayor Emanuel Cleaver, Bishop Buchanan and Hospital President Matheny, the first shovelful of earth was turned. A barbecue lunch followed for the several hundred celebrants. Saint Luke's would provide health services for the Bishop Spencer residents, including monitoring at the facility's clinic, home health care, consultant services, and medical direction for assisted living.

Health care "reform" as proposed by the Clinton Administration was dead, or at least moribund; congressional supporters abandoned their efforts.

The issue of sweeping change in health care would have to be revisited later; significant problems with the existing system required adjustment. Meanwhile, private-sector attempts to address costs continued. It was clear that health care would not revert to what it was; managed care was here to stay, and Saint Luke's constantly grappled with the resultant pricing issues.

John T. Russell now chaired the marketing and public-affairs committee, and the Saint Luke's Health System hosted a group of business representatives at a meeting to hear presentations and engage in discussions of joint efforts by health care providers and employers to balance costs of care and quality of service. Participants received a computer disk designed to assist in appraising the quality and value of health benefits offered by the various providers. It depicted the travels of a quaint little military-type character, "Major Medical," through the health care jungle. High tech at Saint Luke's was not limited to medical care—it had reached the marketing department as well.

If the public can be apprised of the facts concerning costs and quality, Saint Luke's will continue to fare well. Medicare data indicate that the "value" of what Saint Luke's has to offer from the standpoint of caseload, acuity, length of stay, mortality, and costs is superior to that provided by other hospitals.

• • • • •

Charles Lindstrom, now 66 years of age, expressed a wish to retire effective January 1, 1995. His twenty-eight eventful and effective years in office represent the longest tenure of any administrative head of the hospital. At a special meeting on October 7, the board appointed G. Richard Hastings, Lindstrom's able second-in-command and colleague for eighteen years, his successor as CEO of Saint Luke's Health System. Lindstrom's service was lauded in an appreciative board resolution.

• • • • •

Construction began in the fall of 1994 on renovation of the hospital's emergency and surgery departments. The project increased the size of each surgery room from an average of 364 to 600 square feet. The number of treatment stations in the emergency area increased from fourteen to nineteen, and the total size of the emergency area doubled from 6,600 square feet to 14,740 square feet. Total cost: $28 million. The emergency area had need of the new facilities—in the course of 1993 more than 20,000 persons were treated by the Saint Luke's Emergency Services Department.

Dr. Michael Weaver, who headed emergency services at Saint Luke's and served on the Saint Luke's board, was recognized as one of Kansas City's most influential African Americans. *The Kansas City Business Journal* named him one of the city's top twenty-five "up and comers."

The continuing commitment to emergency care without regard to ability to pay at Saint Luke's was in sharp contrast to the performance of many other American hospitals. Federal law forbade hospitals accepting Medicare patients to deny for nonmedical reasons treatment of any emergency-room patient. These hospitals were required to screen each ER patient and render whatever aid was necessary to stabilize his medical condition. In particular, delaying treatment in order to check on health insurance coverage was a violation. But despite the law, some hospitals transferred to other hospitals—"dumped"—patients who were uninsured or who could not pay for their medical care. If a "pocket book biopsy" disclosed no insurance, there was a temptation to transfer.

A consumer group, Public Citizens' Health Research Group, reported in October, 1994, that eighty-six hospitals in twenty-two states were cited for illegal refusals during 1993 and the first quarter of 1994.

• • • • •

Meanwhile, ordinary patient care, performed in extraordinary fashion, continued to be the primary business of Saint Luke's. A patient's October 12 letter to the editor of *The Kansas City Nursing News* praised the quality of that care:

> "When someone does an exceptional job, it should be commended and reported to his superiors and to the community. In this case, an entire crew did an outstanding job, and in a very difficult, critical-care situation.
>
> "I moved to Saint Luke's hospital on August 5 from another hospital. I was greeted from the start by the cheeriest, most accommodating staff I have ever encountered in any situation, let alone a hospital environment. And until my release on August 26, a full three weeks later, the quality of attitude and professional care never wavered. From the most menial to the most specialized of nursing tasks, I was treated with unparalleled professionalism, a caring staff of people."

G. Richard Hastings was authorized to sign a letter of intent permitting Saint Luke's to join the other Health First hospitals in due-diligence efforts over a ninety-day period as the formation of Health First went forward.

On November 2, at a joint meeting of the hospital directors and the foundation trustees, the campaign recommended by Robert Hartsook was approved. Medical education at Saint Luke's Hospital would be endowed, in order to relieve heavy dependence on patient-care dollars and government subsidies. The campaign established a $50 million goal in current and deferred gifts, to be committed by December 31, 1997. The campaign was led by banker J. Thomas Burcham as general chairman, with Dr. Gerald F. Touhy and Albert C. Bean Jr. serving as co-chairmen.

A significant component of the campaign effort was the endowment of chairs in several specialties, including cardiology, anesthesiology, internal medicine, and neuroscience. The price per chair: $2.2 million—one-half to be supplied by the University of Missouri in matching grants.

At a November meeting of the Vanguard Club, a breakfast club of influential Kansas Citians, Dr. Max Berry—now a sprightly 85 years of age—recommended to his receptive audience a "Montana lowball" consisting of three ounces of bourbon whiskey taken neat. It is a health measure learned by Dr. Berry at his father's knee.

• • • • •

At a regular meeting of the hospital board on November 18, the 1995 budget for Saint Luke's Health System was adopted. The system included Saint Luke's Hospital, Saint Luke's Northland Hospital (both campuses) and related subsidiaries, Crittenton, Saint Luke's Health Ventures, Saint Luke's Medical Associates, Saint Luke's Medical Development Corporation, and the system's share of operating gains and losses of various joint ventures.

The system budget projected patient revenue of $458,197,000, producing an operating margin of $2,268,000; and nonoperating revenue of $8,898,000. The operating margin was achieved largely through the profitability of Saint Luke's Hospital, which carried the rest of the Saint Luke's system financially. The system also relied heavily on nonoperating revenue derived from investment income to provide a reasonable reserve for growth and development.

An exhibit to the budget reflected the hospital's commitment to community service for the ensuing year, a total of $24,026,594. The lion's share of these expenditures were education related, including medical education costs and write-offs, Saint Luke's College, charity care and clinical services. Medicaid losses were a major item as well.

The budget indicated the financial impact of changes in health care—the most profound since the inception of Medicare in 1966. The changes were characterized by a dramatic shift in payment incentives and strong pressure for reduction in utilization of hospital services. Outpatient volume at Saint Luke's continued to grow but was outpaced by declining inpatient revenue growth. In this environment, adherence to the hospital's mission as exemplified by the community service budget presented a formidable challenge—but one to which the hospital board was totally committed. As *The New England Journal of Medicine's Special Report* of August 8, 1996, would conclude:

> "If nonprofits are to retain their claim to fiscal and moral difference, they will need not only to match the chains lawyer for lawyer, ad for ad, market strategy for market strategy, and cost saving for cost saving, but also to be clearer about their own mission."

A study released by the National Committee for Quality Health Care revealed the vital role that medical technology played in reforming the health care system and how it improved the quality of care, lowered costs, expanded access and made the system more efficient. *The Arthur Andersen Washington Healthcare News Letter* described the committee's conclusions as follows:

> "The report refutes the claim that medical technology is responsible for driving up healthcare costs, citing, for example, that investment in research and development by pharmaceutical companies has saved $141 billion and 1.6 million lives between 1940 and 1990 from the treatment of diseases like tuberculosis, cardiovascular disease and strokes. The group believes that the problem is not medical technology, but the inappropriate use of technology. The study encourages continued private and public investment in medical technology ... It maintains that everyone in the healthcare system—healthcare providers, insurers and patients—has a responsibility to support and make the best use of medical technology."

A 1994 NRC *Health Care Market Guide* survey confirmed the public perception of Saint Luke's technological superiority in comparison with other area hospitals, a byproduct of its status as a major teaching hospital.

NRC surveyors also identified a public preference for Saint Luke's in terms of critical-care services and nursing care, and high ratings for overall quality and physicians.

The sixteenth Holly Ball was held on December 3, with Kitty Wagstaff serving as honorary chairman of the gala event.

• • • • •

An Associated Press article on December 15 reported the results of a Duke University study:

> "If the doctor says you need an angioplasty, here's some advice: Go to a hospital that does a lot of them.
>
> "A new study shows that the chances of surviving this common procedure are considerably better at hospitals where angioplasties are routine ... the death rate is about one-third higher at hospitals that perform only one or two a week."

Saint Luke's consistently was among the top five hospitals worldwide in the number of angioplasties performed annually.

An article in *The Kansas City Star* reported that the American Heart Association and the American College of Cardiology recommend that hospitals performing angioplasties do at least 200 procedures a year. It noted that Saint Luke's averaged almost 2,000 angioplasties annually, whereas eight Kansas City hospitals fell short of the 200 minimum in either 1993 or 1994.

Saint Luke's patients could take comfort in the fact that the "practice makes perfect" maxim applied to more than angioplasties. The Associated Press article went on to note:

> "Studies of other kinds of care have reached similar conclusions. For instance, researchers have found that hospitals doing large numbers of hip replacements have lower death rates, as do those that frequently perform heart-bypass operations and other blood-vessel surgery."

It was the hospital's practice to send calendars to its constituents at Christmas, featuring photographs taken by Saint Luke's personnel. These always elicited grateful responses from recipients scattered over the region. 1994 was no exception; one respondent enclosed a check for $100 and an expression of thanksgiving "for saving my son's life."

A year-end summary of the Stroke Center reported that 339 patients were discharged from that facility following its opening a year earlier. Development of the center allowed the hospital to participate in national clinical-research protocols, and the National Stroke Association took an active interest in the center's development. The center's goal was recognition as the regional leader in stroke care and the only regional facility where aggressive new therapies were available.

On December 31, an agreement was entered into between Saint Luke's and Anderson County Hospital of Garnett, Kansas, permitting the two institutions to explore merger in an integrated health care delivery system.

THIRTY-EIGHT
1995

Robert H. West ... quality recognized ...
lung reduction ... Stroke Center achievements

A January 4, 1995 article in *The New York Times* was headlined: "Hospitals Are Tempted but Wary As For-Profit Chains Woo Them." The reporter noted that nonprofit hospitals provide much more charity care than do for-profit hospitals, and that in Kansas City "the board of Saint Luke's, concerned about maintaining the hospital's services in the community, rejected an overture from Columbia/HCA ... ." The article quoted Edward Matheny's explanation:

> "We do a lot of things in the community that don't make any sense whatever from a dollar-and-cents standpoint."

On January 9, a CON authorized a $10.9-million expansion at the Northland Hospital's Barry Road campus. The first of March, all medical, surgical, and other acute-care procedures were consolidated by the Northland board of directors at the Barry Road facility, reflecting a considerable discrepancy in volume between the two institutions ... surgeries at Barry Road had increased to 3,650 per year, whereas those at the Smithville campus had gradually declined to 485. The changes were not popular with many Smithville residents, producing a number of irate letters to the press. Local pride was offended, but as one Northland Hospital director remarked: "I can read the numbers as well as the next person." At a time when the escalating cost of health care was a matter of national concern, the numbers did not support duplication at Smithville.

The "practice makes perfect" maxim applied here as well. Patients could anticipate better care at the busy Barry Road facility than in the echoing halls at Smithville. And with continued population growth in their area, the citizens of Smithville could anticipate resumption there of many services in the future. Meanwhile, the two campuses were separated by only twelve miles of highway.

Harry D. Cleburg, CEO of *Fortune* 500's Farmland Industries, succeeded Frank Halferty as one of the Northland representatives on the Saint Luke's Board, and banker Paul Shy replaced Mack Porter as the other.

The merged HealthNet organization (now called HealthNet Excel) contracted to provide health care for Aetna Insurance Company patients, a gain of 38,000 persons for HealthNet participants.

• • • • •

Edward T. Matheny Jr. reached the mandatory retirement age fixed by the hospital's bylaws. At the annual meeting of the hospital board on January 20, 1995, Robert H. West was elected to succeed Matheny as president of Saint Luke's Hospital. Chairman and CEO of Butler Manufacturing Company, West was eminently qualified to lead Saint Luke's into a new millennium. He served for many years as treasurer of the hospital, and chairman of both the Finance Committee and the Audit Committee. He also replaced Mr. Matheny as ex-officio chairman of the Foundation. West was succeeded as hospital treasurer by Warren W. Weaver, vice chairman of bank holding company Commerce Bancshares, Inc.

• • • • •

The VFW Senior Championship attracted a stellar field of senior golfers to Loch Lloyd Country Club in early August. Despite a rain-shortened tournament, Crittenton benefited substantially from the PGA charity event. Professional golfer Bob Murphy was the popular winner.

In October, 1995, Missouri Governor Mel Carnahan presented the Excellence In Missouri Foundation's "Missouri Quality Award" to Saint Luke's, the first hospital to be so recognized. (The other 1995 recipient was the University of Missouri-Rolla.)

Saint Luke's budget, adopted for the following year, anticipated patient revenues approaching a half billion dollars but an operating margin of a scant $3 million. A major reason for this was the 1996 community-service commitment (medical education, charity care, etc.) in excess of $30 million.

Saint Luke's pulmonary-medicine specialists Scott A. Lerner and Vincent M. Lem introduced a successful new procedure for treatment of emphysema—lung reduction; paradoxically, removal of part of the diseased lung by thoracic surgeon Jeffrey M. Piehler brought significant relief in breathing to selected emphysema patients.

The Stroke Center's second year of operation demonstrated that Saint Luke's stroke program was unique and innovative. One of ten programs selected by the National Stroke Association to develop guidelines for stroke centers, it was the only one based in a community hospital ... the others were at major academic centers. The Saint Luke's program balanced a community-hospital patient base with the resources to conduct sophisticated clinical research.

The Stroke Center was also the only midwestern site for a trial sponsored by the National Institutes of Health of the clot buster tPa ... the results of which were reported in the lead article of *The New England Journal of Medicine* (December 14, 1995).

Dr. Marilyn Rymer was elected president of the medical staff, becoming the first women to head the physician organization.

The prestigious American College of Surgeons verified Saint Luke's status as a Level One Trauma Center, the only one in Kansas City caring for both adult and pediatric cases. Dr. Thomas S. Helling, medical director for the trauma center, deserved much of the credit for this achievement.

The Charles N. Kimball Cardiovascular Education Center, named for the former board member and Heart Institute champion, was dedicated on December 7.

THIRTY-NINE
1996

skybridge ... campaign progress ... new emergency room
... bone-marrow transplantation ...
Saint Luke's-Shawnee Mission Health System

*I*n January, 1996, Saint Luke's was runner-up for the "National Quality Health Care Award" presented by the National Committee for Quality Health Care. (The winner was Intermountain Health Care of Salt Lake City, and the other runner-up was Ohio State University Hospital.) And on April 15, 1996, at the 1996 VHA Leadership Conference in Philadelphia, Pennsylvania, Saint Luke's CEO G. Richard Hastings accepted for the hospital VHA's "Quality Leadership Award for Clinical Effectiveness" ... Saint Luke's finished ahead of Boston's Massachusetts General Hospital and Baylor Medical Center.

Dean James J. Mongan of the UMKC School of Medicine was named president of Massachusetts General Hospital—the premier hospital administrative position in the country and one that Dr. Mongan found impossible to decline. Saint Luke's president Robert H. West joined a university search committee to select Mongan's successor. Meanwhile, Dr. J. Stuart Munro of Truman Medical Center became interim dean.

The board in March approved a skybridge across Wornall Road, connecting the Medical Plaza buildings and Saint Luke's Hospital at a point immediately south of the Peet Center. The funding was in place, thanks largely to Donald H. Chisholm and Dick Woods, trustees of the Victor and Caroline Schutte Foundation. Don Chisholm was persuaded of the need for such a connection when transported by wheelchair from the hospital to the medical offices during a cloudburst; Chisholm was handed an umbrella to ward off the rain.

Everett P. O'Neal, Saint Luke's director from 1969 to 1996, died on April 14, 1996, a loss observed by the board at its May meeting.

• • • • •

With suitable ceremony and celebration Bishop Spencer Place was dedicated April 27- 28, the culmination of decades of hopes and dreams. The retirement center offered sixty independent-living apartments, thirty assisted-living suites, and a fifty-seven bed skilled-nursing facility.

At a banquet of the Saint Luke's Hospital Foundation on May 9, foundation president William L. Atwood announced that $32.7 million had been pledged to date for the campaign to endow medical education and research at the hospital. The community was responding to the hospital's need; much of the credit for the campaign's success was due to the effort and skill of the foundation's executive director, Harold J. Schultz, Ph.D.

The auxiliary underwrote continuation of a program providing teddy bears for children in the Ambulatory Surgery Center, and the hospital supported a teen-parent center in partnership with the Kansas City School District.

New, expanded, state-of-the-art emergency room facilities had their grand opening on May 29, 1996. Visitors were welcomed by a beaming Dr. Michael L. Weaver, who pointed out the four spacious ambulance bays and the street-level ambulance entrance on J.C. Nichols Parkway; cardiac hill and its stretcher bearers were ancient history.

Inpatient admissions through May exceeded the budget by 13.5 percent and the prior year by 8.3 percent, leading to net operating revenue for the period of $102.4 million … as opposed to a budgeted $94.8 million. *The Kansas City Business Journal* listed Saint Luke's as first in the area in number of admissions and second in revenue.

The Stroke Center continued to serve as a model for stroke-center development across the country, with a nursing staff certified in the use of the stroke scale developed by the National Institutes of Health. The Saint Luke's stroke team presented a summary of the hospital's clinical tools at the June meeting of the National Stroke Association in Colorado Springs

... Dr. Marilyn Rymer was a member of the National Stroke Center steering committee for stroke center development and networking.

Dr. Robert B. Geller was recruited to develop and direct a bone-marrow transplant program at Saint Luke's. He brought with him, from Emory University in Atlanta, Georgia, expertise in leukemia therapy and marrow transplantation.

Another open-heart surgery program was under consideration by a local hospital. The Kansas City area would now rival the entire nation of Canada in the number of its open-heart programs.

John A. Ovel, president of Boatmen's Trust Company for a five-state area, succeeded William L. Atwood as president of the Saint Luke's Hospital Foundation.

• • • • •

On June 12, 1996, the community was advised that "the area's two largest and most preferred health care providers" had formed the Saint Luke's-Shawnee Mission Health System. Shawnee Mission Medical Center ranked second only to Saint Luke's in admissions, outpatient procedures, and public perception. In 1995, the two hospitals, their subsidiaries and their physicians served 47,522 inpatients, 502,767 outpatients, and 82,474 emergency patients.

The Saint Luke's board earlier had resisted subordinating Saint Luke's Hospital to a holding company. But now there was need for a separate governance structure to operate the new system, and an umbrella board was appointed consisting of ten representatives from Saint Luke's, seven from Shawnee Mission, two Saint Luke's physicians, and one physician from Shawnee Mission. The new board directed the joint system operating company ... under the chairmanship of Saint Luke's Robert H. West. Shawnee Mission chairman Charles Sandefur was vice chairman. Bishop Buchanan, Saint Luke's board chairman, was an ex-officio member of the system board.

The system was led by G. Richard Hastings as its chief executive officer. Shawnee Mission CEO James W. Boyle was the chief operating officer of the new operating company, and Saint Luke's Ronald K. Bremer was its chief financial officer.

With the advent of the new system there dawned a new era at Saint Luke's, assuring even better health care for the Kansas City metropolitan area.

EPILOGUE

*D*uring its 113 years, Saint Luke's has witnessed enormous change in the role of acute-care hospitals. They have been transformed from custodians of the indigent sick to temples of healing.

Saint Luke's own history in many respects parallels that of the country's many thousand community hospitals ... the same struggles with wars, economic depression, managed care and group insurance, Medicare and Medicaid, unions, minimum wage ... all of the trials and tribulations of nonprofit health care providers sustained by unpaid, public-spirited volunteers.

As a major teaching hospital it also has much in common with a smaller, more elite group of institutions belonging to the Association of American Medical Colleges ... offering sophisticated, cutting-edge, high-tech care in centers of excellence, much of it charity care provided in a Level One trauma center and in residents' clinics.

But there are many aspects of the hospital's history that combine to make it unique: one of the world's busiest, most experienced balloon-angioplasty practices; the first artificial kidney machine used in a private hospital setting; the first hyperbaric bed in the United States; pioneer work in cardiology and in cardiac research, benefited by the world's largest angioplasty data bank; expert care for victims of polio, influenza, AIDS, and other disasters; a division of experimental medicine performing basic research; and, one year, the second-most-profitable hospital in the country ... profits returned to the community in many forms.

Saint Luke's is what it is today because of the dedication of thousands of people, largely anonymous. No history of the hospital could identify an appreciable number of these innovators and supporters, particularly among the medical staff, any more than it could recount the daily episodes of drama, humor and heartbreak that constitute the real story of Saint Luke's.

Saint Luke's relationship to the Episcopal Church is ambiguous. It is an "institution" of the Church ... its articles of incorporation provide that if the hospital ceases to exist, its assets shall revert to the Diocese of West Missouri. But Saint Luke's is not owned by the church. It is owned by the community at large—by everybody and by nobody.

The hospital is a voluntary, not-for-profit, comprehensive teaching and referral institution committed to "serve all who seek our services regardless of their socio-economic status."

The mission of Saint Luke's Hospital is "to ensure the highest levels of excellence in providing health care services to all patients in a caring environment."

The hospital today remains true to its mission in a highly competitive environment. Health maintenance organizations and insurance companies demand discounts. Government financial assistance waxes and wanes. Intrusion by for-profit institutions threatens. But Saint Luke's perseveres, the flagship of a system that will endure as long as there is need for "the presence of care."

APPENDICES

APPENDIX A

Leaders of Saint Luke's Hospital

Herman E. Pearse, M.D. . . . . Founder - 1902-1903
The Rev. Percy B. Eversden . . . . Founder - 1902-1903
William A. Rule . . . . Founder - 1902-1903
William B. Clarke 1904-1905
Robert B. Middlebrook 1905-1906
John F. Harding 1906-1908
M.G. Harmon 1908-1909
John T. Harding 1909-1917
A.C. Stowell 1917-1923
George B. Richards 1923-1927
A.W. Peet 1927-1952
David T. Beals Jr. 1952-1963
H.O. Peet 1963-1965
Robert W. Wagstaff 1965-1980
Edward T. Matheny Jr. 1980-1995
Robert H. West 1995-

APPENDIX B

Bishops of the Diocese of West Missouri
Who Have Served As Leaders of the Board of Directors

The Rt. Rev. Edward Atwill 1904-1911
The Rt. Rev. Sidney C. Partridge 1911-1930
The Rt. Rev. Robert N. Spencer 1930-1950
The Rt. Rev. Edward R. Welles II 1950-1972
The Rt. Rev. Arthur A. Vogel 1972-1989
The Rt. Rev. John C. Buchanan 1989-

APPENDIX C

Presidents of Saint Luke's Foundation
for Medical Education and Research

Ferdinand C. Helwig, M.D. 1963-1967
Richard H. Kiene, M.D. 1968-1970
Mark Dodge, M.D. 1971-1976
Christopher Y. Thomas Jr., M.D. 1977-1981
Raymond W. Stockton, M.D. 1981-1983
Thomas T. Crouch, M.D. 1983-1985
David H. Hughes 1985-1990
William L. Atwood 1990-1996
John A. Ovel 1996-

APPENDIX D

Presidents of Saint Luke's Hospital Auxiliary

Mrs. Andrew S. Buchanan 1908-1911
Mrs. Sidney C. Partridge 1911-1916
Mrs. L.G. Byerly 1916-1917
Mrs. Eugene Blake 1917-1919
Mrs. A.W. Peet 1919-1925
Mrs. George English 1925-1926
Mrs. William R. Jacques 1926-1928
Mrs. A.W. Peet 1928-1930
Mrs. Henry Burr 1930-1932
Mrs. William B. Nichols 1932-1934
Mrs. Wilbur A. Cochel 1934-1936
Mrs. Brown Harris 1936-1939
Mrs. Harry Rapelye 1939-1941
Mrs. Carl D. Matz 1941-1943
Mrs. Richard Bower 1943-1945
Mrs. Kearney Wornall 1945-1947
Mrs. Ashe Lockhart 1947-1949
Mrs. Edward D. Claycomb 1949-1951
Mrs. Paul R. Powell 1951-1953
Mrs. Thomas A. Peterson 1953-1955
Mrs. L.J. O'Kane 1955-1957
Mrs. Robert Amick 1957-1959
Mrs. Francis Wornall 1959-1961
Mrs. Robert W. Wagstaff 1961-1963
Mrs. Richard H. Kiene 1963-1965
Mrs. Milton B. Leith 1965-1967

APPENDIX D (CONT.)
Presidents of Saint Luke's Hospital Auxiliary

Mrs. Kenneth M. Dubach 1967-1969
Mrs. Marshall Bliss 1969-1971
Mrs. Maxwell G. Berry 1971-1973
Mrs. Don M. Jackson 1973-1975
Mrs. Frank W. Koger 1975-1977
Mrs. Clifford R. Hall 1977-1979
Mrs. Frank R. Williams 1979-1981
Mrs. Floyd E. Doubleday III 1981-1983
Mrs. Carter H. Kokjer 1983-1985
Mrs. Larry L. McMullen 1985-1987
Mrs. William W. Larue 1987-1989
Mrs. John L. Barnard 1989-1991
Mrs. Kenneth I. Fligg Jr. 1991-1993
Mrs. Frank W. Koger 1993-1995

APPENDIX E
Presidents of Saint Luke's Hospital Medical Staff

Arthur E. Hertzler, M.D. 1917-1920
H.P. Kuhn, M.D. 1920-1922
John G. Hayden, M.D. 1923
Logan Clendenning, M.D. 1924-1925
E. Lee Miller, M.D. 1926-1927
H.A. Breyfogle, M.D. 1928-1929
O. Jason Dixon, M.D. 1930
Virgil W. McCarty, M.D. 1931-1933
Ralph R. Wilson, M.D. 1934-1935
Frank D. Dickson, M.D. 1936-1937
Harvey P. Boughnou, M.D. 1938-1939
F.I. Wilson, M.D. 1940-1941
Theodore A. Aschman, M.D. 1942-1943
Carl B. Schutz, M.D. 1944-1945
Rex L. Diveley, M.D. 1946-1947
Paul A. Gempel, M.D. 1948-1949
Lawrence P. Engel, M.D. 1950-1951
Harvey P. Boughnou, M.D. 1952-1953
Maxwell G. Berry, M.D. 1954-1955
Richard H. Kiene, M.D. 1956
Ernest L. Glasscock, M.D. 1957
Irwin S. Brown, M.D. 1958

APPENDIX E (CONT.)

Presidents of Saint Luke's Hospital Medical Staff

Cameron Marshall, M.D. 1959
M. Donald McFarland, M.D. 1960
Frank S. Hogue, M.D. 1961-1962
Eugene O. Parsons, M.D. 1963
Phillip L. Byers, M.D. 1964
William C. Mixon, M.D. 1965
Andrew D. Mitchell, M.D. 1966
Paul W. Meyer, M.D. 1967
Mark Dodge, M.D. 1968
James E. Keeler, M.D. 1969
Robert E. Allen, M.D. 1970
Blaine Z. Hibbard, M.D. 1971
Raymond W. Stockton, M.D. 1972
Gerhard W. Schottman, M.D. 1973
John F. McDonnell, M.D. 1974
Christopher Y. Thomas Jr., M.D. 1975
Wallace P. McKee, M.D. 1976
Leonard A. Wall, M.D. 1977
Arthur W. Robinson, M.D. 1978
Mario J. Guastello, M.D. 1979
Richard T. O'Kell, M.D. 1980-1981
Fred D. Fowler, M.D. 1982-1983
John L. Barnard, M.D. 1983-1984
Harold W. Voth, M.D. 1985-1986
Paul G. Koontz Jr., M.D. 1987-1988
Thomas T. Crouch, M.D. 1989-1990
John Layle, M.D. 1991
Joseph A. Pinkerton, M.D. 1992
Gerald Touhy, M.D. 1993
Warren L. Johnson Jr., M.D. 1994
G. David Dixon, M.D. 1995
Marilyn Rymer, M.D. 1996

APPENDIX F

Directors of Nursing Education

Lou Eleanor Keely 1903-1916

Clara Tulloss. 1916-1920

Cecelia Calpernia French 1920-1942

Helen B. Valentine 1942-1944

Virginia R. Harrison. 1944-1946

Helen B. Valentine. . . . . February - July 1946

M. Alicia Sayre. 1946-1952

Vernetta W. Todd and Ruth Schubert 1952-1954

M. Jeanne Stickels 1954-1966

Peggy Windes, R.N., M.E. 1966-1968

Rose Marie Hilker, R.N., M.A. 1968-1984

Patricia Teager, R.N., M.S. 1984-1994
   Director of Nursing Education
   Provost, Saint Luke's College

Helen Anna Jepson, Ed.D., R.N. 1994-
   Dean, Chief Education Officer

INDEX

ACKNOWLEDGEMENTS
& BIBLIOGRAPHY

Paul Starr introduces the Acknowledgements section of his authoritative work, *The Social Transformation of American Medicine* (Basic Books, Inc., New York, 1982) with the sentence:

"This book was written in the old-fashioned way: the lone scholar pecking away at his word processor."

While less scholarly, this history of Saint Luke's Hospital of Kansas City is of similar origin. However, the writer is indebted to many persons for *The Presence of Care.*

The primary source, by far, was the archives of Saint Luke's Hospital, particularly minutes of board meetings, hospital publications and oral histories (interviews of physicians, nurses and administrators). Hospital archivist Ferne Malcolm Welles brought order out of chaos among the documents and photographs and also generated many of the interviews—ably assisted by the Saint Luke's Photography Service (Dean Shepard and Michael Kerns) and Margaret Sails.

Carol Ratelle Leach of Minneapolis, Minnesota, provided invaluable counsel and editorial assistance in the early stages of the manuscript, as did Edward T. Matheny III, who also encouraged me to proceed with the project.

My manuscript was reviewed for accuracy and anecdotal additions by the Right Reverend Arthur A. Vogel, retired Bishop of West Missouri, and hospital board chairman for seventeen years; Harold J. Schultz, Ph.D., historian and executive director of the Saint Luke's Foundation; Charles C. Lindstrom, retired CEO of Saint Luke's Hospital and my partner for the fifteen years during which I served as the hospital's president; and medical doctors Arthur W. Robinson, R. Don Blim, Christopher Y. Thomas, and Maxwell G. Berry.

The professional editing of Frederic Hron and his staff at Prime Media, Inc., was complicated by my predilection for split infinitives, but their advice and expertise made the final preparation of the manuscript most enjoyable and satisfying.

The law firm of Blackwell Sanders Matheny Weary & Lombardi provided support services in the production and reproduction of my manuscript, with particular bows to Linda Benso, Beth Johnson, Jan Normandin, Mary Meyer, Jenna Grey, Trudy Goff, and Marie Davis.

The Kansas City Star graciously permitted access to the newspaper's library.

And several publications provided important information and background materials concerning the history of medicine and the environment in which Saint Luke's has existed and prospered, notably, *The Pioneering Surgeons of Saint Luke's Hospital: 1889-1919*, by Ferne Malcolm Welles (1983); *The Social Transformation of American Medicine*, by Paul Starr (Basic Books, Inc., New York, 1982); *Governing America*, by Joseph A. Califano Jr., (Simon and Schuster, New York, 1981); *From Shamans to Specialists*, by Barbara M. Gorman, Richard D. McKinzie, Theodore A. Wilson (Jackson County Medical Society, 1981); *Take Wing*, by E. Grey Dimond, M.D., (The Lowell Press, Kansas City, Missouri, 1991); *American Academy of Pediatrics: The First 50 Years*, by James G. Hughes, M.D. (American Academy of Pediatrics, 1980); *The Haunting of Kansas City*, by Ann Lowry and Tom Ramstack (*Kansas City Magazine*, October, 1984); and *J.C. Nichols and the Shaping of Kansas City*, by William S. Worley (University of Missouri Press, Columbia, Missouri, 1990).

Without the support and encouragement of Robert West and Rich Hastings, this book would never have seen the light of day, and it is a particular pleasure to acknowledge their goodwill and generosity.

POSTSCRIPT

national recognition

*A*s this book was going to press, Saint Luke's Hospital of Kansas City was named the 1997 winner of the prestigious National Quality Health Care Award.

Presented by the National Committee for Quality Health Care and *Modern Healthcare* magazine, the award recognizes hospitals that excel in five areas: leadership, quality health outcomes for patients, integrated delivery of care, financial management systems, and satisfying community health needs.

"We always have perceived that we had quality," said G. Richard Hastings, president and CEO of Saint Luke's-Shawnee Mission Health System, "but this honor certifies that others in our field recognize the outstanding health care Saint Luke's provides."

This national award is the culmination of a century-long commitment by Saint Luke's doctors, nurses, medical technicians and staff members to establish the highest standards of care and create the most effective delivery systems.

The National Committee praised Saint Luke's Hospital for its accomplishments in several areas:

- Commitment to Quality initiatives throughout all areas of the hospital;
- consistently high patient satisfaction scores;
- strategic alliances to achieve the organization's mission;
- Saint Luke's Collaborative Care program;
- community partnerships, outreach programs and charity care;
- Saint Luke's financial stability;
- and the hospital's risk-sharing with physicians and managed care plans.

The National Quality Health Care Award was created in 1993. Prior recipients include: Henry Ford Health System, Detroit; Evanston (Illinois) Hospital Corp., a member of the Northwestern Healthcare Network; and Intermountain Health Care, Salt Lake City.

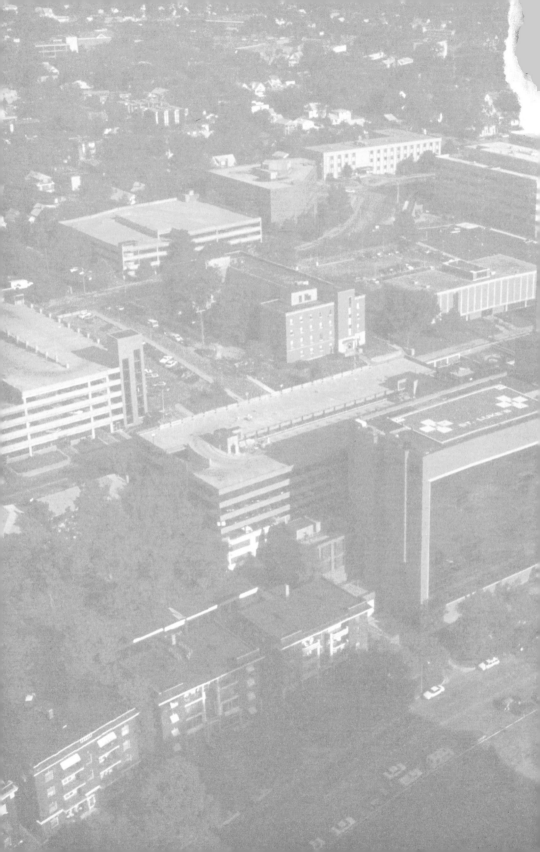